# ADDICTION AND THE LAW

# ADDICTION AND THE LAW

Elie G. Aoun, M.D.
Debra A. Pinals, M.D.
Laurence M. Westreich, M.D.

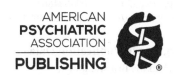

AMERICAN
PSYCHIATRIC
ASSOCIATION
PUBLISHING

**Note:** The authors have attempted to ensure that all information in this book is accurate at the time of publication and consistent with general psychiatric and medical standards, and that information concerning drug dosages, schedules, and routes of administration is accurate at the time of publication and consistent with standards set by the U.S. Food and Drug Administration and the general medical community. As medical research and practice continue to advance, however, therapeutic standards may change. Moreover, specific situations may require a specific therapeutic response not included in this book. For these reasons and because human and technical errors sometimes occur, we recommend that readers follow the advice of physicians directly involved in their care or the care of a member of their family, or any legal professionals involved in legal issues. The content of this book also involves rapidly evolving state and federal laws and regulations, so readers should be mindful of current legal and regulatory language in interpreting the content of this book..

Books published by American Psychiatric Association Publishing represent the findings, conclusions, and views of the individual authors and do not necessarily represent the policies and opinions of American Psychiatric Association Publishing or the American Psychiatric Association.

If you wish to buy 50 or more copies of the same title, please go to www.appi.org/specialdiscounts for more information.

Copyright © 2024 American Psychiatric Association Publishing
ALL RIGHTS RESERVED
First Edition
Manufactured in the United States of America on acid-free paper
28  27  26  25  24     5  4  3  2  1

American Psychiatric Association Publishing
800 Maine Avenue SW, Suite 900
Washington, DC 20024–2812
www.appi.org

**Library of Congress Cataloging-in-Publication Data**
Names: Aoun, Elie G., author. | Pinals, Debra A., author. | Westreich, Laurence
    Michael, author. | American Psychiatric Association, issuing body.
Title: Addiction and the law / Elie G. Aoun, Debra A. Pinals, Laurence M. Westreich.
Description: First edition. | Washington, DC : American Psychiatric Association
    Publishing, [2025] | Includes bibliographical references and index.
Identifiers: LCCN 2024004663 (print) | LCCN 2024004664 (ebook) | ISBN
    9781615374014 (paperback ; alk. paper) | ISBN 9781615374021 (ebook)
Subjects: MESH: Substance-Related Disorders | Legislation as Topic | Alcoholics--
    legislation & jurisprudence | Drug Users--legislation & jurisprudence | Behavior,
    Addictive | Addiction Medicine--legislation & jurisprudence | United States
Classification: LCC RC569.5.C63 (print) | LCC RC569.5.C63 (ebook) | NLM
    WM 33 AA1 | DDC 616.86--dc23/eng/20240522
LC record available at https://lccn.loc.gov/2024004663
LC ebook record available at https://lccn.loc.gov/2024004664

**British Library Cataloguing in Publication Data**
A CIP record is available from the British Library.

# Contents

# About The Authors

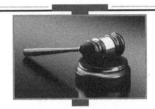

**Elie G. Aoun, M.D.,** is an assistant professor of clinical psychiatry in the Division of Law, Ethics and Psychiatry at Columbia University.

**Debra A. Pinals, M.D.,** is an adjunct clinical professor of psychiatry and director of the Program in Psychiatry, Law, and Ethics at the University of Michigan Medical School; clinical adjunct professor at the University of Michigan Law School; and senior medical and forensic advisor and editor-in-chief for the National Association of State Mental Health Program Directors.

**Laurence M. Westreich, M.D.,** is a clinical associate professor of psychiatry in the Department of Psychiatry at the New York University School of Medicine.

## Disclosures

The authors stated that they had no competing interests during the year preceding manuscript submission.

# FOREWORD

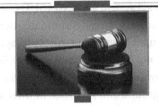

Over the past several years, the practice of addiction psychiatry and addiction medicine has received increased attention because of improving awareness of the dual diagnoses of substance use disorders (SUDs) and co-occurring mental illnesses and because of the recent U.S. opioid crisis. Moreover, medical practices are, out of necessity, expanding to incorporate substance use treatment as part of mainstream clinical care.

Anyone who works with people with SUDs knows that there are innumerable interface issues between SUDs and the law. Individuals with SUDs face the legal system through arrest, incarceration, driving-under-the-influence offenses, child custody disputes, employment issues, or court-ordered drug testing. Administrative, regulatory, and legal systems often play a critical role in how substance problems are addressed, and the result is often quite difficult, given the awkward fit between current scientific and medical views and the black-and-white provisions of often-outdated laws. Only by understanding the basics of both SUDs and governing laws can the practitioner navigate both systems in a manner that is both informed by evidence and relevant to the matter at hand.

Because of the growing demand for attention to SUDs and the imperative for effective substance use treatment to save lives, new questions are emerging about legal matters that arise in practice. This book is designed as an overview of the many areas in which SUDs and the law overlap. It also provides a guide to 1) the specific ways in which SUDs are treated in the U.S. legal system; 2) important SUD-related factors for judges, juries, human resources professionals, employment administrators, and others to consider; and 3) the ways in which health care providers, forensic practitioners, and legal professionals can render opinions and even advise their patients and clients, respectively. With these aims in mind, we hope that this book will appeal to all mental health clinicians, including treating clinicians and forensic psychiatrists, as well as other forensic mental health professionals, legal professionals, and advocates who encounter cases in which the medical management of addictive disorders intersects with the law.

In **Part 1: Introduction and Overview**, we explore the philosophical underpinnings of how the legal system addresses SUDs, with an emphasis on how the present legal stances toward drug decriminalization and other trends flow from historical phenomena. The current (although rapidly changing) legal regulation of substance use and SUD treatment is described in Chapters 1 and 2. Practitioners must be aware of the legal parameters for their practice, and Chapter 3 provides background and guidance in these domains.

Common civil legal issues that arise with SUDs are described in **Part 2: Civil Issues.** This section begins with the challenges of employment law (Chapter 4). Although the Americans With Disabilities Act (ADA) demands respectful treatment of the employee with disabilities, there is a complex interplay among the ADA, employee engagement in problematic drug or alcohol use, and employer rights and obligations. These employer obligations include the need to maintain a safe workplace, implement reasonable accommodations for employees (while not being mandated to implement unreasonable accommodations), and present a positive environment for customers. Employment-related legal matters often focus on the accuracy and fairness of drug and alcohol testing. We address this topic in Chapter 5, which describes the basics of such testing and how test results can be presented effectively in both the legal and clinical spheres. SUDs become even more complicated in the context of family law and family planning, which forms the basis of Chapter 6. In that chapter, issues related to child custody, child welfare, and even criminalization of pregnant women engaged in substance use are discussed. A variety of civil case matters, such as personal injury cases, child custody disputes, and professional malpractice, are addressed in Chapter 7.

In **Part 3: Criminal Issues,** we review the present legal standards used in SUD-related criminal case evaluations as well as the practical aspects of those standards (Chapter 8). In addition to reviewing the legal aspects of crimes committed while the accused is intoxicated, in withdrawal, or seeking substances, Chapter 9 discusses the various interventions that can help redirect people from criminal case processing toward treatment through prearrest diversion, jail diversion, drug courts, reentry services, and other alternative options. The ongoing shift of SUD treatment into our nation's jails and prisons is reviewed, along with suggestions for improving the evaluation, treatment, and follow-up for criminally involved individuals who access that treatment. Chapter 10 covers correctional practices and standards to help readers understand the basic background to correctional behavioral health care.

In **Part 4: Special Topics,** we address some SUD-related legal issues in Chapter 11 that do not fit neatly into the other sections. Among them, we discuss the effects of ongoing cannabis legalization and decriminalization, the changing regulation of buprenorphine during the COVID-19 pandemic, and the legal regulation of therapeutic hallucinogenic substances.

We have aimed to write practical, up-to-date chapters on relevant aspects of SUDs as they relate to the legal regulation of SUD treatment, aspects of statutes and regulations that can affect evaluations performed in forensic contexts, and other areas of interface between SUDs and the civil and criminal legal system. By reading this book, we hope that practitioners will gain a better fund of knowledge to assist their patients, inform their forensic opinions, and provide a greater depth of understanding to answer legal and regulatory questions that arise in their practice about approaches to SUDs.

We have discussed the ideas in this book with many colleagues and friends, and we are particularly grateful to Elizabeth Sinclair Hancq for her organizational skills and copy editing and to Veronica Tadros and Rachel E. Blume for their assistance with the legal citations. Finally, we thank our editor, Erika Parker, for her faith in this book and her insistence on clarity and relevance.

Elie G. Aoun, M.D.
Debra A. Pinals, M.D.
Laurence M. Westreich, M.D.

# PART I

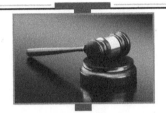

# INTRODUCTION AND OVERVIEW

# CHAPTER 1

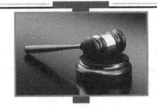

# SUBSTANCE USE DISORDERS IN THE CONTEXT OF LAW AND SOCIETY

## Introduction

Substance use disorders (SUDs) as a concept are facing an identity crisis, as they have over centuries. Movements from sympathetic, medicalized understanding to less sympathetic and more punishment-oriented criminalization have been part of the dialectic around SUDs. For many (albeit not all) physicians, SUDs are a diagnosable brain disorder that is influenced by genetics and other factors and is associated with specific brain changes seen on imaging and in pathology examinations. By contrast, SUD representations in the popular media, as driven by the recent opioid crisis, often present one such disorder—opioid use disorder (OUD)—simply as a condition caused by physician overprescribing of opioids. For many in our society at large and in the legal system, SUDs are conceptualized as a moral failure on the part of individuals who are viewed as unable or unwilling to control their self-indulgent urges.

On July 18, 1990, following the passing of a joint congressional resolution on March 8, 1989, President George H.W. Bush issued a formal declaration to designate the 1990s as the Decade of the Brain. This declaration came with research funding for neuroscience that led to major scientific developments, including the following (American Presidency Project 1999):

- Elucidating the neurobiology of alcohol use disorder and the brain's reward pathway
- Developing novel antidepressant and antipsychotic medications
- Expanding the understanding of neural development and neural plasticity
- Developing functional MRI and brain imaging research
- Laying the foundation for the field of computational neuroscience

In his book celebrating the fiftieth anniversary of the National Institute of Neurological Disorders and Stroke, the late neurologist Lewis Rowland wrote the following of the Decade of the Brain:

> As a public relations gambit, the Decade was a success. As a way of engaging scientists, legislators, and leaders of voluntary agencies, it was a success. As an education program it successfully mirrored the wonderful scientific and technological advances. As part of the preparation for the bipartisan doubling of the neuroscience budget, the Decade was a clear success. We cannot be certain the Decade had anything to do with these advances, which might well have come without the public hue, but the advances and the education marched together. (Rowland 2003, p. 144)

Such brain research accelerated scientific advances in the field of addictive disorders, contributing findings that shaped our conceptualization of SUDs as a brain disease and helped lead to the development of effective medical treatments.

Despite these scientific advances, SUDs remain extremely stigmatized. Effective treatments for many SUDs remain elusive, and most people who would benefit from treatment either cannot access it or do not think they need it. Similarly, legal responses to addiction are often untethered from advancing medical knowledge in the field, leading those with SUDs to cycle continuously through the courts and detention centers without receiving the treatment that they need, and furthering the burdens on the legal system.

In this context of vastly different views of SUDs, their causes, and approaches to overcoming them, a multitude of federal agencies are focused on addressing prescription and nonprescription drug and alcohol use. These agencies include the U.S. Drug Enforcement Administration, the FDA, the Substance Abuse and Mental Health Services Administration, the Office of National Drug Control Policy, the National Institute on Drug Abuse, the National Institute on Alcohol Abuse and Alcoholism, and the Bureau of Alcohol, Tobacco, Firearms and Explosives. Each plays a role regarding 1) access to specific substances that can lead to addiction or 2) access to medications that can treat SUDs. Thus, these agencies play either a direct or peripheral role in SUD access, treatment, and law—whether by promulgating regulations, establishing policy, or supporting research, prevention, or treatment strategies. With the numerous entities involved in this space, there is a confusing landscape in terms of how drug and alcohol use are conceptualized and handled in the regulatory and legal systems. In this chapter, the social context related to SUDs is explored.

## FORENSIC DILEMMA

An attorney argues that her stockbroker client should not receive a probation violation and subsequent return to jail for a urine drug screen (UDS) positive for cocaine because the client is not addicted to cocaine. The attorney, based on the opinion of a hired expert, points out that the single positive UDS does not meet DSM-5 (American Psychiatric Association 2013) criteria for cocaine use disorder and, in fact, her client has no other symptoms meeting criteria for that diagnosis. Because the original jail sentence was for dealing a small amount of heroin and the probationer is receiving treatment for OUD, the attorney says, the one-time use of cocaine is entirely irrelevant to the matter and only came to light because the probation officer had chosen an unfairly broad "fishing expedition" 10-panel drug screen. The probation officer defines the cocaine use as a problem because, they assert, the conditions of probation require regular negative drug screens generally, not a specific diagnosis, and all addictions are connected. The use of cocaine, the probation officer says, is illegal, is dangerous to the probationer and the public, and constitutes a violation of probation.

Consider the following:

1. Which definition is correct for cocaine use: DSM-5 criteria or cocaine use as a legal problem?
2. Should parolees and probationers undergo UDSs for many substances? Or only for the substances with which they are associated?

Both definitions are correct, but in different parts. Although DSM-5 criteria for an SUD comprise the gold standard for diagnosis, individuals can certainly come to harm even if their symptoms do not meet criteria for an SUD. By contrast, in the legal sphere, sanctions can be imposed only under specific circumstances, one of which might be the use of a particular substance even absent a person's symptoms meeting full criteria for a DSM-5 diagnosis: definitions used for legal purposes are different from definitions in DSM-5. Similarly, the individual may have an SUD but may not have a positive drug test result. DSM-5 includes a cautionary statement that a diagnosis itself is not to be confused with what is required to meet a legal standard.

Parolees and probationers are usually subjected to broad drug screens if authorities want to find use of other addictive substances. Thus, use of other alternative substances would potentially be identified on these drug screens.

Although a person with an SUD for a particular substance is certainly vulnerable to addiction to multiple substances or at least to problems with a second substance, fundamental fairness in a judicial situation demands that the testee at least know what they are being tested for.

In this Forensic Dilemma, the judge decides not to sanction the probationer and return him to jail. Two weeks later, the probationer is slightly injured while driving under the influence of alcohol. The probation officer again issues a citation for violation of probation because of the probationer's evident addictive behavior. The probationer's attorney argues against this violation on the basis that 1) the use of alcohol is not illegal and 2) adjudication of the charge of driving under the influence is several months away, meaning that her client has, of course, not been convicted of any crime. Although the probation officer acknowledges that alcohol use has not been banned as a condition of probation, they argue for the violation both as a sanction and as a way to get the probationer into mandated addiction treatment. Consider the following questions:

3.  Are all addictions connected?
4.  Does mandated addiction treatment work?

The probation officer is correct in saying that a person with an addiction to one substance is vulnerable to addiction to a second substance. However, in the legal sphere, consequences must be tied to specific actions. The probation officer is also correct in asserting that managed addiction treatment—which the probationer may be able to receive in jail—demonstrates effectiveness similar to treatment that is voluntary in nature (Werb et al. 2016).

## The Many Names of SUDs

The term *addiction* relates to its Latin root, in which the verb *addico* means "giving away." Greek civilizations used this term to refer to slaves, and Roman law coined *addictus* as a reference to people who did not pay their debts and were consequently traded as slaves. It was not until the nineteenth century, when opium use rose in Europe and the United States and Asians were blamed as the drug's source, that this term began to be used to refer to people who used drugs or drank alcohol excessively. In that context, addicts were seen as individuals who depended on their continued use of alcohol or illicit drugs to feel "normal." Since then, numerous descriptive terms have been used to refer to people with maladaptive patterns of alcohol or drug use. Consequently, laws and regulations use many terms inconsistently when referring to people with SUDs, without a clear definition of each such term. Instead, the courts and legislatures have relied on different methods for clarifying the meaning of the terms used, which often vary between jurisdictions and relate to the illness severity and the specific substance used (with alcohol use being commonly treated differently from drug use). In both civil and criminal laws, such distinctions can play a major role because the disposition of a case may hinge, at least in part, on a finding of specific substance use or specific SUD.

Medical terminology for SUDs has, in part, tracked parallel to the framework of the scientific conceptualization of medical conditions marked by the maladaptive patterns of alcohol or drug use, as evidenced in the successive DSM editions. Indeed, in DSM-I (American Psychiatric Association 1952), addiction, subdivided into alcoholism and drug addiction, is listed as a personality disorder of the sociopathic personality disorder type. Subsequent DSM editions, starting with DSM-III (American Psychiatric Association 1980), relied on a different diagnostic conceptualization of addictive disorders based on the distinction between substance abuse and substance dependence diagnoses (excluding the term *addiction*). DSM-5 (American Psychiatric Association 2013) eliminated this distinction of abuse and dependence in favor of a single SUD diagnosis, with severity determined by the number of symptoms present that meet criteria. In addition, the term *substance abuse* more recently has been viewed as stigmatizing because it conveys a negative choice on the part of the "abuser." Thus, many systems, laws, and organizations have stricken that term in favor of *substance use disorder*. Although *substance misuse* is still used, it is thought by some advocates to convey a choice of wrongly using a drug or substance. These complexities in language use are important as the field further recognizes SUDs as illnesses. DSM-5-TR (American Psychiatric Association 2022) continues to eschew the term *addiction* for diagnostic determination, but it reflects that SUDs connote severe problems related to compulsive and habitual use of drugs and alcohol. Although this is important, the term *addiction* will be used at times in this book to convey broad principles.

Forensic psychiatry is a subspecialization focused on the intersection of law and psychiatry and covers the legal regulation of psychiatric practice. This field seeks to use language as clearly and unambiguously as possible. Therefore, inconsistency in terms referring to people with SUDs in legal statutes, legal definitions, and explanations of their use in case law complicate an already thorny issue. This inconsistency highlights the question of whether the legal system, which is not as nimble in terms of updates to statutes with new scientific advances, can be seen as using various terms like *addiction* and *SUD* and even older terms like *substance dependence* interchangeably. Epidemiological researchers find that most people who receive a substance dependence diagnosis have symptoms that meet diagnostic criteria for an SUD that is at least moderate in severity (Beckson and Tucker 2014; Compton et al. 2013; Dawson et al. 2013), or *moderate SUD* or *severe SUD* could be considered the legal equivalent in most cases when laws or case law cite the term *substance dependence* (Norko and Fitch 2014). As one examines laws surrounding SUDs, therefore, it is important to keep in mind the legal definitions and their application to modern medical understanding.

# Reframing SUDs

Stigma related to SUDs is a major factor that contributes to the evolution of legal analyses, laws, and resultant policies shaping society's response to them. It is common for people with nonpsychiatric medical conditions to be nonadherent to prescribed treatments. For example, some patients with diabetes are inconsistent with their medication use or engage in self-defeating behaviors that lead to diabetes-related complications. Nonadherence is often experienced by clinical professionals as a source of frustration and by the public as a reflection of the severity of the person's illness. Yet systems of support are typically put in place to help individuals with chronic illness achieve greater stability. In contrast, for a person with an SUD, using substances or engaging in substance-related behaviors is often seen as a reflection of their lack of moral values and a willful hedonistic choice to relapse or even get high, despite the consequences to themselves and others in their lives.

Society-wide reasons for the stigma surrounding addiction are complex and only dimly understood. One important aspect of this stigma, however, relates to the nature of behaviors associated with substance use and the addicted person's apparent associated disregard for others. One hallmark of SUDs is continued compulsive substance use despite negative consequences, such as being on probation under conditions that require abstaining from substance use, disregarding the consequences and risks associated with driving while intoxicated, prostituting for access to drugs, or forgoing food for drugs. When a person with an SUD continues to use drugs despite these negative consequences, it may seem like they do not care for their marriage, relationships, freedom, or the safety of others or even themselves. If that were true, there would certainly be a solid case to argue that SUD-related behaviors reflect the person's coldness to others and dispassion about their own well-being. Given our understanding of phenomenological processes in SUDs, however, such assertions are naive and incorrect.

Scientific understanding of the brain, behavior, and role of substances necessitates a reframe away from such stigmatizing conceptualizations of SUDs, and relapses associated with SUDs, as a moral failing or judgment of the individual's intentions or motives. Beyond the superficial aspect of SUDs marked by using substances, a deeper conceptualization of such disorders involves understanding how these disorders affect a person's brain-based decision-making abilities. One commonly discussed associated rationale suggests that self-medicating to numb or mask negative emotional states despite any potential consequences is a primary driver of repeated substance use; yet this, too, is somewhat simplistic.

It appears that as individuals develop addictive disorders and the disorder severity increases, their valuation of the addictive substance increases while that of nonaddictive processes decreases. In other words, after the initial positive reinforcement associated with drug or alcohol use increases for people with SUDs, there is a related subsequent concomitant avoidance of negative reinforcement associated with the absence of substances. The individual is thus less likely to find comfort or relief when engaging in activities that they used to value positively. Of course, tracing the roots of SUDs to one's actions of using a substance in the first place raises a host of other philosophical, scientific, and contextual questions. When people first initiate drug or alcohol use voluntarily for recreational purposes and then develop an SUD, there can be debate as to whether they fully grasped the risk of developing an SUD. Taken together, there is much to learn about the problematic nature of stigmatizing first use and repeated substance use. In addition, there is much to learn about the importance of and current trends toward reframing laws and policies to reflect evolving priorities 1) to both prevent and treat SUDs as they are developing or identified and 2) to reflect understanding of the ongoing brain-related changes with chronic patterns of SUDs.

# The Free Will/Determinism Duality in SUDs

In *Robinson v. California* (1962), the U.S. Supreme Court ruled that having an SUD may not be considered a status criminal offense without violating the Eighth Amendment of the U.S. Constitution against cruel and unusual punishment, as incorporated into the Fourteenth Amendment due process clause. The court implicitly acknowledged that for people with SUDs, drug or alcohol use may be driven by predetermined drives (*Robinson v. California* 1962). Conversely, in *Powell v. Texas* (1968), the U.S. Supreme Court concluded that although having an SUD cannot be criminalized as a status for a person with an SUD, behaviors related to using substances are not driven by an "irresistible compulsion" that the person would be "utterly unable to control." The high court ruled that having an SUD does not entirely erase a person's volitional control over their behaviors. These two cases represent a clear example of the free will/deterministic duality for SUDs in constitutional jurisprudence (these cases are further discussed in Chapter 2, "Legal Regulation of Substances and Legal Issues in Substance Use Disorder Treatment," and Chapter 8, "Criminal Case Evaluations in Substance Use Disorders"). This type of duality is reflected in various landscapes where the law attempts to deal with SUDs. Societal discourse about addictive disorders is replete with this debate—looking at factors that are predetermined by neurobiology and modulated by past experiences or open to spontaneous course alteration based on drives and desires. Further, an examination of whether the concepts of SUDs as a brain disease or volitional phenomenon is fraught, given that this can become a key issue in legal determinations. It is important in legal cases of relevance for the fact finder to understand the dialectic between *blaming* and *understanding* individuals with SUDs for the behavior of substance use. Some arguments about these views and the complexity of the science distinguishing willful choice and biological drive are explored next. These arguments, in turn, are reflected in complex laws that must examine whether an individual has engaged in or will engage willfully in further at-risk behavior.

## The Deterministic Argument

To test whether having an SUD predetermines substance-related behaviors and impairs an individual's ability to exert control over such behaviors, one would need to establish that such behaviors are driven entirely by the neurobiology of SUDs as a brain disease shaped by past circumstances, behaviors, and experiences and marked by genetic factors and neurophysiological changes. In that regard, according to the theory of *allostasis* (the motivational processes aiming at achieving a normal homeostatic balance), addictive phenomena are best understood as an "undue influence" whereby biological factors impair the homeostatic balance, leading to imbalance of the brain reward and stress response systems. Substance use and associated behaviors would move the balance closer to *homeostasis*—albeit, temporarily—which makes it predictably likely that individuals will continue to use substances to maintain the homeostatic balance. How this relates to ascribing blameworthiness or the mens rea associated with criminal conduct could then make a difference. In other words, if the externalizing undue influence of the substances leads to the use of an illegal substance, then the individual may or may not be blameworthy.

To understand this argument, it is important to understand some of the science behind it. The supporting scientific evidence comes from the identification of neural circuits involved with SUDs, in states of both intoxication and withdrawal or craving. This argument is further supported by evidence that SUDs respond to pharmacological treatment in a somewhat predictable fashion, as evidenced by FDA approval of medications that target specific neurobiological functions to treat SUDs.

Genetic factors are also known to contribute to the inception of SUDs (Ducci and Goldman 2012). The genetics of SUDs are complex, owing to epistasis and to the diversity of addictive substances, incomplete penetrance, variable expressivity, interactions between genetic and environmental factors, polygenicity, and gene interactions. In some instances, some of these genetic factors also increase or decrease the likelihood of specific substance-related behaviors or even susceptibility to environmental factors or response to treatment for people with SUDs (Ducci and Goldman 2012). Environmental factors are known to interact with one's genetic makeup when certain genotypes correlate with exposure to a given environmental factor or when a person's genotype can influence their exposure to that environmental factor (Caspi and Moffitt 2006).

Evidence of the heritability of SUDs comes from epidemiological data showing that a family history of SUDs is an important risk factor for SUDs (Goldman et al. 2005). Genes coding for neurotransmitter transporters are also thought to play a role in SUDs. For example, mutations affecting serotonin transporter SLC6A4 predict stress-induced cortisol release and increase the risk of SUDs (Enoch et al. 2010; Mueller et al. 2011). Finally, polymorphisms in the gene coding for catechol-O-methyltransferase, which metabolizes dopamine and norepinephrine, are associated with methamphetamine, nicotine, and polysubstance use disorders (Jugurnauth et al. 2011; Vandenbergh et al. 1997).

In summary, if SUDs and associated substance-using behaviors are predetermined by genetics, consideration should be given to the nonvolitional aspect of substance-related behavior and might be looked at differently by the law.

## Incentive Sensitization Theory, Habit Learning Theory, Opponent Process Theory, and Neurobiological Basis of SUDs Driving Behavior

When scientific research methods are applied to investigate and identify the basis of SUDs and related behaviors, the neurobiology of addictive conditions allows for the development of predictable psychological responses to specific cues or triggers among at-risk individuals. Therefore, how much of the behavior of a person with an SUD is truly volitional is an open question, and this question is particularly significant in the forensic sphere. The law may reexamine the way in which responsibility is attributed in such contexts in the future as further scientific data become available.

The incentive sensitization theory posits that repeated and ongoing use of substances hypersensitizes signaling at the mesotelencephalic dopaminergic reward systems. This theory provides insight into the neurobiological changes responsible for the motivational factors causing the disorder. That is, an individual may not be "blamed" for their acts related to ongoing substance use because of understanding that their brains have shifted chemically to be more "hard-wired" to continue using substances despite adverse consequences. The idea behind incentive sensitization theory is that hypersensitization leads to chemically driven inflation of the incentive salience, or the motivation associated with using a given substance at the brain circuit level, which is often referred to as the *a process* (in contrast with the *b process*, which refers to aversive states seen with substance use, including the experience of withdrawal symptoms). Consequently, the incentive salience of substance-associated stimuli and paraphernalia rituals also increases (Berridge and Robinson 2016).

Hypersensitization of reward system signaling causes individuals using a substance to move from liking the subjective effects of the substance to wanting or needing the substance (i.e., incentive salience). This explains, at least in part, why people with SUDs continue to use a substance even when they are no longer deriving a pleasurable effect from it (Everitt and Robbins 2005). This hypersensitization leads to overstimulation of dopaminergic circuits, whereby they may become insensitive to non–substance-related stimuli.

The incentive sensitization model is supported by findings that the intensity of substance-induced euphoria correlates with the strength of the striatal dopaminergic activity (Volkow et al. 2009). Further, animal studies show increased drug self-administration (Vezina 2004) and increased dopaminergic activity in mesolimbic centers, including the striatum (Tindell et al. 2005), following sensitization to a given drug. Following drug sensitization, exposure to the drug even after a protracted period of abstinence increases dopamine release in humans (Boileau et al. 2006).

Building on the incentive sensitization theory, one may conceptualize SUDs as disorders of normal habit learning in which associative learning phenomena are used to demonstrate the basis for one's development of maladaptive substance use patterns. Some maladaptive behaviors (e.g., using an illicit substance) become semiautomatic, driven by associations with specific cues, stressful states, or exposure to the substance of choice (O'Brien et al. 1998). Using a classical conditioning paradigm, it is posited that specific cues, stressful states, or exposures to the substance as a neutral stimulus lead to drug-seeking behavior as the conditioned response. In this pattern of substance use, the neutral stimulus becomes a conditioned stimulus, and the unconditioned response becomes a conditioned response manifesting as a cue or stress or as substance-induced reinstatement of substance use. As these associations are cemented slowly, the person continues engaging in substance-using behaviors when exposed to cues, even in the absence of a perceived reward associated with substance use or if negative consequences occur. At that point, what started as a goal-directed behavior becomes a compulsive act driven by habit-learning processes (Hogarth et al. 2013). However, such stimulus-response habits explain the observed phenomenology of SUDs, rather than the underlying causative factors in the development of SUDs in the first place. Overall, because drug-induced sensitization of the mesocorticolimbic pathways plays a causative role in SUD development in the incentive sensitization theory, Pavlovian behavioral conditioned incentive motivational processes reinforce the person's response to addictive substances by attributing salience.

Beyond this observed phenomenological transition, neurochemical evidence supports this theory. Indeed, marked changes in dopaminergic learning systems are observed, including shifting the control over substance-related behaviors from prefrontal cortical and ventral striatal areas to dorsal striatal areas (Everitt and Robbins 2005; Hyman 2005). Moreover, adding to the data on incentive sensitization, the habit-learning theory further demonstrates that with conditioning, reward-predicting stimuli associated with substance use can significantly increase striatal dopaminergic transmission regardless of the availability of the addictive substance (Schultz 1997). As such, mesolimbic dopaminergic neural circuits demonstrate how even substance-related stimuli become rewarding in their own right.

In addition to the mesotelencephalic dopaminergic reward salience pathway and the memory and habit learning pathway, four additional primarily dopaminergic neural pathways (indirectly controlled by inhibitory γ-aminobutyric acid input, excitatory glutamate input, and other modulatory monoamines) are thought to moderate SUD-related behaviors. These pathways include brain circuitry controlling motivation, interoception, aversion avoidance, and executive function, including inhibitory control (Volkow and Baler 2014; Volkow et al. 2016). In people without SUDs, the balanced interaction of these pathways is key to the normal inhibitory control of substance use in the face of cravings. SUDs, in contrast, are marked by disruptions in this normal balance, thus perpetuating the consumption of substances (Volkow et al. 2016).

For example, in people with SUDs, disruptions in the striatal dopaminergic receptors that play a role in the regulation of executive functioning in the prefrontal cortex can lead to impaired inhibitory control of substance use and compulsive alcohol or drug consumption (Volkow and Fowler 2000; Volkow et al. 2009). Such changes evidencing decreased prefrontal cortex activity may explain the loss of control over substance consumption. Furthermore, disruptions of dopaminergic circuits within the nucleus accumbens, orbitofrontal cortex, anterior cingulate cortex, amygdala, ventral pallidum, and dorsal striatum have been associated with changes in motivational aspects of drug or alcohol use (Salamone et al. 2007).

Disruptions in dopaminergic circuits are considered the basis for the phenomenological process of SUD-mediated anhedonia. One notable aspect of SUD presentation is the person's inability to experience pleasure from non–substance-related stimuli; with advanced disease, this expands to substance-related stimuli as well (Wise 2008). The theoretical basis for this phenomenon is best explained through the allostatic model of the brain. Indeed, whereas *allostasis* refers to the motivational processes aiming at achieving a normal homeostatic balance, people with SUDs, by reason of the persistent sequelae of heavy drug and alcohol use known as the *allostatic load*, are thought to function in a chronic state of homeostatic deviation (Koob and Mason 2016). This is further evidenced in findings that people with SUDs often experience relapse even after extended periods of abstinence, suggesting that the neuroadaptive changes caused by addictive disorders lead to dysregulations in the brain reward and antireward systems. Such dysregulations representing the weight of the allostatic load are evidenced by drug-induced anhedonia.

Although examination of the addictive and reward aspects of drugs and alcohol may provide an understanding of impulsivity in SUDs, it does not address the compulsive behaviors noted with increasing illness severity. Indeed, for people with more advanced SUDs, continued substance use is often driven by a need to prevent withdrawal and negative affect and manifests as ongoing purposeless repetitive use-related behaviors (Koob and Le Moal 2001). With the development of physiological dependence, the addictive drive shifts from positive to negative reinforcement (Koob and Le Moal 2005, 2008). The brain antireward system may also play a role in the emergence of compulsivity in SUDs.

Overall, the opponent process theory postulates that the natural drive to prevent or minimize such experiences—a powerful negative reinforcement drive—is key in the emergence of compulsive substance use and is responsible for the maintenance of addictive behaviors. In this context, self-defeating acts are merely collateral damage in the quest to avoid negative emotional states. This conceptualization of addictive processes is the basis for managing acute and protracted withdrawal as a priority in SUD treatment (Koob and Le Moal 2008). In theory, these explanations for use despite negative consequences could inform future case law examining relapse and associated responses that might involve legally justified termination from employment, removal of a child from a parent with an SUD, criminalization, or eviction from housing.

# The "Volitional" Argument

The arguments presented in the previous section contain hypotheses that may explain why people with SUDs engage in self-destructive behaviors as a result of genetic and neurobiological pathway impairments, both of which are internal characteristics of that person. Cognitive factors also play a role in the inception of such behaviors. These factors may include internal cognitive patterns observed among people with SUDs, externally driven cognitive processes, or manifestations of the expected effects of the specific drug or alcohol consumed.

Metacognition or explicit cognitive processes related to SUDs manifest as faulty patterns of executive functioning that are well documented among people with SUDs. They represent nonautomatic patterns of self-regulatory mechanisms failing at controlling one's responses to drug-related urges (Copersino

2017). Mindfulness is one dimension of such cognitive processes comprising self-reflection and appraisal of affective and motivational significance. Here, deficits in self-awareness and nonjudgmental mindfulness states are associated with maladaptive substance use and SUDs (Baer et al. 2006).

Executive function deficits represent another aspect of metacognitive processes thought to play a role in SUDs. Specifically, executive dysfunction that can lead to an inability to override substance-related impulses is a major component in the development of SUDs. Impairments in individual components of executive function, such as self-control, decision-making, and problem-solving, are necessary elements leading to such dysfunction (Spechler et al. 2016; Wasmuth et al. 2015). With SUDs, executive control failures are noted, emanating from factors including attention-deficit or other trait-related impulse control impairments and neurodevelopmental immaturity (Conrod and Nikolaou 2016).

Impulsivity is the third component of internal cognitive processes central to the inception and maintenance of SUDs and relates to executive control failure. Impulsive decision-making manifests as a combination of novelty-seeking, risk-taking, and delayed discounting (Copersino 2017). In SUDs, the combination of the dynamic opposition of self-control and urge-related behavior is thought to best explain observed impulsive substance use behaviors (Bickel et al. 2016).

Alternatively, external cognitive processes relating to neurochemical disinhibition as an expected effect of drugs and alcohol, either directly or indirectly, may provide another facet to further understand these behaviors. Indeed, the direct pharmacological action of drugs and alcohol alters cognition, mood and affect reactivity, impulsivity, inhibition, and the ability to test what is real and what is not (Blanco-Gandía et al. 2015; Gillet et al. 2001; Naranjo and Bremner 1993). Similarly, the impaired cognitive states seen with substance intoxication decrease conscious awareness of the hazards associated with high-risk behaviors (Blanco-Gandía et al. 2015; Hoaken and Stewart 2003). This provides an indirect path for drugs and alcohol to promote acts that are against the person's best interests.

To better illustrate this argument, the following four examples summarize specific clinical encounters:

- A person with OUD injects heroin and is aware of the risks associated with sharing needles and seeks to use clean needles. However, when intoxicated, they are more likely to share needles or use dirty needles.
- A person with methamphetamine use disorder has unprotected sexual intercourse when intoxicated, yet they always use prophylactic measures against sexually transmitted diseases and pregnancy otherwise.

- A woman intoxicated with phencyclidine (PCP) use disorder is arrested after resisting arrest and assaulting a law enforcement officer after using PCP. When sober, she is calm and friendly.
- A man with alcohol use disorder has been in a stable and supportive marriage for 23 years. He starts swearing at and insulting his spouse when he comes home drunk one day and his spouse makes a remark about his drinking.

In all four examples, the individual in question typically only engages in such self-destructive acts when under the influence of the specific substance. Indeed, heroin is known to cause a level of clouded sensorium and to impair a person's judgment, methamphetamine use is associated with high-risk sexual behaviors, PCP is a known cause of aggression, and alcohol causes emotional lability and disinhibition.

The relationship between substance use and high-risk sexual behavior has been studied extensively (Bourne et al. 2015; Sewell et al. 2018). Substances are thought to play different roles, including managing a person's sexual inhibitions and the inhibitory anxiety associated with making oneself intimately and sexually vulnerable, allowing them to disavow a problematic piece of reality or facilitate the expression of sexual fantasies (Ostrow and Shelby 2000). Although these might be desired goals of the person seeking to use alcohol or drugs in a sexual encounter, they can be associated with undesired behaviors or consequences, such as unprotected sex, sexual victimization, sexually transmitted disease, or unplanned pregnancy.

A similar model was proposed to explain the relationship between substance use and criminal behavior. Paul Goldstein introduced a taxonomy framework to examine the temporal and causal relationship between crime and substance use and to identify common driving factors for both (Goldstein 1985). The framework described three patterns:

1. *Economic-compulsive crimes* (or *economic-related crime*): the criminal act serves to generate financial resources to fund the use of substances.
2. *Psychopharmacological crime* (or *use-related crime*): using substances impairs the individual's cognition, resulting in criminally sanctioned behaviors as a direct effect of the substance, or allows the person to become more disinhibited to have the courage to commit the crime.
3. *Systemic crime* (or *system-related crime*): relates to the situation when criminal acts are the direct result of the drug trade (at the production, manufacturing or processing, transportation, or sale levels).

In this model, all three categories of criminal acts are driven primarily by factors intrinsic to the substance use rather than to the person committing the act.

Although all of the explanatory theories just described suggest that the individual's control over substance use and substance-related behaviors is diminished for people with SUDs, it is unsurprising that many argue against that notion. Further, many courts have found that although criminal acts committed under the influence of a substance might be caused directly by the substance, the decision to use the substance that precedes the act is most often made voluntarily by the person (*Powell v. Texas* 1968). Such positions are based on the following assertions: 1) that substance use and SUDs are choices and self-inflicted phenomena and 2) that people with SUDs understand the negative value of their acts, yet choose to engage in them despite that understanding. This latter point is the foundation for the critical stance that holds people with SUDs engaged in substance use as culpable and responsible, thus justifying the external negative consequences they may face for their behavior (e.g., probation violation, conviction).

In older epidemiological studies of people with SUDs, researchers suggested that for many, the severity of substance use decreases significantly as they age, and some even abstain completely from any substance without any treatment or other clinical interventions as they age. These phenomena, known as maturing out or natural recovery, were postulated to be related to the personal sense of responsibility at work or as a parent that makes substance use less appealing or to dying early from the consequences of substance use (Foddy and Savulescu 2006; Granfield and Cloud 1996; O'Malley 2004; Winick 1962). This paradigm suggests that the decision to continue using substances is volitional, driven by a risk-benefit analysis: that is, the person using substances finds that the benefits of substance use outweigh any potential consequences. This would support the moral failure as a basis for substance use. The maturing-out phenomenon has not been replicated in empirical research, however, and is no longer accepted in the scientific community (Barnea and Teichman 1994; Searby et al. 2015). Indeed, although this phenomenon may be observed among recreational drug users, this is not the case among individuals with SUDs; as such, it should no longer be used as evidence of the volitional argument in SUDs. This discussion of the maturing-out phenomenon is included here, even though it is no longer considered scientifically sound, because it is frequently referenced in the legal literature.

Finally, cultural observations and scientific research data show that some people with SUDs can control their substance-related behavior, at least some of the time. Some of these findings are reviewed later in this chapter. The most basic level of such evidence comes from anecdotal and first-person reports about individuals with SUDs deciding to discontinue the use of substances "cold turkey" without any treatment or clinical support (Heyman 2009). Such practices are not clinically advisable, although they have resulted in successful outcomes in many situations. In these cases, one could argue that deciding to abstain—and hence, to use—is volitionally driven.

Behavioral economic analyses have described multiple ways in which the severity of a given substance's use is cost sensitive, supported by reports of people with SUDs choosing to undergo withdrawal to reduce their tolerance and require fewer drugs at a lower cost (Heyman and Mims 2016; Pickard 2017). These findings are similar to those of studies demonstrating reductions in use when the cost of a substance increases (Ainslie 2000; Pickard 2017). Such study populations include recreational drug users and people with SUDs; the former group may bear greater responsibility for the large-scale reduction in substance use than the latter group. These principles have been widely adapted in SUD research examining interventions in which people with SUDs would choose alternative reinforcers, such as cash, over drugs or alcohol (Haass-Koffler et al. 2018; Hart et al. 2000; Kenna et al. 2009; O'Malley et al. 2002). In such models, investigators note that alternative reinforcers provide a sensitive assessment of the relative reinforcing value of addictive substances. Similarly, contingency management is a psychotherapeutic modality whereby people with SUDs are rewarded with small amounts of money or other nominal rewards for remaining abstinent; this intervention has been effective in the treatment of several SUDs (McPherson et al. 2018). Here again, the effectiveness of this intervention stems from the relative increased value of alternative reinforcers compared with alcohol or drugs. Finally, positive outcomes seen with physicians with SUDs involved in a physician health program are another example of alternative reinforcers (in this case, the fear of losing one's medical license) promoting recovery in SUDs, which suggests that the decision to use or not use is merely a balancing test of choices.

The basis for such economic models is similar to that of drug courts or conditional release from incarceration with community supervision (parole or probation). In such models, people charged with a crime may be diverted to treatment in lieu of incarceration and are required to abstain from using drugs or alcohol (Bonfine et al. 2018; Munetz and Griffin 2006). The success of such interventions is based on the principle of therapeutic jurisprudence, whereby legal leverage and pressure counterbalance the difficulty of sustaining abstinence (*Commonwealth v. Eldred* 2018; *U.S. v. Miller* 1975).

Overall, these observations support the idea that 1) substance use is not wholly involuntary and 2) people with SUDs are responsive to alternative reinforcers or other incentives to abstain from using. As such, these individuals maintain a degree of control over their substance use, as they often do in the circumstances described earlier. In seeing substance use as a choice (albeit, not fully volitional), people with SUDs can be thought of as responsible and consequently blameworthy for their actions and the consequences, further contributing to stigma but also leaving courts and laws a space to consider when substance use violates societal norms. This apparently volitional use of substances underlies why substance use and substance-related behaviors are not excused socially or legally. Indeed, holding people capable of forming decisions responsible for their actions and their consequences is a foundation of modern jurisprudence. Indeed, free will is an important component of the rule of law, with the recognition that there are many factors that influence free will that are not exculpatory, so questioning it challenges the foundation of many aspects of our legal system.

# A Model for Identity Cohesion for SUDs

An array of theories of behavior as they relate to SUDs are reviewed in this chapter. Indeed, there remain numerous competing and complementary hypotheses in terms of how scientists, philosophers, and legal scholars explain why people with SUDs act in ways seemingly inconsistent with their best interests and what aspects of the conditions are disease based and necessitate treatment or volition based and necessitate civil and criminal legal controls.

This review affirmatively accepts the premise that an SUD is a disease. Building on that premise, theories surrounding the arguments for and against the volitional control that people with SUDs have over their behaviors were investigated in this chapter, recognizing that laws must draw bright lines in determining suitability for benefits, employment provisions, criminal determinations of guilt, and other matters requiring delineation. There is no single overarching theory to distill and answer all such questions. The conceptualization presented first reviews models attributing less volitional control over behavior, such as the role of genetic factors in shaping one's actions, followed by neurobiological changes demonstrated in people with SUDs and their effects on behavioral control. The common thread is that whether individuals are born with a given neurobiological predisposition to engage in SUD-related behaviors or develop neurobiological changes later in life after excessive and uncontrolled substance use, they share common changes in neural pathways explaining their behaviors. Here, SUDs are "end-stage" conditions; this means that at the time the condition is diagnosable, neuroadaptive changes have occurred and cause the observed SUD-related behaviors.

In the second part of this chapter, theories were described that attribute more volitional control over behavior in those with SUDs, including common cognitive patterns and disinhibitory cognitive effects of drugs and alcohol. Although such phenomena are reproducible, they are subject to cognitive-restructuring interventions. Finally, a fully volitional model was presented, whereby SUD-related behaviors are considered controllable, and failure to control them may reflect the person's desires and morals. Although the first section was "data heavy" and the section on the volitional argument was based on observational studies and case reports, this should not be taken to suggest that the former argument is more valid than the latter. Rather, this reflects the nature of the different arguments and the fact that volition and free will are not easily measurable or distinguished and can require nuanced analyses that, in many cases, can assist regulators, administrators, and legal decision-makers in making whatever decisions are before them.

In further understanding why people with SUDs engage in self-defeating behaviors, understanding the role of neural circuits provides at least a partial explanation. Indeed, the incentive salience and the increased valuation of addictive substances (as explained by the incentive sensitization theory) provide the prerequisite foundational basis for dysregulation in motivational circuits (as postulated in the dopamine imbalance theory). Further, pathological learned associations between substance effects and substance-related stimuli and associated behaviors (including behaviors against a person's self-interest) are consistent with the habit learning theory. In this context, what started as goal-directed and hedonistic behavior before the person's substance use became disordered is now semiautomatic and reinforcement driven despite any possible negative consequences. When viewed through this lens, SUD is a chronic, relapsing neurobiological disease marked by compulsive and irresistible substance use and self-defeating acts despite any negative consequences. This perspective, often held by physicians and social justice advocates, promotes a sense of compassion when working with individuals with addictive disorders.

By contrast, the volitional model attributes blame and responsibility to individuals with SUDs. To many, this model is seen as attributing a negative moral valence to those with SUDs. Yet some data suggest that individuals with SUDs who ascribe to the volitional model are less likely to experience relapse to substance use than those who do not (Miller et al. 1996). Indeed, for people with SUDs, the belief that one has some control over one's behavior promotes a sense of agency, empowerment, and personal growth, all of which promote recovery (Lewis 2015). Indeed, agency leads to motivation and stifles the overwhelming weight of addictive processes. On the other hand, the volitional model carries legal implications and is often seen as opposing the use of SUDs as a mitigating or excusing factor in legal responsibility for SUD-related behaviors, which could inadvertently give people with SUD-related problematic behaviors "permission" to do as they please. Regulatory and legal decision-makers are increasingly involving attorneys, judges, and even lay jurors who are gaining more sophisticated understanding of addiction and thereby showing an ability to resist outlandish or simply inaccurate theories about its cause.

## Conclusions

Notwithstanding the definitional complexity of substance use and SUDs in law and policy, it is important to acknowledge that stigma about SUDs shapes public perception of substance-related behaviors and carries myriad social, legal, and political implications. In the unfortunate absence of effective tools to measure volitional control and volitional impairment, it would be naive to separate individuals who were "compelled" to act by their illness from those who have "chosen" to engage in maladaptive substance-related acts. One useful approach, especially in the legal sphere, is to combine these theories using Hanna Pickard's model of responsibility without blame for SUD (Pickard 2017). This model promotes the notion that even when a person with SUD evidently chooses to act in a self-defeating manner despite an understanding of its consequences, and given the evidence that people with SUDs respond to incentives and alternate reinforcers, society at large should choose not to adopt a critical moral stance against these behaviors. Rather than responding to substance-related behaviors with gratuitous blame, advocating for productive and supportive interventions and medical treatment leads to better outcomes for everyone involved. The responsibility without blame model diverges from the wholly volitional model that defines people with SUDs as deliberately inflicting harm on themselves and others, and it also diverges from an entirely nonvolitional model that ignores the brain's neuroplasticity and presents a fatalistic prognosis for SUDs. Rather, Pickard's model suggests that even when SUDs are not to be used as an excuse from responsibility, they ought to be used as an opportunity to mitigate future risk, show compassion, and promote evidence-based treatments. Using this model, SUD-related behaviors reflect *impairments* in volition rather than *total failures* of volitional control. Accepting a role for free will in shaping substance-related behaviors should not prevent advocacy for alternatives to blame and shame and for opportunities such as diversion from criminal case processing, freedoms from employment discrimination, promotion of family structures, and, most importantly, opportunities for access to treatment and social supports necessary to promote recovery and reduce negative consequences of SUDs for the individual and society.

# Key Points

- Medical and legal definitions related to substance use and substance use disorders (SUDs) can vary, and one should use caution in applying clinical definitions to legal decisions and vice versa.
- Although SUDs are ubiquitous in U.S. society, they are seen variously as psychiatric illnesses, moral failings, and illegal acts.
- Nonadherence to treatment for addiction and relapse can be viewed by the legal system as noncompliance or recidivism.

- The legal and regulatory systems that address individuals who engage in substance use often struggle with a duality between free will and deterministic explanations for SUDs.

- Scientific explanations for SUDs, although increasingly well accepted in the medical community, are sometimes unknown in the legal community.

- Moralistic or volitional explanations for SUDs are prevalent in some legal spheres and must be balanced by the scientific evidence available.

# References

Ainslie G: A research-based theory of addictive motivation. Law Philos 19(1):77–115, 2000

American Presidency Project: Proclamation 6158—Decade of the Brain, 1990–1999. July 17, 1999. Available at: https://www.presidency.ucsb.edu/documents/proclamation-6158-decade-the-brain-1990-1999. Accessed October 23, 2023.

American Psychiatric Association: Diagnostic and Statistical Manual: Mental Disorders. Washington, DC, American Psychiatric Association, 1952

American Psychiatric Association: Diagnostic and Statistical Manual of Mental Disorders, 3rd Edition. Washington, DC, American Psychiatric Association, 1980

American Psychiatric Association: Diagnostic and Statistical Manual of Mental Disorders, 5th Edition. Arlington, VA, American Psychiatric Association, 2013

American Psychiatric Association: Substance-related and addictive disorders, in Diagnostic and Statistical Manual of Mental Disorders, 5th Edition, Text Revision. Washington, DC, American Psychiatric Association, 2022, pp 543–665

Baer RA, Smith GT, Hopkins J, et al: Using self-report assessment methods to explore facets of mindfulness. Assessment 13(1):27–45, 2006 16443717

Barnea Z, Teichman M: Substance misuse and abuse among the elderly: implications for social work intervention. J Gerontol Soc Work 21(3–4):133–148, 1994

Beckson M, Tucker D: Commentary: craving diagnostic validity in DSM-5 substance use disorders. J Am Acad Psychiatry Law 42(4):453–458, 2014 25492071

Berridge KC, Robinson TE: Liking, wanting, and the incentive-sensitization theory of addiction. Am Psychol 71(8):670–679, 2016 27977239

Bickel WK, Snider SE, Quisenberry AJ, et al: Competing neurobehavioral decision systems theory of cocaine addiction: from mechanisms to therapeutic opportunities. Prog Brain Res 223:269–293, 2016 26806781

Blanco-Gandía MC, Mateos-García A, García-Pardo MP, et al: Effect of drugs of abuse on social behaviour: a review of animal models. Behav Pharmacol 26(6):541–570, 2015 26221831

Boileau I, Dagher A, Leyton M, et al: Modeling sensitization to stimulants in humans: an [11C]raclopride/positron emission tomography study in healthy men. Arch Gen Psychiatry 63(12):1386–1395, 2006 17146013

Bonfine N, Munetz MR, Simera RH: Sequential intercept mapping: developing systems-level solutions for the opioid epidemic. Psychiatr Serv 69(11):1124–1126, 2018 30185122

Bourne A, Reid D, Hickson F, et al: Illicit drug use in sexual settings ("chemsex") and HIV/STI transmission risk behaviour among gay men in South London: findings from a qualitative study. Sex Transm Infect 91(8):564–568, 2015 26163510

Caspi A, Moffitt TE: Gene-environment interactions in psychiatry: joining forces with neuroscience. Nat Rev Neurosci 7(7):583–590, 2006 16791147

Commonwealth v Eldred, 101 N.E.3d 911 (Mass. 2018) (No. SJC-12279)

Compton WM, Dawson DA, Goldstein RB, et al: Crosswalk between DSM-IV dependence and DSM-5 substance use disorders for opioids, cannabis, cocaine and alcohol. Drug Alcohol Depend 132(1–2):387–390, 2013 23642316

Conrod PJ, Nikolaou K: Annual research review: on the developmental neuropsychology of substance use disorders. J Child Psychol Psychiatry 57(3):371–394, 2016 26889898

Copersino ML: Cognitive mechanisms and therapeutic targets of addiction. Curr Opin Behav Sci 13:91–98, 2017 28603756

Dawson DA, Goldstein RB, Grant BF: Differences in the profiles of DSM-IV and DSM-5 alcohol use disorders: implications for clinicians. Alcohol (Hanover) 37(Suppl 1):E305–E313, 2013 22974144

Ducci F, Goldman D: The genetic basis of addictive disorders. Psychiatr Clin North Am 35(2):495–519, 2012 22640768

Enoch MA, Gorodetsky E, Hodgkinson C, et al: Functional genetic variants that increase synaptic serotonin and 5-HT3 receptor sensitivity additively predict alcohol and drug dependence. Biol Psychiatry 67(9):91S, 2010

Everitt BJ, Robbins TW: Neural systems of reinforcement for drug addiction: from actions to habits to compulsion. Nat Neurosci 8(11):1481–1489, 2005 16251991

Foddy B, Savulescu J: Addiction and autonomy: can addicted people consent to the prescription of their drug of addiction? Bioethics 20(1):1–15, 2006 16680876

Gillet C, Polard E, Mauduit N, et al: [Acting out and psychoactive substances: alcohol, drugs, illicit substances] [in French]. Encephale 27(4):351–359, 2001 11686057

Goldman D, Oroszi G, Ducci F: The genetics of addictions: uncovering the genes. Nat Rev Genet 6(7):521–532, 2005 15995696

Goldstein P: The drugs/violence nexus: a tripartite conceptual framework. J Drug Issues 15(4):493–506, 1985

Granfield R, Cloud W: The elephant that no one sees: natural recovery among middle-class addicts. J Drug Issues 26:45–61, 1996

Haass-Koffler CL, Goodyear K, Zywiak WH, et al: Comparing and combining topiramate and aripiprazole on alcohol-related outcomes in a human laboratory study. Alcohol Alcohol 53(3):268–276, 2018 29281033

Hart CL, Haney M, Foltin RW, et al: Alternative reinforcers differentially modify cocaine self-administration by humans. Behav Pharmacol 11(1):87–91, 2000 10821213

Heyman G: Addiction: A Disorder of Choice. Cambridge, MA, Harvard University Press, 2009

Heyman GM, Mims V: What addicts can teach us about addiction: a natural history approach, in Addiction and Choice: Rethinking the Relationship. Edited by Heather N, Segal G. Oxford, UK, Oxford University Press, 2016, pp 386–408

Hoaken PN, Stewart SH: Drugs of abuse and the elicitation of human aggressive behavior. Addict Behav 28(9):1533–1554, 2003 14656544

Hogarth L, Balleine BW, Corbit LH, et al: Associative learning mechanisms underpinning the transition from recreational drug use to addiction. Ann NY Acad Sci 1282:12–24, 2013 23126270

Hyman SE: Addiction: a disease of learning and memory. Am J Psychiatry 162(8):1414–1422, 2005 16055762

Jugurnauth SK, Chen CK, Barnes MR, et al: A COMT gene haplotype associated with methamphetamine abuse. Pharmacogenet Genomics 21(11):731–740, 2011 21934638

Kenna GA, Zywiak WH, McGeary JE, et al: A within-group design of nontreatment seeking 5-HTTLPR genotyped alcohol-dependent subjects receiving ondansetron and sertraline. Alcohol (Hanover) 33(2):315–323, 2009 19032576

Koob GF, Le Moal M: Drug addiction, dysregulation of reward, and allostasis. Neuropsychopharmacology 24(2):97–129, 2001 11120394

Koob GF, Le Moal M: Plasticity of reward neurocircuitry and the "dark side" of drug addiction. Nat Neurosci 8(11):1442–1444, 2005 16251985

Koob GF, Le Moal M: Addiction and the brain antireward system. Annu Rev Psychol 59:29–53, 2008 18154498

Koob GF, Mason BJ: Existing and future drugs for the treatment of the dark side of addiction. Annu Rev Pharmacol Toxicol 56:299–322, 2016 26514207

Lewis M: The Biology of Desire: Why Addiction Is Not a Disease. New York, Perseus Books Group, 2015

McPherson SM, Burduli E, Smith CL, et al: A review of contingency management for the treatment of substance-use disorders: adaptation for underserved populations, use of experimental technologies, and personalized optimization strategies. Subst Abuse Rehabil 9:43–57, 2018 30147392

Miller WR, Westerberg VS, Harris RJ, et al: What predicts relapse? Prospective testing of antecedent models. Addiction 91(Suppl):S155–S172, 1996 8997790

Mueller A, Armbruster D, Moser DA, et al: Interaction of serotonin transporter gene-linked polymorphic region and stressful life events predicts cortisol stress response. Neuropsychopharmacology 36(7):1332–1339, 2011 21368747

Munetz MR, Griffin PA: Use of the sequential intercept model as an approach to decriminalization of people with serious mental illness. Psychiatr Serv 57(4):544–549, 2006 16603751

Naranjo CA, Bremner KE: Behavioural correlates of alcohol intoxication. Addiction 88(1):25–35, 1993 8448514

Norko MA, Fitch WL: DSM-5 and substance use disorders: clinicolegal implications. J Am Acad Psychiatry Law 42(4):443–452, 2014 25492070

O'Brien CP, Childress AR, Ehrman R, et al: Conditioning factors in drug abuse: can they explain compulsion? J Psychopharmacol 12(1):15–22, 1998 9584964

O'Malley PM: Maturing out of problematic alcohol use. Alcohol Res Health 28(4):202, 2004

O'Malley SS, Krishnan-Sarin S, Farren C, et al: Naltrexone decreases craving and alcohol self-administration in alcohol-dependent subjects and activates the hypothalamo-pituitary-adrenocortical axis. Psychopharmacology (Berl) 160(1):19–29, 2002 11862370

Ostrow DG, Shelby RD: Psychoanalytic and behavioral approaches to drug-related sexual risk taking. J Gay Lesbian Psychother 3:123–139, 2000

Pickard H: Responsibility without blame for addiction. Neuroethics 10(1):169–180, 2017 28725286

Powell v Texas, 392 U.S. 514 (1968)

Robinson v California, 370 U.S. 660 (1962)

Rowland LP: NINDS at 50: An Incomplete History Celebrating the Fiftieth Anniversary of the National Institute of Neurological Disorders and Stroke. New York, Demos Medical Publishing, 2003

Salamone JD, Correa M, Farrar A, et al: Effort-related functions of nucleus accumbens dopamine and associated forebrain circuits. Psychopharmacology (Berl) 191(3):461–482, 2007 17225164

Schultz W: Dopamine neurons and their role in reward mechanisms. Curr Opin Neurobiol 7(2):191–197, 1997 9142754

Searby A, Maude P, McGrath I: Maturing out, natural recovery, and dual diagnosis: what are the implications for older adult mental health services? Int J Ment Health Nurs 24(6):478–484, 2015 26256656

Sewell J, Cambiano V, Miltz A, et al: Changes in recreational drug use, drug use associated with chemsex, and HIV-related behaviours, among HIV-negative men who have sex with men in London and Brighton, 2013–2016. Sex Transm Infect 94(7):494–501, 2018 29700052

Spechler PA, Chaarani B, Hudson KE, et al: Response inhibition and addiction medicine: from use to abstinence. Prog Brain Res 223:143–164, 2016 26806775

Tindell AJ, Berridge KC, Zhang J, et al: Ventral pallidal neurons code incentive motivation: amplification by mesolimbic sensitization and amphetamine. Eur J Neurosci 22(10):2617–2634, 2005 16307604

U.S. v Miller, 549 F.2d 105 (9th Cir. 1975)

Vandenbergh DJ, Rodriguez LA, Miller IT, et al: High-activity catechol-O-methyltransferase allele is more prevalent in polysubstance abusers. Am J Med Genet 74(4):439–442, 1997 9259381

Vezina P: Sensitization of midbrain dopamine neuron reactivity and the self-administration of psychomotor stimulant drugs. Neurosci Biobehav Rev 27(8):827–839, 2004 15019432

Volkow ND, Baler RD: Addiction science: uncovering neurobiological complexity. Neuropharmacology 76(Pt B):235–249, 2014 22688927

Volkow ND, Fowler JS: Addiction, a disease of compulsion and drive: involvement of the orbitofrontal cortex. Cereb Cortex 10(3):318–325, 2000 10731226

Volkow ND, Fowler JS, Wang GJ, et al: Imaging dopamine's role in drug abuse and addiction. Neuropharmacology 56(Suppl 1):3–8, 2009 18617195

Volkow ND, Koob GF, McLellan AT: Neurobiologic advances from the brain disease model of addiction. N Engl J Med 374(4):363–371, 2016 26816013

Wasmuth SL, Outcalt J, Buck K, et al: Metacognition in people with substance abuse: findings and implications for occupational therapists. Can J Occup Ther 82(3):150–159, 2015 26103713

Werb D, Kamarulzaman A, Meacham MC, et al: The effectiveness of compulsory drug treatment: a systematic review. Int J Drug Policy 28:1–9, 2016 26790691

Winick C: Maturing out of narcotic addiction. Bull Narc 14:1–7, 1962

Wise RA: Dopamine and reward: the anhedonia hypothesis 30 years on. Neurotox Res 14(2–3):169–183, 2008 19073424

## CHAPTER 2

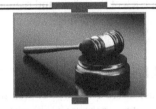

# LEGAL REGULATION OF SUBSTANCES AND LEGAL ISSUES IN SUBSTANCE USE DISORDER TREATMENT

## Introduction

Changing regulations about the special confidentiality of medical records related to substance use disorders (SUDs) perfectly describe the complex way in which U.S. society views, and regulates, addiction and its treatment. Because of the obvious stigma directed toward people with SUDs, legislators have enacted laws and regulations such as 42 C.F.R. Part 2 (Confidentiality of Substance Use Disorder Patient Records) to protect individuals with SUDs by sequestering their medical records from the prying eyes of work supervisors, colleagues, and even family members. However, in one unintended consequence of this segregation of SUD-related medical records and information, those with SUDs receive less comprehensive care *precisely because of* their clinician's lack of relevant medical information about the SUD. Recently, more sophisticated medical records legislation attempts to respect patient privacy but also share relevant medical information with clinicians who need it to deliver appropriate treatment.

In addition to siloed aspects of care, the United States has endured centuries of debate about the regulatory and legal parameters surrounding the legality of addictive substances. For substances that are legal to consume, laws specific to each substance type have been enacted to address distribution, sales, access, and use. Issues pertaining to the fiscal implications of the sales of substances have been debated, including sales taxes on substances that generate revenue for entirely unrelated purposes. Each of these laws and regulations is built on the philosophy that substance use could lead to negative consequences of addiction for society and for individuals.

## FORENSIC DILEMMA

A patient with opioid use disorder (OUD) has been receiving treatment for 5 years in a local opioid treatment program (OTP), where methadone is permitted to be prescribed for this condition. The patient's course has been relatively stable but lately he has seemed increasingly depressed. He does not want anyone to know about his treatment and substance use history. The patient's family physician is seeking information about the patient's treatment but the opioid treatment plan indicates that without a release of information, there is no basis to share information with the provider. The provider says that information sharing is part of the continuity of care.

Consider the following:

1. Can protected health information (PHI) be shared across providers?
2. Can the family provide consent for medical record release on behalf of the patient?
3. Would the situation change if the patient's depression were to lead to suicidal thoughts?

There are different provisions for confidentiality among general medical records, mental health records, and substance-use-specific treatment records. SUD treatment records must be maintained as confidential under the Code of Federal Regulations (42 C.F.R. Part 2), whereas the privacy of mental health records is typically governed by the Health Insurance Portability and Accountability Act of 1996 (HIPAA) and by state laws, which can be more but not less stringent than HIPAA. Privacy obligations for SUDs have historically been much more stringent than those for mental health records, including stricter penalties for violations. In recent years, there have been efforts to make the regulations more clinically helpful, given that there may be critical factors in information sharing across providers, as the case example in the Forensic Dilemma shows.

A family member cannot consent on a patient's behalf to release substance use treatment records or any PHI, unless the family member is the patient's legally authorized representative (e.g., guardian, parent, or power of attorney). If the patient becomes suicidal, there may be an emergency exception allowing certain information sharing, but the information shared should be relevant to resolving the emergency, and the reason for the sharing of information should be documented with a rationale for the emergency exception. Until recently, OTPs did not report information about methadone to state prescription drug monitoring programs (PDMPs). A rule promulgated in August 2020 by the federal government gave states the authority to permit, but not require, methadone treatment information to be entered into the PDMP system (American Association for the Treatment of Opioid Dependence 2022). If the patient in this example were being treated in a state where this information is shared with the PDMP, the primary care provider would be able to see it in the PDMP database. However, there are both advantages and disadvantages when methadone treatment information is in the PDMP database, because nonclinicians, including law enforcement, may have access to it as well.

# Historical Overview of the Legal Regulation of Substances

The United States has a complex history of laws related to substances that have addictive potential. This section summarizes some of the salient events and historical markers of legislation related to the legal regulation of substances.

As society was heading into the Roaring Twenties, Congress ratified the Eighteenth Amendment to the U.S. Constitution in 1919 to prohibit the manufacture and sale of alcohol. Section 1 of the amendment, which came into effect in January 1920, follows:

> After one year from the ratification of this article the manufacture, sale, or transportation of intoxicating liquors within, the importation thereof into, or the exportation thereof from the United States and all territory subject to the jurisdiction thereof for beverage purposes is hereby prohibited. (U.S. Const. Amend. XVIII, § 1 1919)

The initial act supporting prohibition reflected concerns largely voiced via the temperance movement, positing that widespread access to alcohol contributed to social problems, including poverty and other ills. After the Eighteenth Amendment came the Volstead Act (the National Prohibition Act of 1919), which defined all liquor, wine, and beer as qualifying for prohibition. One unintended consequence was that prohibition led to an illegal underground movement of alcohol sales, leaving the public more opposed to prohibition. Thirteen years after the Eighteenth Amendment was ratified, it was repealed with the Twenty-First Amendment, making alcohol legal again. To date, the Eighteenth Amendment is the only amendment to the U.S. Constitution that has ever been repealed.

Although alcohol is a legal substance in the United States, several aspects of regulation remain that limit and monitor alcohol sales and access. The Bureau of Alcohol, Tobacco, Firearms and Explosives is the federal law enforcement agency within the U.S. Department of Justice that is responsible for identifying and eliminating criminal activities associated with trafficking of liquor and contraband tobacco across state lines.

In colonial times, alcohol consumption by children was not prohibited in the United States. However, alcohol laws that limit the age of alcohol purchase and consumption have since evolved. With passage of the Twenty-First Amendment repealing prohibition, Congress gave states the authority to control alcohol sales, import, distribution, and possession laws. With the Uniform Minimum Drinking Age Act (1984), the federal government set the minimum legal drinking and possession age for alcohol at 21 years. Despite this age restriction, in the 2020 National Survey on Drug Use and Health (SAMHSA 2021), approximately 9.2% of people ages 12–20 years reported binge drinking in the last month, and 16.1% of underage individuals reported any alcohol use in the past month. In addition, 6.4% of the adult population surveyed reported heavy alcohol use in the past month. Of youth ages 12–17 years, 2.8% qualified as having alcohol use disorder (SAMHSA 2021).

Alcohol-related fatalities remain high in the United States, with 31% of motor vehicle fatalities involving alcohol (U.S. Department of Transportation 2015). The World Health Organization (2014) described the public health import of regulation and restrictive alcohol policies in part to reduce harmful effects of alcohol. This report also indicated that more countries reported stricter blood alcohol levels for legal limits to drive a vehicle in 2012 compared with 2008.

The negative outcomes associated with alcohol use continue to drive regulatory and legal shifts. For example, driving laws related to alcohol consumption represent a complicated area of intersection. With state variations and a range of policies and legislative efforts, impaired driving remains an area of major concern. Several policy efforts are posited to have had positive effects on reducing impaired driving and associated risks: these include sobriety checkpoints, random breath testing, legal blood alcohol concentration limits for driving being lowered to 0.05 g/dL, driving-under-the-influence courts, mandatory alcohol ignition car locks, and routine alcohol monitoring (Fell 2019).

Another example of an effort to limit problematic alcohol usage among vulnerable populations through rules and policy includes the reduction of binge drinking on college campuses. Binge drinking is attributed to many tragic deaths and injuries each year. Krieger et al. (2018) reported that binge drinking among college-age youth occurs at a frequency as high as 30%–40%. Efforts to regulate college binge drinking through policy development are increasing (Toomey and Wagenaar 2002). Other areas of regulatory and legal influence include employment rules related to alcohol use and evaluation of fitness, covered in Chapter 4. As clinical and scientific understanding related to reducing alcohol use and its problematic aspects increases, laws and policies will evolve to meet the challenge of harm avoidance.

The legal regulation of opioids and cocaine has followed a different pathway from that of alcohol. Cocaine has an interesting history, because it was once used as an anesthetic and was included in the recipe for Coca-Cola beverages until its removal from those products in 1903 (History.com Editors 2018; Redman 2011). By the mid-1800s, morphine, an opioid, was being used in the United States to treat a variety of conditions, including pain, anxiety, and tuberculosis. At the end of the Civil War, it was clear that many veterans were experiencing morphine addiction. German chemical company Bayer produced another opioid, heroin, as a "nonaddictive" substitute for morphine. Heroin was marketed for several purposes, from cough suppression to pain treatment and even for detoxification for individuals experiencing morphine addiction (Netherland and Hansen 2017).

Congress enacted the Harrison Narcotics Tax Act (1914), which required taxation of the production and distribution of opiates and cocaine products. In *United States v. Doremus* (1919), the U.S. Supreme Court determined that Congress exceeded its federal authority over states by imposing a law that included 1) taxing the sale or distribution of opioids and limiting sales to areas related to prescribing and dispensing and 2) requiring special forms to track these transactions. By 1924, heroin was deemed illegal, as it became increasingly clear that it was an addictive substance (Michaels House n.d.). Subsequently, several court cases limited prescription of opioids in an effort to curb addiction. The Drug Abuse Control Amendments (1965) were passed to help limit the risks of abuse. Title II of the Comprehensive Drug Abuse Prevention and Control Act (1970), commonly known as the Controlled Substances Act (CSA), considers opioids as addictive agents, and places them on a schedule of addiction. Across the schedule of substances, the most addictive drugs are not available even by prescription, as described later in this chapter (42 C.F.R. Part 8 [2001], Medication Assisted Treatment for Opioid Disorders).

Other substances perceived as contributing to addiction and crime were also regulated. With the evolution of the 1980s crack cocaine epidemic, Congress passed the Anti-Drug Abuse Act (1986), which incorporated mandatory sentences for possession of certain amounts of crack or powdered cocaine. As discussed later in this chapter, there were many racial implications to the strict criminalization of crack cocaine, especially as the epidemic was clearly affecting Black and low-income communities disproportionately.

Marijuana policies and laws have also evolved, and the professional cultivation of marijuana is not new. Marijuana was used in early U.S. history because the hemp plant was known for its strong fibers for rope and cloth. During the nineteenth century, many states had marijuana plantations for these purposes, and marijuana was used medicinally until the late 1930s. Its recreational use was based in part on smoking hashish and other methods of use, which increased after the Mexican Revolution (1910–1920). During prohibition and as the price of alcohol increased, some considered marijuana a replacement substance. The Marijuana Tax Act (1937) criminalized the drug; later, there were even stricter rules with mandatory minimum sentences related to its use (Public Broadcasting Service 2022). As more White populations began using marijuana, concern grew and the Comprehensive Drug Abuse Prevention and Control Act (1970) provided for certain mandatory penalties for drug-related offenses to be removed. From there, the adoption of separate standards for marijuana compared with opioids or cocaine evolved (Public Broadcasting Service 2022).

More recently, the legalization of marijuana for medicinal and recreational purposes has been a rapidly advancing area of law. As of January 2022, 19 states have fully legalized marijuana, with about 10 additional states allowing its use for medical purposes, authorizing its decriminalization, or both (DISA 2022). At the federal level, marijuana may be shifted to a Schedule III drug, based on proposed changes that were promulgated in 2024 (DEA 2024). Uncertainty and controversy remain regarding whether legalization ultimately increases or decreases the prevalence of marijuana use or addiction (Wilkinson et al. 2016). With the changing legal landscape, clinicians should be cognizant of areas of importance, such as driving while intoxicated, the potential for secondary ingestion by children and other bystanders, the potential complications and prevalence rates of comorbid polysubstance use, and the potential for health problems, including potential psychosis (Wilkinson et al. 2016). The effects of marijuana legalization on public health require ongoing surveillance. In a study highlighting significant increases in U.S. cannabis use, researchers using U.S. National Survey on Drug Use and Health data showed that from 1992 to 2022, the per-capita rate of daily or near-daily cannabis use rose 15-fold. Although use of alcohol remained more prevalent than that of cannabis, the average cannabis user reported using 15–16 days per month, whereas the average drinker reported alcohol use on 4–5 days per month. The study was based on self-report, excluded some populations, and could not directly tie cannabis policy changes to the increase in use, but the authors concluded that "…whichever way causal arrows point, cannabis use now appears to be on a fundamentally different scale than it was before legalization." (Calkins 2024)

The stimulant amphetamine has been available for almost 150 years. It was used medicinally in the 1920s to assist with blood pressure and other ailments, but its misuse became problematic when the drug began to be marketed over the counter. During World War II, amphetamine was used for soldiers to fight fatigue and enhance mood and endurance; later, it was used to treat depression (Rensberger 1972). The illegal and underground use of amphetamine became popular for individuals who needed to stay awake for long periods and for students attempting to enhance study performance. Injectable forms of amphetamine were used and sold by pharmacies. In a *New York Times* article, Rensberger (1972) described amphetamine use for weight loss and the increased use of "speed," which led the U.S. Department of Justice Bureau of Narcotics and Dangerous Drugs to try to limit the number of amphetamines that pharmaceutical companies could manufacture.

Private production of amphetamine products, including crystal methamphetamine, often called ice, has further changed the landscape and has contributed to countless deaths associated with the opioid crisis (Drug Addiction Treatment Act 2000). In Oregon, possession of small amounts of any illegal substance, including methamphetamine, was decriminalized in 2020. This legislation also was intended to direct individuals with possession of these substances into treatment (State of Oregon Legislative Policy and Research Office 2020). At the same time, amphetamines remain a mainstay of treatment for conditions such as ADHD and even narcolepsy.

Another set of historical markers and trends regards the legal regulation related to benzodiazepines (Wick 2013). Chlordiazepoxide was identified in 1955 by a chemist at Hoffmann-La Roche and was marketed shortly thereafter as Librium; diazepam was introduced subsequently. Because they were considered a safer alternative to barbiturates, benzodiazepines gained great popularity as an effective and safe sedative and anxiolytic. By the 1970s, benzodiazepines were among the most frequently prescribed medications. But as these medications gained popularity, so did recognition of their potential for misuse and addiction. The use of benzodiazepines concomitantly with opioids has raised a further specter of concern related to the opioid epidemic, so the regulation of benzodiazepines continues to be relevant.

Ketamine emerged in the 1950s as an anesthetic agent. Evolving out of experimentation with phencyclidine, which has a similar mechanism of action, ketamine became recognized as a safe medication that could be used as a surgical anesthetic (Li and Vlisides 2016; Mion 2017). Despite its effectiveness and safety profile for anesthesia, ketamine's psychedelic effects made it a popular drug of misuse. At low doses, ketamine creates a stimulant effect, along with mild dissociation and hallucinations as well as perceptual distortions; at higher doses, it can have effects that mimic schizophrenia-type symptoms. Data have emerged suggesting that long-term ketamine use can induce more persistent neuropsychiatric symptoms (Liu et al. 2016). Still more recent data led to the approval of esketamine for the treatment of refractory depression in 2019, with tight regulatory parameters making it available only in a certified doctor's office or clinic (U.S. Food and Drug Administration 2019).

Finally, psychedelic drugs, also well known for their addictive potential, have recently emerged with new considerations regarding their legal regulation. Beginning in 2019, Denver, Colorado, followed by Oakland and Santa Cruz, California, shifted away from attaching criminal penalties to the use or possession of psychedelic drugs, which has extended to numerous other cities in the United States. In November 2020, Oregon became the first state to decriminalize personal possession of small amounts of all illegal drugs through Measure 110 (State of Oregon Legislative Policy and Research Office 2020). The law reduced the level of violation from a criminal misdemeanor to a new violation (Class E felony) punishable by a $100 fine, which could be waived by participating in a health assessment at an addiction recovery center. Substance use treatments related to this law were to be funded by marijuana sales taxes. The possession of large amounts and the commercialization of drug sales were not legalized. A noteworthy aspect of the Oregon law is that the Oregon Health Authority was also charged with developing and instituting regulations related to the clinical usage and licensure of psychedelic treatment services by 2022 through the help of an advisory board (Smith and Appelbaum 2021). Although Smith and Appelbaum (2021) reported that some studies have shown promise related to psychedelic use in the treatment of depression (see also Davis et al. 2021), PTSD, suicidal thoughts, and substance use, concerns about their risks remain in regard to worsening psychosis and other issues. Also, as Smith and Appelbaum (2021) pointed out, serotonergic psychedelics and substances such as entactogen MDMA (3,4-methylenedioxymethamphetamine) do not have the same mechanism of action and yet are linked together in the legalization advocacy. The authors noted the importance of proceeding with caution with these types of legalization measures.

# Legal Regulation of Substances and the Intersection With Social Determinants and Race and Ethnicity

Substance use and its ties to race and ethnicity, socioeconomic status, and disparities in access to care are notable throughout history. Some have posited that racist views catalyzed the passage of the Harrison Narcotics Tax Act of 1914 partly to limit Black users of cocaine who were increasingly seen as dangerous (History.com Editors 2018). At the same time, China was one of the major growth spots for opium. In 1919, a commission established an international effort to work with the government of China to cease opium manufacturing and distribution. One of the resulting social effects was that individuals of Chinese descent were generally blamed for their exportation of opium-related products (International Opium Commission 1909).

In more recent times, the Anti-Drug Abuse Act of 1986 has received much public scrutiny on the racial and ethnic equity front. The law has significant racial implications because smaller amounts of crack cocaine were criminalized but powdered cocaine was not, and it was clear that crack cocaine users were more likely to be Black (Vagins and McCurdy 2006). The American Civil Liberties Union issued a report calling attention to this issue through its advocacy efforts (Vagins and McCurdy 2006), noting that since the passage of this legislation, the sentencing duration for Black Americans had increased by a factor of more than four. This discrepancy was addressed—to some degree—by the Fair Sentencing Act (2010), which made the ratio of penalty between crack and powder cocaine more appropriate (from 100:1 to 18:1, meaning that 5 g of crack cocaine would receive the same punishment as 500 g of powder cocaine). There remains debate as to whether the shift was retroactive to individuals sentenced under the old laws. In 2018, the First Step Act (2018) called for retroactive sentence reduction if the crack cocaine offense triggered a mandatory minimum sentence (Foster and Lampe 2021).

More recently, the U.S. Supreme Court addressed the amount of a substance that would lead to conviction in *Terry v. United States* (2021). Terry asserted that he should have been eligible for a sentence reduction of his 2008 conviction related to possession and intent to distribute an unspecified amount of crack cocaine. The court ruled that although the sentence reduction would have been appropriate under the First Step Act for a crack cocaine offense that had triggered a mandatory minimum sentence, Terry's offense did not qualify because he was sentenced as a career offender with an unspecified amount of crack cocaine that later was identified as just under 4 g (*Terry v. United States* 2021). However, in her concurring opinion, Justice Sonia Sotomayor commented on the consequences of the court's decision. She noted that the construction of the preceding laws and sentencing commission guidelines allowed "street-level crack dealers to receive significantly longer sentences than wholesale importers of powder cocaine" and that "Black people bore the brunt of this disparity. Around 80% to 90% of those convicted of crack offenses between 1992 and 2006 were Black, while Black people made up only around 30% of powder cocaine offenders in those same years" (*Terry v. United States* 2021). Justice Sotomayor added that Terry was labeled a career offender for drug-related offenses committed as a teenager. In her conclusion, Justice Sotomayor noted that others like him would be left out of the opportunity for a more balanced sentence and that Congress "had numerous tools to right this injustice" (*Terry v. United States* 2021), a fact reported in the news media after the ruling (Totenberg 2021).

The Equal Justice Initiative (2019) reported that despite a more compassionate view of opioid use in the United States, there continued to be an uneven distribution across racial lines in how drug enforcement is executed. Goudsward (2019) found that arrests related to cocaine offenses were four times greater than those related to heroin in 2016, and White individuals were more likely to be involved in the heroin-related offenses. The report from Goudsward (2019) and findings from many others have demonstrated a significant difference in funds flowing to states for public health measures to address the opioid epidemic, which disproportionately affected White populations initially. This is contrary to the legal world's response to the crack cocaine epidemic, which focused mostly on mandatory minimum sentences.

Separate from laws related to the criminalization of drug possession and distribution, important findings pertaining to the regulatory requirements of certain substances have contributed to unequal distribution of treatment program types. For example, in a study of U.S. counties in 2016, those with dense Black or African American and Hispanic or Latino populations had more facilities that provided methadone (i.e., heavily regulated and separated OPTs), whereas population centers with a higher proportion of White individuals were more likely to have facilities and clinical services available that provided buprenorphine (Goedel et al. 2020). The authors concluded that a shift in regulatory requirements, like those described in the next section, may reduce racial disparities in access to treatment.

# Legal Authority, Medical Basis, and Public Policy for Scheduling and Controlling Substances

During their long history, efforts to legalize addictive substances and their use have provoked widely different opinions. In some cases, public interest in broader access to particular substances, efforts to reduce the ranks of those incarcerated for SUDs, and potential for tax revenue and economic aspects of commercialization have all generated advocacy for legalization (Smith and Appelbaum 2021). As with psychedelics, different city ordinances, state laws, and federal laws may operate related to possession and use of such substances. Because of the shifting legal landscape, it can be challenging for practitioners to keep track of relevant laws when treating a patient who is using substances. Nevertheless, it is important for clinicians to understand the local legal landscape regarding addictive substances. The federal statute known as the CSA was signed into law in 1970 to help regulate the manufacturing, sales, and security of specific substances being developed by pharmaceutical industries. As described earlier in this chapter, Title II of the CSA provided legislative contours

**Table 2–1.**     Factors used for drug schedule classification

The factors for the determination of drug schedule classification are listed in Section 201(c), [21 U.S.C. § 811(c)] of the CSA as follows:

1.  Its actual or relative potential for abuse

2.  Scientific evidence of its pharmacological effect, if known

3.  The state of current scientific knowledge regarding the drug or other substance

4.  Its history and current pattern of abuse

5.  The scope, duration, and significance of abuse

6.  What, if any, risk there is to the public health

7.  Its psychic or physiological dependence liability

8.  Whether the substance is an immediate precursor of a substance already controlled under this subchapter

to help combat drug abuse and created five drug classifications, known as schedules, to regulate certain substances used for various purposes. Both the FDA and the U.S. Drug Enforcement Administration (DEA) have the authority to review substances, determine the schedule to which substances should be assigned, and revise this determination as warranted.

Various elements are used to determine the proper scheduling of substances, including their potential for abuse, medical use, and international and distribution regulations and agreements. Schedule I drugs have high abuse potential, whereas Schedule V drugs have the lowest abuse potential.

The eight factors delineated in Table 2–1 relate to how particular substances are analyzed to determine their schedule classification. The five drug schedules for controlled substances include the following (Pottle and Parisi 2023; U.S. Drug Enforcement Administration 2018):

- *Schedule I drugs* include those with no defined medical purpose, with the highest potential for abuse, and with no accepted safety for use under medical supervision. Examples include heroin, hallucinogens, marijuana (per federal rules), and MDMA. On May 21, 2024, the DEA published in the Federal Register a proposed rule changing marijuana from Schedule I to Schedule III. After a 2-month period of public comment, the DEA administrator may request a hearing in front of an administrative law judge, who will make the ultimate rescheduling determination. If marijuana is indeed changed to a Schedule III substance, there will be substantial implications in easing restrictions on research with THC and eliminating the nationwide ban on cannabis use, which has already been increasingly undercut by state laws allowing medical and recreational use of cannabis (DEA 2024).

- *Schedule III drugs* include those with moderate to low abuse potential (lower than Schedule I and Schedule II), currently accepted medical use, and low to moderate potential for physical or psychological dependence. Examples include anabolic steroids and testosterone, codeine, buprenorphine, and ketamine.
- *Schedule IV drugs* include those that have accepted medical use and a lower potential of abuse compared with Schedule III substances. Examples include benzodiazepines, dextropropoxyphene, zolpidem, tramadol, eszopiclone, and zaleplon.
- *Schedule V drugs* include those with the lowest potential for abuse. Examples include prescription medications to control symptoms of fibromyalgia and irritable bowel syndrome as well as cough medications with low amounts of codeine (e.g., Robitussin AC).

At times, research has suggested further consideration of a particular substance's scheduling. For example, Johnson et al. (2018) argued that psilocybin should be moved to Schedule IV based on their analysis of the eight factors and their views of the putative beneficial effects of psilocybin-assisted therapies.

According to the CSA, a valid prescription of a controlled substance must be issued for "legitimate medical purposes by a registered practitioner acting in the usual course of sound professional practice" (21 C.F.R. 1306 [2022]). Prescribers must be registered with the DEA or must be exempt from registration. For each prescription, providers must enter specific information, including date, DEA number, prescriber name and address, patient name and address, drug name, drug strength and dosage, quantity prescribed, directions for use, and any refill information. The pharmacist must review the prescriptions and ensure that they are being prescribed for true medical reasons (Gabay 2013). The manner of the prescription (e.g., telephone, fax, or electronic) is regulated as well. Also, not all prescriptions for scheduled substances can be refilled. DEA numbers are generated by an automatic formula. A particular hospital or health care institution may have an institutional DEA number that can be used with the institution's authority.

States also have their own controlled substance laws, in addition to federal laws, which can create some confusion. Legalization of marijuana is one example in which state laws and federal laws conflict, which can be challenging for practitioners. They may wish to consult with risk management specialists before prescribing or recommending controlled substances differently than the federal law requires, although this may shift if marijuana is moved to Schedule III. Programs that receive federal funds will generally require adherence to federal laws. Finally, states may require a separate controlled substance prescription authorization within the state that is separate from the DEA number required by prescribers.

Administrative rules provide authoritative paradigms, in addition to state and federal laws, for substance use treatment. For example, rulemaking within states includes requirements for licensure of particular substance use treatment services, oversight responsibilities of agencies, and even qualifications of particular staff, including the medical director overseeing these programs. It is important for individuals in these roles to be familiar with local requirements. Laws, regulations, and policies that may relate to SUD treatment as a whole also have separate provisions for particular aspects of care, such as those revolving around particular treatments. With the opioid epidemic drawing increased attention to the need to make access to care a top priority, many states have examined their rule set to try to remove barriers to care. To highlight this further, the following section addresses medications that are highly regulated for the treatment of OUDs.

# Methadone and Buprenorphine Regulation for the Treatment of Opioid Use Disorders

As the opioid crisis was becoming increasingly apparent, initial examination of overdose deaths pointed attention to prescription opioid use as a major contributor (Soelberg et al. 2017). Several notable areas of policy and law have been based on this observation, designed to stem the tide of opioid prescribing and increase access to addiction treatment. Major litigation against manufacturers of drugs like oxycodone (OxyContin) have resulted in settlement dollars distributed across various governmental entities (American Bar Association 2019). Prescribing practices have been shifting, with more oversight and requirements for prescription drug monitoring. Although these changes have curtailed prescription drug overdoses to some extent, there has since been a shift to overdoses related to heroin and fentanyl.

Federal agencies involved in the regulation and investigation of aspects of opioids include the DEA, the FDA, and the U.S. Department of Justice (DOJ) (Soelberg et al. 2017). The DEA, in partnership with the DOJ, began to identify and track "pill mills," which involved physicians illegally prescribing narcotics under the guise of treatment (Soelberg et al. 2017). The DEA also invested in enhanced use of state PDMPs, which provide information regarding any use of Schedule II or III medications through prescription. In response to the opioid epidemic, mandates for use of PDMPs prior to prescribing increased around the country (Soelberg et al. 2017). Prescription limit laws and oversight of physician practices in which opioid prescription seemed excessive also have been enacted. In a systematic review of these interventions, Lee et al. (2021) found that these types of state policies generally were associated with reduced misuse of prescription opioids, but they may have also unintentionally siphoned individuals with OUDs toward accessing illegal drugs and thereby increasing mortality. Other examples of anti-opioid addiction laws include required increases in naloxone access and revised good Samaritan laws, which were designed to decrease the risk of prosecution to individuals who called for rescue of an individual experiencing an opioid overdose but who themselves may have been using illegal substances (McClellan et al. 2018). At least one study reported that these laws were associated with reduced opioid mortality (McClellan et al. 2018). Other relevant laws enacted in response to the opioid epidemic include those that add specific requirements for informed consent when a patient is being prescribed particular opioid-containing pain medications. For example, these laws may require a particular form of opioid to be used, in which there is an acknowledgment that the patient receives information about the danger of opioid addiction (Public Act 246 2017).

Access to buprenorphine and methadone in the United States is regulated separately from the prescription of other medications, which has profoundly affected access to care. In particular, 42 C.F.R. Part 8 governs the accreditation and certification of OTPs. These treatment plans were formerly referred to colloquially as methadone clinics; more recently, language has shifted to refer to them as OTPs, in part due to the stigma of the former label. The Substance Abuse and Mental Health Services Administration (SAMHSA) is responsible for overseeing the standards and certification processes of these programs. Besides the oversight by multiple agencies and requirements involved in being authorized as an OTP, zoning restrictions can add barriers to setting up these clinics in particular communities (McBournie et al. 2019).

OTP accreditation contains many components, including a program sponsor and a designated medical director who assumes responsibility for administering all medical services performed by the OTP and ensuring its adherence to local, state, and federal laws and regulations. These programs are required to have continuous quality improvement, initial and maintenance treatment program components, special services for pregnant patients, counseling services, drug abuse testing services, appropriate record keeping and patient confidentiality protocols, medication administration, dispensing and use protocols, and strict parameters related to unsupervised or take-home methadone use (21 U.S.C. § 823; 42 U.S.C. § 257a; Department of Human Services 2024). There were expanded take-home allowances for Methadone that were adopted by SAMHSA in 2023 after experience with the pandemic and advocacy to minimize burdens to accessing methadone care (SAMHSA 2024). those were interim, then there were permanent take-home guidelines (Facher 2024; Foley & Lardner LLP, 2024): see Federal Review 2024. The medical director must factor in a number of issues to determine the appropriateness of the take-home methadone dosage (Table 2–2), including the following: absence of recent drug misuse (including alcohol), clinic attendance, behavioral problems at the clinic,

**Table 2–2.** Take-home dosing authorized in 42 C.F.R. 8.12(i)(3)(i) for opioid treatment programs

| Duration in treatment | Take-home allowance |
| --- | --- |
| Days 1–14 | Up to 7 doses |
| Days 15–30 | Up to 14 doses |
| Days 31+ | Up to 28 doses |

recent criminal activity, the stability of patient's home environment and relationships, length of time in treatment, safe storage of take-home medications, and whether the rehabilitative benefit of take-home dosing outweighs the benefit of clinic attendance and balances the potential risk of the drug being diverted for misuse (42 C.F.R. 8.12[h]).

This strict dosing schedule shifted during the COVID-19 pandemic, allowing greater flexibility for take-home dosing of methadone. In one study, researchers found that individuals with concomitant methamphetamine use were provided with take-home doses similar to those of people who had not used methamphetamine in the context of the pandemic, whereas previously they had not been allowed similar take-home dosing (Amram et al. 2022). Even with this flexibility, OTPs faced several challenges as a result of the pandemic, including maintaining service levels and dealing with limitations posed by federal guidance (SAMHSA 2021).

Other countries do not regulate methadone for OUD to the extent that it is regulated in the United States (McBournie et al. 2019). In June 2021, new DEA rules authorized mobile units to extend access to narcotic treatment programs outside of clinic settings (U.S. Drug Enforcement Administration 2021). Thus, given the ongoing strain on the treatment system and data regarding the relentless and persisting high death rates pertaining to the opioid crisis, there have been new efforts to improve access to medications for OUD. In December 2022, SAMHSA introduced new provisions that would increase the flexibility of methadone prescribing, partly adopting lessons learned from the pandemic response (SAMHSA 2021). Then in February 2024, a final rule made those flexibilities permanent. This makes further access broader and creates changes to the legal regulation of methadone prescribing.

Buprenorphine, a synthetic opioid, was developed in the 1960s and is a Schedule III drug that can be administered in an office-based setting to treat OUD. Legislation was enacted in the Drug Addiction Treatment Act (2000) that permitted its access in office-based settings, but only by prescribers who had received additional training on the drug and how to prescribe it before they could treat patients (Kumar et al. 2021). Initially, physicians were allowed to manage treatment for only 30 patients receiving buprenorphine, which could be extended to 100 patients after the first year of prescribing at the 30-patient limit. These provisions marked a strict regulatory framework for the treatment of OUDs in office-based settings. On the plus side, they also allowed for the first time a highly regulated substance to be used outside of a designated OTP for the treatment of OUD. As a response to the COVID-19 pandemic, the DEA announced substantially decreased requirements for buprenorphine prescribing (SAMHSA 2021).

With the increased mortality rates related to opioid overdose deaths, several other legislative advances have been made to increase access to treatment while still attempting to balance risks of misuse and diversion of medications for unauthorized distribution. The Comprehensive Addiction and Recovery Act (2016) expanded qualifying buprenorphine prescribers to include nurse practitioners and physician assistants who meet particular criteria. In July 2016, SAMHSA released a final rule that went into effect on August 6, 2016, which was designed to increase access to medication-assisted treatment with buprenorphine in office-based settings (Medication Assisted Treatment for Opioid Use Disorders, 42 C.F.R. § 8 2016). This final rule allowed individual practitioners, as authorized under the CSA, to dispense or prescribe FDA-approved Schedule II, IV, or V controlled substances by filing an initial notification of intent to treat a maximum of 30 patients at a time, followed 1 year later by a notification of intent to treat up to 100 patients at a time. Eligible practitioners could then request approval to treat up to 275 patients under the CSA. The SUPPORT for Patients and Communities Act (2018) further added clinical nurse specialists, certified registered nurse anesthetists, and certified nurse midwives to the categories of eligible prescribers of buprenorphine to treat OUD. The act also allowed qualified practitioners to treat up to 100 patients instead of 30 in the first year of authorization, in particular circumstances (National Association of State Alcohol and Drug Abuse Directors 2022).

With the strict regulations related to both buprenorphine and methadone treatments for OUDs, policymakers were faced with the dilemma of countless individuals unable to access care during the COVID-19 pandemic if some rules were not shifted. Thus, in an unprecedented fashion, SAMHSA, the DEA, and other federal agencies rallied to make adaptations. For example, although a full physical evaluation was still required for admission to an OTP, SAMHSA granted an exemption such that new patients treated with buprenorphine did not require an in-person physical examination if the authorizing health professional determined that an adequate evaluation of the patient could be accomplished through telehealth (SAMHSA 2021). The buprenorphine waiver requirement itself was slowly weakened. In the Consolidated Appropriations Act (2023), the requirement for the data waiver was removed entirely. Practitioners across the board are required to receive certain opioid-related training, but there is no additional specific requirement for prescribing buprenorphine as of early 2023 (SAMHSA 2021). This is a major policy change that will hopefully yield increased access to this medication.

# Confidentiality Rules for Substance Use Treatment Services

The confidentiality of treatment records is of critical importance across medical care—all the more so for records about addiction and its treatment. HIPAA was enacted in 1996. Although it was passed for many reasons related to transfer of insurance coverage and simplification thereof, with this new law, the U.S. Department of Health and Human Services created the HIPAA Privacy and Security Rules, in which specifically defined PHI was ruled impermissible to disclose unless patients gave their authorization or other exceptions existed (HIPAA Journal 2019). The Enforcement Rule was introduced in 2006, allowing for the investigation of covered entities that might be violating the Privacy Rule and authorizing the U.S. Department of Health and Human Services Office for Civil Rights to bring criminal charges against persistent offenders who did not invoke corrective measures within 30 days; individuals were also permitted to pursue independent civil legal action related to confidentiality breaches that caused them "serious harm" (HIPAA Journal 2019). For practitioners trying to understand the landscape of privacy laws, it is important to realize that states also have their own state-enforced privacy protection laws, which can be stricter than HIPAA but cannot be less strict. Thus, to determine allowances for information sharing related to those areas covered under HIPAA, the clinician must often look to both state and federal laws and seek guidance on interpretation when needed.

Separate from HIPAA, the Code of Federal Regulations (particularly 42 C.F.R. Part 2) has an important place in the governance of privacy related to SUD treatment (SAMHSA 2021). Disclosure of records for patients with SUDs is specified in 42 C.F.R. Part 2. This regulation was first promulgated in 1975 and was developed in reaction to the potential use of SUD information in nontreatment settings, such as administrative or criminal hearings, related to the patient. It was designed to protect patients in SUD treatment from adverse consequences in legal matters such as criminal, child custody, divorce, or employment proceedings. It applies to what are called "Part 2 programs or other lawful holder" of patient information related to a Part 2 consent. Because clinicians treat people with co-occurring disorders, it can be confusing to know where Part 2 applies. A program under Part 2 provisions has a specific definition:

> A "program"... is an individual, entity (other than a general medical facility), or an identified unit in a general medical facility, that "holds itself out" as providing

and provides diagnosis, treatment, or referral for treatment for an SUD. Medical personnel or other staff in a general medical facility who are identified as providers whose primary function is to provide diagnosis, treatment, or referral for treatment for an SUD are also Programs.

Thus, SUD-specific treatment programs generally qualify. However, even separate from what is covered for SUD-specific programs, an individual must consent to sharing information that they have an SUD, and Part 2 requires specific information on consent forms, including specificity about the individuals authorized to receive or disclose the information as well as the "amount and kind" of information permissible to disclose and the purpose of the disclosure (42 C.F.R. § 2.31). Whereas HIPAA allows for the disclosure of PHI without patient consent in certain circumstances, such as treatment, payment, or health care operations, 42 C.F.R. Part 2 does not contain such allowances (SAMHSA 2021). Although this legislation was written with the intent to protect patients, one study based in Oregon raised concerns that the strict elements of Part 2 and the legal confusion associated with the rules and challenges in obtaining patient consent resulted in greater barriers to care coordination and integration (McCarty et al. 2017).

In 2016, SAMHSA released a proposed rule to update the 42 C.F.R. Part 2 regulations and facilitate information exchange while reducing administrative burdens (Marbury 2016). The final rule, announced in August 2020, clarified and modified several areas of Part 2. Specifically, it required that treatment records created by non–Part 2 providers based on their patient encounters are not covered by Part 2, unless SUD records from Part 2 programs are contained in those records. It also allowed a patient with an SUD to consent to disclosure of their Part 2 treatment records to an entity (e.g., the Social Security Administration) without having to name a person who would be the recipient of the information. The rules further allowed disclosures of information to PDMPs and such central registries (and permitted OTPs to enroll in PDMPs as consistent with state law), and they defined medical emergencies that would allow disclosures (SAMHSA 2021). Still, one study found that electronic health systems used various techniques, such as sensitive note designation, limited role-based access for providers, and "break the glass" technology, among others, to enhance intrainstitutional communication and care coordination related to substance use treatment (Campbell et al. 2019). Despite these approaches, the authors opined that the amendments to 42 C.F.R. Part 2 had not adequately addressed information-sharing needs.

SAMHSA has made several attempts to clarify for the public some of the provisions of 42 C.F.R. Part 2 and HIPAA to enhance care coordination capabilities (SAMHSA 2022c). Also, in part catalyzed by the COVID-19 pandemic, the Coronavirus Aid, Relief, and Economic Security Act (2020) attempted to align aspects of HIPAA and Part 2 for the purpose of treatment, payment, and operations, which became law in March 2020 and required SAMHSA to release new regulations to implement it as of 2021 (American Psychiatric Association 2022). Through the experiences with COVID-19 and the opioid crisis, there is more discussion about what may need changing or clarifying in terms of the legal regulation of privacy for SUD treatment, and practitioners should stay abreast of this evolving landscape.

# Legal Regulation Related to Substance Use Treatment

The Mental Health Parity and Addiction Equity Act (2008; MHPAEA) was enacted through the advocacy of legislators Paul Wellstone and Pete Domenici, and it prevents health insurance companies from providing mental health or SUD benefits that are limited compared with those benefits for medical or surgical care (Centers for Medicare and Medicaid Services 2023). The MHPAEA was further amended by the Affordable Care Act to broaden its application to individual health care coverage in addition to group plans. Although the law is complex in terms of its applicability, in essence it built on the Mental Health Parity Act (1996), which provided for prohibitions on annual or lifetime dollar limits on mental health benefits that disadvantage individuals more than benefits for medical or surgical interventions. The MHPAEA extends the parity requirements to SUDs. The act does not require benefits to be covered for mental health and SUDs, but it requires group health plans that cover these benefits to provide benefits no less favorable than medical or surgical benefits.

Before passage of the Affordable Care Act and the MHPAEA, both of which expanded health insurance coverage for mental health and SUD treatment, 2% of the population with employer-sponsored health insurance had coverage that excluded mental health benefits and 7% had coverage that entirely excluded substance use treatment benefits (Frank et al. 2014). Discretion can vary by state in terms of how these benefits are covered across Medicaid programs (Burns 2015). In a more recent review of data for 2005–2018 from the National Survey on Drug Use and Health, 37.6% of privately insured individuals with a drug use disorder did not know whether their plan covered drug use treatment, and this finding was consistent over the study years (Mojtabai et al. 2020). Of the individuals who knew about their coverage, they reported modest increases in coverage. However, the authors noted that even when individuals had substance use treatment coverage, only 13.4% received treatment. Although the parity law is a critical step forward, numerous challenges remain to ensure that it is implemented across all sectors and applied rigorously.

Separate from the parity issues, in *Wit v. United Behavioral Health* (2019), a Ninth Circuit judge ruled that guidelines used by United Behavioral Health were improper in determining the level of care needed by beneficiaries and cited that the guidelines deviated from recognized and accepted published criteria of the American Society of Addiction Medicine. Following this finding, thousands of beneficiaries were entitled to financial relief. However, the decision was overturned on technical grounds, creating vocal advocacy about the reversal and calling for a rehearing at the time of this writing (The Kennedy Forum 2022). The case has continued to be litigated, but the original opinion has not been overturned as of this writing. Although this case has implications that reach beyond substance use services, it represents another step forward in ensuring health care coverage appropriate to conditions including SUDs.

# Landmark Case Evolution Related to Drug and Alcohol Use

As seen in the information presented in this chapter, there is a long and complex relationship among substance use, criminalization, and treatment laws. Two landmark legal cases that made some of these distinctions were decided by the U.S. Supreme Court decades ago (*Powell v. Texas* 1968; *Robinson v. California* 1962), and the issues they raised are reflected in current debates.

In *Robinson v. California* (1962), Robinson was stopped by a police officer who observed needle tracks on Robinson's arms from his intravenous heroin use. At the time, a California statute made it a misdemeanor to be addicted to narcotics. Upon his conviction, Robinson was sentenced to 90 days of incarceration and appealed his conviction up to the U.S. Supreme Court. Robinson died before the case was decided, although the justices were unaware until afterward and determined that the ruling was not moot. Still, in its ruling, the U.S. Supreme Court found that it was a violation of the Eighth Amendment prohibition against cruel and unusual punishment to punish an individual for being addicted to narcotics. Justice Stewart noted that "one day in prison for the 'crime' of having a common cold, would be cruel and unusual" (*Robinson v. California* 1962).

*Powell v. Texas* (1968) was decided 6 years later. Texas had on the books a statute that criminalized public intoxication. The defendant, Powell, was arrested and ultimately convicted on a charge of public intoxication under the Texas statute. Although Powell had been so convicted many times before, his attorney appealed this conviction and the case went all the way up to the U.S. Supreme Court. The court's opinion sided with Texas, noting that Powell had not been convicted of alcoholism; rather, he was convicted for being publicly intoxicated and therefore engaging in behavior that could be considered criminal. Thus, his conviction was not viewed as a similar violation of the Eighth Amendment as seen in *Robinson*. In its finding in *Powell*, the court noted that the American Medical Association (AMA) had designated alcoholism as a "major medical problem," although the AMA had not agreed on what it meant to refer to it as a disease.

The recognition of alcohol use disorder as an illness set the stage for future cases. For example, in *Traynor v. Turnage* (1988), two veterans sued the U.S. Veterans Administration regarding a regulation that defined alcoholism as willful misconduct. The regulation meant that these two veterans with primary alcohol use disorder were unable to access particular educational benefits. In *Traynor*, the U.S. Supreme Court, relying in part by briefs submitted by the AMA and the American Psychiatric Association (APA), ruled that the Rehabilitation Act (1973) was meant to include people with alcoholism (also included in the Americans With Disabilities Act 1990), so the veterans should have been allowed to use these educational benefits (Henry 2019).

In a review, Slater (2018) noted that the U.S. Supreme Court now considers scientific findings about brain development and culpability for certain offenders. For example, the neurological underpinnings of chronic alcohol use disorder may warrant a similar shift when analyzing the criminalization of alcoholism. Slater (2018) called into question the constitutionality of a Virginia habitual drunkard statute.

In another case, *Montana v. Egelhoff* (1996), the U.S. Supreme Court left under the state's purview the determination of whether a jury could be prevented from considering intoxication evidence to mitigate intent in a criminal act. In this case, Egelhoff was convicted of homicide after he was found intoxicated in a vehicle next to his gun and two people who were determined to have died from gunshot wounds. He was charged with deliberate homicide, which requires purposefully and knowingly causing the death of another person. His defense attorney asserted that Egelhoff's intoxication prevented him from establishing *mens rea*, the required mental state for the particular crime. A Montana statute limited the consideration of voluntary intoxication in determining the existence of this *mens rea*. Upon his conviction, Egelhoff's attorneys argued that the Montana statute violated his constitutional right to due process. As noted, the U.S. Supreme Court decided against Egelhoff, emphasizing that intoxication may not be a factor in mitigating a conviction but that states can decide how to address these issues.

*Commonwealth v. Eldred* (2018) addressed whether an individual with addiction could be found to have violated their probation for use of drugs, given that drug use is a factor in the disease of SUD. Although the U.S. Supreme Court ruled siding with the state in this case, the ruling articulated the importance of balancing rehabilitation and public safety concerns. One commentary on the case observed that removing a mechanism allowing the court to monitor and enforce abstinence might make courts less likely to provide opportunities for defendants to remain in their communities with specific conditions of release pertaining to substance use treatment (MacLean and Packer 2019). Other commentators argued that the court had too narrow of a take on the matter in light of emerging addiction science, and that it focused on the status-act dichotomy of *Robinson* and *Powell* but ultimately missed the opportunity to view addiction as a status as seen in *Robinson* (Harvard Law Review 2019).

Taken together, these cases reflect confusion within the legal system about the underlying meaning of SUDs and how best to address them. There has been a vacillating construct of addiction as both a matter of will and a matter of illness, although more attention has been paid to findings from the medical community regarding addictions. Ideally, case law will evolve over time in tandem with better scientific understanding of addiction.

# Civil Commitment for Addiction

Civil commitment is an approach that traditionally has involved court-ordered involuntary hospitalization of individuals who are adjudicated, as a result of mental illness, to pose a risk of harm to themselves or others or to be substantially unable to care for themselves. There are mental health commitment laws actively utilized in every jurisdiction in the United States, and the parameters for civil commitment are narrowly defined in statutory criteria, usually in mental health laws on a state-by-state basis. These laws vary in several aspects, ranging from the overall criteria to the specific processes in place to execute a civil commitment (SAMHSA 2021). For a variety of reasons, including research that emerged in this arena (Swartz and Swanson 2004), civil commitment to outpatient care for people with mental illness, also known as *assisted outpatient treatment*, has become more widely used, with several states enacting laws to expand such access (SAMHSA 2021). On the basis of the principles of parens patriae and police powers, in which the government can intrude on one's liberty in acting almost as a parent to the people or protect people from harm, there have been years of case law and scholarly discussion about the contours, due process rights, and specifics of the effects of such commitments.

Civil commitment for SUDs, theoretically resting on the same premise that an individual poses a risk of harm to self or others but owing to some SUD as opposed to mental illness, has also been recognized in law but with wide variation across states (Christopher et al. 2015). Specifically, states vary as to whether such laws exist, whether and how existing laws are utilized, and whether they are linked to mental health laws or separate from them (Williams et al. 2014). These statutes are difficult to categorize because they may be found in public health or mental health laws, and they are moving targets, with some states enacting recent laws in the wake of the opioid crisis. As of 2012, 33 states had civil commitment for SUD statutes, but the commitments ranged from a few cases per year to thousands of individuals committed annually (Christopher et al. 2015). The duration of commitment ranged from less than 1 month to more than 1 year, and the criteria required for commitment (with dangerousness being most common) and which substances were or were not subsumed under the statute varied across states (Christopher et al. 2015).

The roles of these laws have raised several questions. For example, Israelsson and colleagues (2015) reviewed European laws and raised questions about the potential for civil rights infringements due to limited safeguards against unlawful detention related to these laws. Some researchers have raised similar ethical concerns about these laws in the United States, calling for more studies to determine their effectiveness (Jain et al. 2018). It is also important to note that these laws are related to civil commitment, which is separate from use of court orders, drug courts, and other legal strategies in criminal contexts.

Christopher and colleagues (2018) conducted several studies related to civil commitment for SUDs, finding that opioid users who have been civilly committed can have a high risk of overdose. Positive associations of an individual's experience of commitment, in addition to linkage to medication upon discharge, were associated with longer postcommitment abstinence, according to the study results.

In 2019, the APA became a leading voice on this issue, with a position statement that called for adequate access to high-quality SUD treatment and noted that there is no generalizable research to date that shows the effectiveness of civil commitment for SUDs (American Psychiatric Association 2019). Although the APA position represents one professional organization's viewpoint, Messinger and Beletsky (2021) called on addiction care providers to challenge the use of coercive practices to get people with SUDs into treatment. Survey data on physician attitudes for civil commitment for SUDs are varied, with one study reporting that approximately 60% of addiction medicine providers were in favor of civil commitment for SUDs (Jain et al. 2021). Although advocates have been pushing for court-mandated treatment, especially in the face of the opioid crisis, there remains much controversy over these laws, in no small part because of the challenges in implementing civil commitment programming for people with SUDs. Nonetheless, practitioners should be familiar with practices and requirements related to SUD civil commitment if it is legally permissible in their own jurisdictions.

## Conclusions

The legal regulations and statutes related to substances with addiction potential cover several areas, including allowing or limiting access to treatment, parity of treatment benefits for individuals with SUDs, privacy protections, and civil commitment of individuals who meet substance use criteria. Given the evolving attitudes related to SUDs, the opioid crisis, and the more recent recognition of the high mortality associated with methamphetamine use, there is ample room for advocacy to help shape future policy related to substance use laws. Moreover, given the tight regulations related to substances with addiction propensities, it is important for SUD treatment providers and forensic evaluators to understand local laws that can affect practice and outcomes. This chapter highlighted some of those key areas for consideration.

# Key Points

- Enhanced patient confidentiality obligations regarding medical records related to substance use disorders (SUDs) were introduced initially to protect patients but are now being revised to facilitate effective treatment.
- Shifting regulatory stances toward alcohol in the United States over the last 100 years presaged the present chaotic legal state of affairs with cannabis.
- Attitudes and legal perceptions of SUDs are profoundly influenced by socioeconomic status and race and ethnicity.
- Federal regulation of methadone and buprenorphine has seriously affected individuals with SUDs, and the COVID-19 pandemic necessitated quick changes in those regulations.
- Legal responses to SUDs are often formulated according to principles delineated by the U.S. Supreme Court decisions *Robinson v. California* (1962) and *Powell v. Texas* (1968), which conceived of addiction as a disease but held the individuals responsible for their unlawful acts.

# References

American Association for the Treatment of Opioid Dependence: AATOD PDMP Policy Guidance Statement for OTPs. Available at: http://www.aatod.org/advocacy/policy-statements/aatod-pdmp-policy-guidance-statement-for-otps/. Accessed January 30, 2022.
American Bar Association: Opioid lawsuits generate payouts, controversy. 2019. Available at: https://www.americanbar.org/news/abanews/aba-news-archives/2019/09/opioid-lawsuits-generate-payouts-controversy/. Accessed October 29, 2023.

American Psychiatric Association: Position statement on civil commitment for adults with substance use disorders. 2019. Available at: https://www.psychiatry.org/getattachment/00976942-2f44-4f6d-9a19-edc9a344bd8e/Position-Civil-Commitment-for-Adults-with-SUD.pdf. Accessed April 14, 2024.

American Psychiatric Association: Final rule: 42 CFR Part 2, confidentiality of substance use disorder patient records. Available at: https://www.psychiatry.org/psychiatrists/practice/practice-management/hipaa/42-cfr-part-2. Accessed January 30, 2022.

Americans With Disabilities Act of 1990 (P.L. 101–336), 104 Stat. 328 (codified as amended at 42 U.S.C. §§ 12101–12213 [2008])

Amram O, Amiri S, Thorn EL, et al: Changes in methadone take-home dosing before and after COVID-19. J Subst Abuse Treat 133:108552, 2022 34304950

Anti-Drug Abuse Act of 1986 (P.L. 99–570), 100 Stat. 3207

Burns ME: State discretion over Medicaid coverage for mental health and addiction services. Psychiatr Serv 66(3):221–223, 2015 25554852

Calkins JP: Changes in self-reported cannabis use in the United States from 1979 to 2022. Addiction 2024. Available at: https://doi.org/10.1111/add.16519. Accessed June 21, 2024.

Campbell ANC, McCarty D, Rieckmann T, et al: Interpretation and integration of the federal substance use privacy protection rule in integrated health systems: a qualitative analysis. J Subst Abuse Treat 97:41–46, 2019 30577898

Centers for Medicare and Medicaid Services: The Mental Health Parity and Addiction Equity Act (MHPAEA). September 6, 2023. Available at: https://www.cms.gov/marketplace/private-health-insurance/mental-health-parity-addiction-equity#Fact_Sheets_and_FAQs. Accessed June 4, 2024.

Christopher PP, Pinals DA, Stayton T, et al: Nature and utilization of civil commitment for substance abuse in the United States. J Am Acad Psychiatry Law 43(3):313–320, 2015 26438809

Christopher PP, Anderson B, Stein MD: Civil commitment experiences among opioid users. Drug Alcohol Depend 193:137–141, 2018 30384320

Commonwealth v Eldred, 101 N.E.3d 911 (Mass. 2018)

Comprehensive Addiction and Recovery Act of 2016 (P.L. 114–198), 130 Stat. 695 (codified at 42 U.S.C. § 201 note)

Comprehensive Drug Abuse Prevention and Control Act of 1970 (P.L. 91–513), 84 Stat. 1236

Consolidated Appropriations Act of 2023 (P.L. 117–328)

Coronavirus Aid, Relief, and Economic Security Act of 2020, S.3548, 116th Cong.

Davis AK, Barrett FS, May DG, et al: Effects of psilocybin-assisted therapy on major depressive disorder: a randomized clinical trial. JAMA Psychiatry 78(5):481–489, 2021 33146667

Department of Human Services: Medications for the Treatment of Opioid Use Disorder Final Rule. 42 CFR 8 89 FR 7528, 2024. Available at: https://www.federalregister.gov/documents/2024/02/02/2024-01693/medications-for-the-treatment-of-opioid-use-disorder. Accessed June 14, 2024.

DISA: Map of marijuana legality by state. Available at: https://disa.com/map-of-marijuana-legality-by-state. Accessed January 2022.

Drug Enforcement Administration: 21 CFR Part 1308 Docket No. DEA-1362; A.G. Order No. 5931-2024. Schedules of Controlled Substances: Rescheduling of Marijuana. Available at: https://www.dea.gov/sites/default/files/2024-05/Scheduling%20NPRM%20508.pdf. Accessed May 25, 2024.

Drug Abuse Control Amendments of 1965 (P.L. 89–74), 79 Stat. 226 (codified as
    amended at 21 U.S.C. § 301, note)

Drug Addiction Treatment Act of 2000, H.R. 2634, 106th Cong.

Equal Justice Initiative: Racial double standard in drug law persists today. December 9,
    2019. Available at: https://eji.org/news/racial-double-standard-in-drug-laws-
    persists-today/. Accessed October 29, 2023.

Facher L: Methadone treatment gets first major update in over 20 years. Available at:
    https://www.statnews.com/2024/02/01/opioid-addiction-methadone-clinic-regu-
    lations. Accessed July 25, 2024.

Fair Sentencing Act of 2010 (P.L. 111–220)

Federal Review. Medications for the Treatment of Opioid Use Disorder. National Ar-
    chives, 2024. Available at: https://www.federalregister.gov/documents/2024/02/02/
    2024-01693/medications-for-the-treatment-of-opioid-use-disorder. Accessed July
    25, 2024.

Fell JC: Approaches for reducing alcohol-impaired driving: evidence-based legislation,
    law enforcement strategies, sanctions, and alcohol-control policies. Forensic Sci
    Rev 31(2):161–184, 2019 31270060

First Step Act of 2018 (P.L. 115–391)

Foley & Lardner LLP. Opioid Treatment Programs: SAMHSA Makes Permanent Regu-
    latory Flexibilities. Health Care Law Today, 2024. https://www.foley.com/insights/
    publications/2024/02/opioid-treatment-programs-samhsa-regulatory-flexibilities/
    . Accessed July 25, 2024.

Foster M, Lampe JR: Crack cocaine offenses and the First Step Act of 2018: overview and
    implications of Terry v. United States. Congressional Research Service, LSB10611.
    June 22, 2021. Available at: https://crsreports.congress.gov/product/pdf/LSB/
    LSB10611. Accessed October 29, 2023.

Frank RG, Beronio K, Glied SA: Behavioral health parity and the Affordable Care Act. J
    Soc Work Disabil Rehabil 13(1–2):31–43, 2014 24483783

Gabay M: Federal Controlled Substances Act: controlled substances prescriptions. Hosp
    Pharm 48(8):644–645, 2013 24421533

Goedel WC, Shapiro A, Cerdá M, et al: Association of racial/ethnic segregation with
    treatment capacity for opioid use disorder in counties in the United States. JAMA
    Netw Open 3(4):e203711, 2020 32320038

Goudsward AJ: Crack vs. heroin: 5 takeaways from our investigation into the role of race
    in drug battle. Asbury Park Press, December 2, 2019. Available at: https://
    www.app.com/in-depth/news/investigations/2019/12/02/crack-heroin-five-
    takeaways-our-investigation-black-race-arrests-inequities-sentencing/
    4302777002/. Accessed October 27, 2023.

Harrison Narcotics Tax Act of 1914, Ch. 1, 38 Stat. 785

Harvard Law Review: Commonwealth v Eldred: Massachusetts Supreme Judicial Court
    holds drug-free probation requirement enforceable for defendant with substance
    use disorder. May 10, 2019. Available at: https://harvardlawreview.org/2019/05/
    commonwealth-v-eldred/. Accessed October 29, 2023.

Henry TA: Court listened to AMA on defining alcoholism as a disease, not a crime.
    AMA Public Health, August 16, 2019. Available at: https://www.ama-assn.org/
    delivering-care/public-health/court-listened-ama-defining-alcoholism-disease-
    not-crime. Accessed on February 17, 2022.

HIPAA Journal: HIPAA history. 2019. Available at: https://www.hipaajournal.com/
    hipaa-history/. Accessed January 30, 2022.

History.com Editors: Cocaine. August 21, 2018. Available at: https://www.history.com/topics/crime/history-of-cocaine. Accessed October 27, 2023.

International Opium Commission: Report of the International Opium Commission, Vol I, Report of the Proceedings, February 1 to February 26, 1909. Available at: https://archive.org/details/cu31924032583225/page/n31/mode/2up. Accessed October 27, 2023.

Israelsson M, Nordlöf K, Gerdner A: European laws on compulsory commitment to care of persons suffering from substance use disorders or misuse problems: a comparative review from a human and civil rights perspective. Subst Abuse Treat Prev Policy 10:34, 2015 26316067

Jain A, Christopher P, Appelbaum PS: Civil commitment for opioid and other substance use disorders: Does it work? Psychiatr Serv 69(4):374–376, 2018 29607774

Jain A, Christopher PP, Fisher CE, et al: Civil commitment for substance use disorders: a national survey of addiction medicine physicians. J Addict Med 15(4):285–291, 2021 33989260

Johnson MW, Griffiths RR, Hendricks PS, et al: The abuse potential of medical psilocybin according to the 8 factors of the Controlled Substances Act. Neuropharmacology 142:143–166, 2018 29753748

The Kennedy Forum: Wit v. United Behavioral Health. 2022. Available at: https://www.thekennedyforum.org/wit/#:~:text=Wit%20vs.,for%20mental%20health%20and%20addiction. Accessed December 29, 2022.

Krieger H, Young CM, Anthenien AM, et al: The epidemiology of binge drinking among college-age individuals in the United States. Alcohol Res 39(1):23–30, 2018 30557145

Kumar R, Viswanath O, Saadabadi A: Buprenorphine. StatPearls, 2021. Available at: https://www.ncbi.nlm.nih.gov/books/NBK459126/. Accessed February 17, 2022.

Lee B, Zhao W, Yang KC, et al: Systematic evaluation of state policy interventions targeting the US opioid epidemic, 2007–2018. JAMA Netw Open 4(2):e2036687, 2021 33576816

Li L, Vlisides PE: Ketamine: 50 years of modulating the mind. Front Hum Neurosci 10:612, 2016 27965560

Liu Y, Lin D, Wu B, et al: Ketamine abuse potential and use disorder. Brain Res Bull 126(Pt 1):68–73, 2016 27261367

MacLean N, Packer IK: Requiring abstinence from substance use as a condition of probation. J Am Acad Psychiatry Law 47(3):365–367, 2019

Marbury D: Proposed HHS rule could modernize 42 CFR Part 2 at last. Behav Healthc 36(1):32–33, 2016 27328564

Marijuana Tax Act of 1937 (P.L. 75–238)

McBournie A, Duncan A, Connolly E, et al: Methadone barriers persist, despite decades of evidence. Health Affairs Forefront, September 23, 2019. Available at: https://www.healthaffairs.org/content/forefront/methadone-barriers-persist-despite-decades-evidence. Accessed October 27, 2023.

McCarty D, Rieckmann T, Baker RL, et al: The perceived impact of 42 CFR Part 2 on coordination and integration of care: a qualitative analysis. Psychiatr Serv 68(3):245–249, 2017 27799017

McClellan C, Lambdin BH, Ali MM, et al: Opioid-overdose laws association with opioid use and overdose mortality. Addict Behav 86:90–95, 2018 29610001

Mental Health Parity Act of 1996 (P.L. 104–204)

Mental Health Parity and Addiction Equity Act of 2008 (P.L. 110–343), 122 Stat. 3881 (codified as amended 42 U.S.C. § 201 note)

Messinger J, Beletsky L: Involuntary commitment for substance use: addiction care professionals must reject enabling coercion and patient harm. J Addict Med 15(4):280–282, 2021 33989262

Michaels House: The history of opiates. n.d. Available at: https://michaelshouse.com/opiate-rehab/history-of-opiates. Accessed June 20, 2024.

Mion G: History of anaesthesia: the ketamine story—past, present and future. Eur J Anaesthesiol 34(9):571–575, 2017 28731926

Mojtabai R, Mauro C, Wall MM, et al: Private health insurance coverage of drug use disorder treatment: 2005–2018. PLoS One 15(10):e0240298, 2020 33035265

Montana v Egelhoff, 518 U.S. 37 (1996)

National Association of State Alcohol and Drug Abuse Directors: Buprenorphine patient limits: history and overview. Available at: https://nasadad.org/wp-content/uploads/2019/01/Buprenorphine-Patient-Limits-1.pdf. Accessed January 30, 2022.

Netherland J, Hansen H: White opioids: pharmaceutical race and the war on drugs that wasn't. Biosocieties 12(2):217–238, 2017 28690668

Pottle Z, Parisi T: Controlled Substances Act and scheduling. Addiction Center, April 17, 2023. Available at: https://www.addictioncenter.com/addiction/controlled-substances-act-and-scheduling/. Accessed April 17, 2023.

Powell v Texas, 392 U.S. 514 (1968)

Public Act 246 of 2017, Michigan (codified at Mich. Comp. Laws §§ 333.7303b–333.730c, 333.16221, and 333.16226)

Public Broadcasting Service: A social history of America's most popular drugs. Frontline. Available at: https://www.pbs.org/wgbh/pages/frontline/shows/drugs/buyers/socialhistory.html. Accessed on January 30, 2022.

Redman M: Cocaine: what is the crack? A brief history of cocaine as an anesthetic. Anesth Pain Med 1(2):95–97, 2011 25729664

Rehabilitation Act of 1973 (P.L. 93–112), 97 Stat. 355 (codified as amended at 29 U.S.C. § 701)

Rensberger B: Crackdown on a drug that maims and kills. The New York Times, February 27, 1972. Available at: https://www.nytimes.com/1972/02/27/archives/crackdown-on-a-drug-that-maims-and-kills-amphetamines.html. Accessed October 30, 2023.

Robinson v California, 370 U.S. 660 (1962)

Slater M: Is "Powell" still valid? The Supreme Court's changing stance on cruel and unusual punishment. Virginia Law Review, May 15, 2018. Available at: https://virginialawreview.org/articles/powell-still-valid-supreme-courts-changing-stance-cruel-and-unusual-punishment/. Accessed October 30, 2023.

Smith WR, Appelbaum PS: Two models of legalization of psychedelic substances: reasons for concern. JAMA 326(8):697–698, 2021 34338743

Soelberg CD, Brown RE Jr, Du Vivier D, et al: The US opioid crisis: current federal and state legal issues. Anesth Analg 125(5):1675–1681, 2017 29049113

State of Oregon Legislative Policy and Research Office: Measure 110 (2020): background brief. 2020. Available at: https://www.oregonlegislature.gov/lpro/Publications/Background-Brief-Measure-110-2020.pdf. Accessed October 26, 2023.

Substance Abuse and Mental Health Services Administration; U.S. Department of Health and Human Services: Medication final rule. Fed Regist 81(131):44711–44739, 2016.

Substance Abuse and Mental Health Services Administration: Disclosure of Substance Use Disorder Patient Records: Does Part 2 Apply to Me? Rockville, MD, Substance Abuse and Mental Health Services Administration, May 2018. Available at: https://www.samhsa.gov/sites/default/files/does-part2-apply.pdf. Accessed October 30, 2023.

Substance Abuse and Mental Health Administration: Civil Commitment and the Mental Health Care Continuum: Historical Trends and Principles for Law and Practice. Rockville, MD, Substance Abuse and Mental Health Services Administration, 2019. Available at: https://www.samhsa.gov/sites/default/files/civil-commitment-continuum-of-care.pdf. Accessed October 30, 2023.

Substance Abuse and Mental Health Services Administration: Opioid Treatment Programs Reported Challenges Encountered During the COVID-19 Pandemic and Actions Taken to Address Them. Rockville, MD, Substance Abuse and Mental Health Services Administration, November 2020a. Available at: https://oig.hhs.gov/oas/reports/region9/92001001.pdf. Accessed October 30, 2023.

Substance Abuse and Mental Health Services Administration: Fact Sheet: 42 CFR Part 2 Revised Rule. Rockville, MD, Substance Abuse and Mental Health Services Administration, July 13, 2020b. Available at: https://www.samhsa.gov/newsroom/press-announcements/202007131330. Accessed October 30, 2023.

Substance Abuse and Mental Health Services Administration: Key Substance Use and Mental Health Indicators in the United States: Results From the 2020 National Survey of Drug Use and Health (HHS Publ No PEP21–07–01–003, NSDUH Series H-56). Rockville, MD, Substance Abuse and Mental Health Services Administration, October 25, 2021. Available at: https://www.samhsa.gov/data/sites/default/files/reports/rpt35325/NSDUHFFRPDFWHTMLFiles2020/2020NSDUHFFR1PDFW102121.pdf. Accessed October 30, 2023.

Substance Abuse and Mental Health Services Administration: SAMHSA Proposes Update to Federal Rules to Expand Access to Opioid Use Disorder Treatment to Help Close Gap in Care. Rockville, MD, Substance Abuse and Mental Health Services Administration, December 13, 2022b. Available at: https://www.samhsa.gov/newsroom/press-announcements/20221213/update-federal-rules-expand-access-opioid-use-disorder-treatment. Accessed October 30, 2023.

Substance Abuse and Mental Health Services Administration: Substance Abuse Confidentiality Regulations. Rockville, MD, Substance Abuse and Mental Health Services Administration, January 14, 2022c. Available at: https://www.samhsa.gov/about-us/who-we-are/laws-regulations/confidentiality-regulations-faqs. Accessed October 30, 2023.

Substance Abuse and Mental Health Services Administration: Waiver Elimination (MAT Act). Rockville, MD, Substance Abuse and Mental Health Services Administration, 2023. Available at: https://www.samhsa.gov/medication-assisted-treatment/become-buprenorphine-waivered-practitioner. Accessed January 7, 2023.

Substance Abuse and Mental Health Services Administration: Methadone Take-Home Flexibilities Extension Guidance. SAMHSA, 2024. Available at: https://www.samhsa.gov/medications-substance-use-disorders/statutes-regulations-guidelines/methadone-guidance#:~:text=In%20treatment%200%2D14%20days,be%20provided%20to%20the%20patient. Accessed July 25, 2024.

SUPPORT for Patients and Communities Act of 2018 (P.L. 115–271)

Swartz MS, Swanson JW: Involuntary outpatient commitment, community treatment orders, and assisted outpatient treatment: what's in the data? Can J Psychiatry 49(9):585–591, 2004 15503729

Terry v United States, 141 S. Ct. 1858 (2021)

Toomey TL, Wagenaar AC: Environmental policies to reduce college drinking: options and research findings. J Stud Alcohol Suppl 14(14):193–205, 2002 12022725

Totenberg N: Race, drugs, and sentencing at the Supreme Court. National Public Radio, June 14, 2021. Available at: https://www.npr.org/2021/06/14/1006264385/race-drugs-and-sentencing-at-the-supreme-court. Accessed October 30, 2023.

Traynor v Turnage, 485 U.S. 535 (1988)

Uniform Minimum Drinking Age Act of 1984 (P.L. 98–363)

United States v Doremus, 249 U.S. 86 (1919)

U.S. Const. Amend. XVIII, § 1 (1919)

U.S. Department of Transportation: Traffic safety facts: 2014 crash data key findings. National Highway Traffic Safety Administration (DOT-HS-812-219). November 2015. Available at: https://crashstats.nhtsa.dot.gov/Api/Public/ViewPublication/812219. Accessed October 24, 2023.

U.S. Drug Enforcement Administration: Drug scheduling. July 10, 2018. Available at: https://www.dea.gov/drug-information/drug-scheduling. Accessed October 27, 2023.

U.S. Drug Enforcement Administration: DEA finalizes measure to expand medication-assisted treatment. Press Release, June 28, 2021. Available at: https://www.dea.gov/press-releases/2021/06/28/dea-finalizes-measures-expand-medication-assisted-treatment. Accessed October 27, 2023.

U.S. Food and Drug Administration: FDA approves new nasal spray medication for treatment-resistant depression: available only at a certified doctor's office or clinic. Press Release, March 25, 2019. Available at: https://www.fda.gov/news-events/press-announcements/fda-approves-new-nasal-spray-medication-treatment-resistant-depression-available-only-certified. Accessed October 27, 2023.

Vagins DJ, McCurdy J: Cracks in the system: twenty years of the unjust federal crack cocaine law. American Civil Liberties Union, October 2006. Available at: https://www.aclu.org/wp-content/uploads/document/cracksinsystem_20061025.pdf. Accessed October 27, 2023.

Wick JY: The history of benzodiazepines. Consult Pharm 28(9):538–548, 2013 24007886

Wilkinson ST, Yarnell S, Radhakrishnan R, et al: Marijuana legalization: impact on physicians and public health. Annu Rev Med 67:453–466, 2016 26515984

Williams AR, Cohen S, Ford EB: Statutory definitions of mental illness for involuntary hospitalization as related to substance use disorders. Psychiatr Serv 65(5):634–640, 2014 24430580

Wit v United Behavioral Health, Case No. 14-cv-02346-JCS (N.D. Cal. Feb. 28, 2019)

World Health Organization: Global Status Report on Alcohol and Health. 2014. Available at: https://www.who.int/publications/i/item/global-status-report-on-alcohol-and-health-2014. Accessed October 29, 2023.

# CHAPTER 3

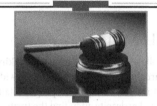

# LEGAL STRUCTURES FOR TREATING PATIENTS WITH ADDICTIONS

## Introduction

Treatment of patients with substance use disorders (SUDs) presents serious medicolegal challenges to the treating clinician, even when compared with the treatment of general psychiatric illness. Stigma directed against people with SUDs can complicate engagement and may even lead clinicians to reject these patients, which may constitute patient abandonment. Further medicolegal complications include the sometimes less-than-voluntary nature of treatment, pressures exerted on the patient by family or friends, the propensity of people with SUDs for denying or lying about their substance use, and management of nonadherence to recommended treatment. Another issue rests in prescribing legitimate medications, only to find that some of those medications are being diverted or otherwise used inappropriately. Another fraught area relates to having a patient experience relapse or die from an overdose of illicit or prescribed medication while receiving treatment. The occasional diversion of medications can also represent a malpractice threat to the treating clinician, as can concerns that a clinician might be accused of malpractice if a patient with SUD harms another person while intoxicated. Clinicians, therefore, are often understandably concerned about potential increased liability associated with treating patients with SUDs. This chapter provides background on areas of risk related to treating patients with SUDs and issues pertaining to the standard of care, while being mindful of the inherent medicolegal challenges of working in the field of SUD treatment.

## FORENSIC DILEMMA

A 22-year-old female college senior who has been drinking daily for more than a year experiences a seizure the morning after a campus-wide party. An initial treatment attempt at a local intensive outpatient program failed because the patient continued to drink every day despite attending the treatment program 3 days per week. She has wildly fluctuating pulse and blood pressure measurements, cannot quantify how much she is drinking, and appears to be hallucinating about bugs in her dorm room. After consultation with the student health center psychiatrist, the patient is referred to a nearby inpatient treatment center that has detoxification facilities and a 2-week rehabilitation program. The patient agrees to go, but on her second day in the withdrawal management unit, her health insurance company notifies the facility and the patient that no insurance reimbursement will be provided because the treatment is not medically necessary.

Consider the following:

1. In responding to the situation in this Forensic Dilemma, what negotiating options do the treating clinicians and inpatient facility have?
2. Are the American Society of Addiction Medicine (ASAM) patient placement criteria (PPC) relevant to the medicolegal situation?

Unfortunately, clinicians and addiction treatment facilities often need to advocate for their patients when health insurance companies deny payment for necessary services that are, in fact, covered by the health insurance contract. Although pursuing remedies under the Mental Health Parity and Addiction Equity Act (2008; MHPAEA) is the province of attorneys and often a matter of public policy rather than individual application, clinicians can start the discussion by mentioning this federal legislation. The MHPAEA generally requires insurance companies to treat mental illnesses, such as SUDs, in much the same way as they treat other medical illnesses or conditions requiring surgery (Mental Health Parity and Addiction Equity Act 2008). Similarly, the ASAM PPC can be used to demonstrate that the patient's level of need necessitates an inpatient detoxification admission (American Society of Addiction Medicine 2013). With third-party payers, a demonstration of widely accepted and printed standards in the medical literature is generally more effective than the clinician's description of what may be an obvious clinical need. Furthermore, lack of insurance funding for treatment is not a justification for dereliction of one's duty of care to a patient. Thus, if the patient is discharged due to insurance limits but the clinician feels that more treatment is needed and harm ensues, then the clinician can be sued for negligent discharge. Therefore, it is critical to understand appropriate levels of care and even work with administrators to ensure that patients receive the treatment required for their condition or that there is an appropriate transfer to another provider.

# Therapeutic Prescription of Potentially Addictive Medications

President Richard Nixon signed the Comprehensive Drug Abuse Prevention and Control Act (1970) as the legal foundation of the federal government's goal to address aspects of addiction in the United States. The act requires the pharmaceutical industry to implement strict security requirement for certain types of drugs. Title II of this act, the Controlled Substances Act (CSA), established federal policies regulating the manufacturing, importation, possession, use, and distribution of various drugs. Furthermore, the CSA established a classification of drugs under five schedules based on every substance's potential for abuse, safety, addictive potential, and accepted medical uses. Congress tasked the U.S. Drug Enforcement Administration (DEA) and the FDA with jointly implementing the CSA. Since it was signed into law, Congress has amended the CSA 11 times to account for newly introduced drugs. Alcohol and tobacco are excluded from the CSA (21 U.S.C. § 811).

The CSA classification of drugs significantly affects physicians' willingness and ability to prescribe these compounds, and it also limits research into their potential effects. For example, substances such as marijuana or peyote, classified under Schedule I, are identified as having high abuse potential, having no accepted medical use, and being unsafe to use under medical supervision. Proposed changes to the CSA classification, if successful, will likely increase both clinical use and research studies of marijuana (DEA 2024). In contrast, substances such as pregabalin or cannabidiol, classified under Schedule V, are identified as having low abuse potential relative to other substances identified in the CSA and as having low potential for physical or psychological dependence; they are currently accepted for medical use in the United States. Table 3–1 summarizes the primary characteristics of the five CSA classification schedules.

**Table 3–1.** Controlled Substances Act classification schedules

| | Schedule I | Schedule II | Schedule III | Schedule IV | Schedule V |
|---|---|---|---|---|---|
| Abuse potential | High | High | Lower than Schedule I or II | Lower than Schedule III | Lower than Schedule IV |
| Accepted medical use | None | Accepted with severe restrictions | Accepted | Accepted | Accepted |
| Safety for use | Unsafe for use under medical supervision | Abuse may lead to severe physical/psychological dependence | Abuse may lead to mild/moderate physical/psychological dependence | Abuse may lead to limited physical/psychological dependence vs. Schedule III | Abuse may lead to limited physical/psychological dependence vs. Schedule IV |
| Notes | Cannot be prescribed by a medical provider Subject to production quotas by the Drug Enforcement Administration | Requires written or electronic prescription Original prescription required (not faxed or oral) May not include refills | Requires written, electronic, or oral prescription May not include more than five refills | Requires written, electronic, or oral prescription May not include more than five refills | Requires written, electronic, or oral prescription May include refills |
| Examples | Cathinone (khat); dimethyltryptamine; heroin; γ-hydroxybutyrate; LSD; marijuana; ibogaine; MDMA; mescaline/peyote; psilocybin | Amphetamines; barbiturates (short acting); cocaine; codeine; fentanyl; hydrocodone; hydromorphone; methadone; methamphetamine; morphine; oxycodone | Anabolic steroids; barbiturates (intermediate acting); buprenorphine; dronabinol (Marinol); ketamine | Benzodiazepines; nonbenzodiazepine hypnotics (Z drugs); barbiturates (long acting); carisoprodol; modafinil; suvorexant; tramadol | Cough suppressants with small amounts of codeine; cannabidiol; pregabalin |

# Statutes, Regulations, and Case Law Affecting SUD Treatment

## FEDERAL RULES RELATED TO TREATING OPIOID USE DISORDERS

Addiction treatments are complex, and there is a great deal of interest in identifying effective approaches to reduce SUD-associated morbidity and mortality. The landscape, however, is fraught with regulatory and legal requirements that can be confusing and present medicolegal risks for treating clinicians. States have specific statutes that can affect prescribing, licensing, and related rules for certain SUD treatment services, and federal laws and rules also impact the treatment of SUDs.

Use of a controlled substance to treat opioid use disorder (OUD), for example, raises several challenges. In fact, OUD is the only SUD with FDA-approved medication treatments that involve controlled substances (methadone and buprenorphine). For example, γ-hydroxybutyrate is used in parts of Europe to treat alcohol use disorder, but no controlled substances are FDA approved for the maintenance treatment of alcohol use disorder in the United States.

Methadone may be dispensed to individuals with OUD through opioid treatment programs (OTPs). These programs are regulated through Title 42 of the Code of Federal Regulations (Medication Assisted Treatment for Opioid Disorders, 42 C.F.R. 8 [2001]), which sets standards for the specific methadone formulations permitted, safeguards against abuse or misuse, some dosing guidelines, other components of the treatment, and OTP recordkeeping. The federal government certifies and accredits OTPs (42 C.F.R. 8). The Substance Abuse and Mental Health Services Administration (SAMHSA) oversees this process, and state opioid treatment authorities are responsible for ensuring compliance with federal opioid treatment regulations in their state or territory.

Buprenorphine prescribing to individuals with OUD is regulated through the Drug Addiction Treatment Act (2000). This act allows for office-based OUD treatment using Schedule III, IV, and V medications that are FDA approved for that indication. Currently, buprenorphine is the only such medication that falls under these provisions (methadone is classified as Schedule II). In essence, the Drug Addiction Treatment Act allows physicians to apply for a waiver to prescribe buprenorphine for OUD treatment upon meeting certain requirements, such as carrying a valid state license and DEA registration and participating in additional training (Drug Addiction Treatment Act 2000). Physicians who qualify for the waiver are assigned a second DEA number beginning with the letter X (commonly referred to as an *X-waiver*). The Drug Addiction Treatment Act and its subsequent amendments (discussed later in this chapter) regulate the number of patients that a given physician can treat using buprenorphine.

As a result of the COVID-19 pandemic, the federal government considerably loosened prescribing rules for buprenorphine in an attempt to stem the rising tide of opioid overdoses and deaths attributable, in part, to difficulties in delivering appropriate treatment (Spetz et al. 2022). In April 2021, buprenorphine prescribers who were already licensed and had DEA certificates were only required to file a Notice of Intent to prescribe buprenorphine with the federal government, rather than receive buprenorphine training. Clinicians who wanted to prescribe for more than 30 patients were still required to receive training. Certain face-to-face evaluations were not required to initiate treatment, allowing for telehealth and virtual approaches to expand. How the regulatory landscape will shift as the COVID-19 public health emergency wanes remains to be seen.

## LEGAL PARITY REQUIREMENTS AND SUD TREATMENT

The MHPAEA aims to prevent health insurance providers from limiting mental health or SUD treatment benefits beyond the limits imposed on nonpsychiatric medical or surgical benefits (Mental Health Parity and Addiction Equity Act 2008). Specifically, the act requires a general equivalence between mental health benefits (including SUDs) and medical or surgical benefits, including equivalency at the level of financial requirements (e.g., copayments and deductibles), treatment limits (e.g., number of visits or number of treatment days), and out-of-network benefits. The act requires that denial of coverage be subject to the same medical necessity determination review as for medical or surgical benefits, and it requires insurance providers to disclose the reasons for any denial of benefits for mental health, including SUD treatment services. Although the MHPAEA is a federal law, states may have their own laws related to parity that make parity even more enforceable. However, these laws continue to expand because of the number of loopholes and challenges in actually having parity be realized. Thus, as noted in the Forensic Dilemma at the start of this chapter, clinicians may experience challenges in accessing benefits for their patients even when the response seems disparate from what it would be for medical or surgical conditions.

## PATIENT PROTECTION AND AFFORDABLE CARE ACT OF 2010

In 2010, President Barack Obama signed the Patient Protection and Affordable Care Act (ACA). Although the intent of the act extends far beyond SUD treatment, with the goal of decreasing the number of uninsured individuals, its provisions require reimbursement for the treatment needs of people with SUDs (Patient Protection and Affordable Care Act 2010). Historically, public and private insurance providers presented significant limitations and restrictions with regard to covering the full range of SUD treatments; the ACA delivered major coverage expansions, ensuring greater access to SUD care.

The ACA has expanded insurance access through Medicaid expansion and state health insurance exchanges, benefiting millions of previously uninsured individuals. The act also allows adult children to remain on their parent's insurance plans up to age 26 years, and it prohibits insurance companies from denying coverage to people with preexisting conditions, including SUDs. Millions of Americans with SUDs who previously could not access medical care for SUD treatment became eligible for such services (Wen et al. 2015).

The ACA requires insurance plans to cover screening and brief intervention for SUDs and includes SUD treatment under the essential health benefits that even the most basic plans are required to cover. One limitation of the ACA is that it does not specify what types of SUD treatment must be included, leaving it up to the states to make such determinations.

Further, the ACA includes changes in regulatory procedures requiring that SUD treatment be included in existing health insurance plans, strengthening the MHPAEA protections (Abraham et al. 2017). The ACA requires all insurance plans, including those offered on the state exchanges and plans made available through the expansion of Medicaid, to cover SUD treatment at the same level as medical or surgical conditions.

Finally, the ACA promotes innovative models of care, such as collaborative care models, health homes, and accountable care organizations. These models facilitate the integration of SUD treatment in the general medical care that patients receive by allowing generous and novel reimbursement models that incentivize service integration and coordination of care for individuals with complex needs. This will have a tremendous effect on access to care for people with SUDs who may not be motivated to seek out SUD-specific treatment services but are likely to welcome it if delivered through the same organization where they receive care for the rest of their medical needs (Croft and Parish 2013).

# COMPREHENSIVE ADDICTION AND RECOVERY ACT OF 2016

In 2016, President Obama signed the Comprehensive Addiction and Recovery Act (CARA) in the context of the opioid epidemic. The act seeks to promote a coordinated response to SUDs, including prevention, treatment, recovery, law enforcement, criminal justice reform, and overdose reversal (Comprehensive

Addiction and Recovery Act 2016). Further, CARA specifically promotes the use of medications for OUD.

CARA amends the CSA to facilitate the prescribing of buprenorphine for the treatment of OUD. The act increases the total number of patients any given prescriber can treat using the medication and excludes patients who are directly administered the medication through a hospital (e.g., in an emergency department or on an inpatient unit) or an OTP from counting toward the patient limit set. Additionally, it expands prescribing privileges to midlevel practitioners such as nurse practitioners and physician assistants. Nurse practitioners and physician assistants are required to complete 24 hours of training (in contrast with the 8 hours of training required by physicians) and must be supervised by or work in collaboration with a physician who is qualified to prescribe the medication. These requirements were relaxed during the COVID-19 pandemic, as noted earlier in this chapter.

CARA allocates funding for naloxone prescribing programs meant to cover the cost of purchasing naloxone, offset copayments, and train providers to identify opioid overdoses and use naloxone to reverse them. Additionally, the act authorizes and funds programs for pharmacists to dispense the medication pursuant to statewide standing orders. It expands the availability and promotes the use of naloxone by law enforcement agencies and first responders. CARA also allocates funding to programs specifically aiming at addressing OUDs for pregnant and postpartum women. With regard to justice-involved populations, CARA endorses collaborations with criminal justice stakeholders to expand and promote the screening, assessment, and treatment of SUDs among incarcerated individuals.

Finally, CARA promotes educational programs and grants to expand medical education curricula focused on SUDs. In addition, the act sponsors community-based awareness and educational programs aimed at youth, parents, and older adults, among other demographics, focused on SUD prevention, methamphetamine use disorder and OUD, and overdose reversal. Moreover, it seeks to support states in developing and maintaining prescription drug monitoring programs (PDMPs).

# CORONAVIRUS AID, RELIEF, AND ECONOMIC SECURITY ACT OF 2020

The Coronavirus Aid, Relief, and Economic Security Act (CARES Act) of 2020 made several changes to the confidentiality for SUD treatment records regulated under 42 C.F.R. Part 2 to align more closely with HIPAA (Confidentiality of Substance Use Disorder Patient Records 2020; Coronavirus Aid, Relief, and Economic Security Act 2020). Following passage of the CARES Act, SAMHSA issued updated rules regulating the implementation of these changes. The final rules issued by SAMHSA allow for the disclosure of covered treatment records upon receipt of a consent for release of such records for the provision of care and coordination of treatment, payment, and general operations of health care. Only after patients submit a written consent to release covered health information are clinicians permitted to disclose such records (up until the consent is revoked by the patient). The SAMHSA final rules demonstrate that patients are permitted to restrict the use and disclosure of their SUD records, and clinicians are required to make every reasonable effort to accommodate these restrictions. The final rules allow for the disclosure of SUD records to public health authorities as long as these records are deidentified. However, the final rules bar the use of any such records in legal proceedings against an individual unless the release of the records is permitted by the patient or properly ordered by a court. There are strict breach notification requirements in the event that protected information is accessed inappropriately, and fines and penalties are listed to punish the improper release of protected information and deter such releases (Confidentiality of Substance Use Disorder Patient Records 2022). The basis for this enactment was an attempt to minimize stigma in the treatment of SUDs by addressing privacy barriers to seeking such treatment.

# The Practice of Medicine in Treating Individuals With SUDs

As mentioned in Chapter 1, SUDs are often highly stigmatized, sometimes even by health care professionals. It is important to note, however, that patients with SUDs are gaining increased attention, especially in light of the opioid epidemic. The weight of the morbidity and mortality associated with drug and alcohol use is significant and is increasingly recognized as a health care priority. Clinicians from every specialty interact with patients with SUDs, and drug and alcohol use disorders are among the most commonly encountered conditions in medical practice, particularly given the wide range of associated comorbidities, both psychiatric (mood or psychotic disorders, accidents, suicides, or violence) and nonpsychiatric (e.g., cerebrovascular, cardiac, hepatic, or renal disorders). However, SUDs remain inadequately diagnosed and poorly managed in the health care system. From a forensic perspective, the stigma and irrationality directed toward SUDs often requires explanation to judges, juries, and hearing officers. So, it is incumbent on forensic experts to understand both the science and the clinical realities of SUDs as well as the ways in which stigma and misunderstandings affect the person with SUDs.

To provide adequate care to patients with SUDs, clinicians should seek knowledge, training, and experience in identifying both direct and indirect manifestations of SUDs in their early and advanced stages. It is important to maintain a positive attitude toward patients with SUDs and to develop adequate communication skills and increase familiarity with psychotherapeutic, social, and pharmacological treatment options for various addictive disorders to best address the complex needs of the population. In addition, it is critical to be able to refer patients to specialized treatment services whenever needed.

Health care providers should understand that SUDs are more than merely disorders of using "too much" of a substance. Rather, SUDs are disorders of thinking that involve impairments in executive and cognitive functions as they relate to the decision-making process of using an intoxicating substance. Even though people with SUDs use excessive amounts of drugs or alcohol, one cannot conclude that all people who use excessive amounts of drugs or alcohol have an SUD. As is the case with other psychiatric disorders, an SUD diagnosis is made when a patient's symptoms meet the phenomenological diagnostic criteria threshold listed in DSM-5 (American Psychiatric Association 2013). The diagnostic criteria can be subdivided into three categories as follows:

1. Loss of control
2. Adverse consequences
3. Physiological dependence (the state resulting from repeated use of a substance marked by tolerance, withdrawal symptoms, or both)

DSM-5 is the industry standard and defines the scope of mental conditions, including SUDs, treated by clinicians. As noted in the following section, DSM-5 defines SUDs as a maladaptive pattern of substance use leading to significant impairment or distress that is met when the patient carries at least 2 of the following 11 diagnostic criteria within a 12-month period:

## Loss of Control

1. Substance taken in a larger amount or for a longer period than intended
2. Persistent desire or unsuccessful efforts to control or stop substance use
3. Craving or a strong desire or urge to use the substance
4. Use continues despite knowledge of resultant physical or psychological problems
5. Continued use in situations in which it is physically hazardous

## Adverse consequences

1. Great deal of time spent to obtain, use, or recover from effects
2. Use resulting in a failure to fulfill major role obligations
3. Continued use despite recurrent social or interpersonal problems

4. Use resulting in important social, occupational, or recreational activities given up or reduced

**Physiological dependence**

1. Tolerance
2. Withdrawal

*Tolerance* to a given substance is a phenomenon marked by requiring a higher dose of the substance to achieve the same intoxicating effect (alternatively, it can be understood as experiencing a reduced effect at the usual dose). In contrast, *withdrawal* refers to the phenomenon marked by experiencing symptoms that are different from the expected effects of that substance following a discontinuation or reduction of substance use. In patients who experience withdrawal, resuming substance use would reverse withdrawal and relieve these symptoms.

It is important to recognize that for patients medically prescribed a controlled substance for a legitimate medical indication, tolerance and withdrawal are excluded in diagnosing an SUD. There may be exceptions to this when the patient may qualify for a distinct SUD for use of a prescribed substance in a pattern that raises problems and is in excess to what is medically indicated for the underlying condition. Regardless, the severity of an SUD is assessed by the number of diagnostic criteria present (2–3, mild; 4–5, moderate; ≥6, severe).

For individuals with a history of SUDs, the following qualifiers are also available as listed in DSM-5 for SUDs:

- *In early remission:* when a person who previously met diagnostic criteria for an SUD has not met any diagnostic criteria (except for craving) for longer than 3 months
- *In sustained remission:* when a person who previously met diagnostic criteria for an SUD has not met any diagnostic criteria (except for craving) for longer than 12 months
- *On maintenance therapy:* when a person who previously met diagnostic criteria for an SUD has not met any diagnostic criteria (except for tolerance or withdrawal) as a result of being prescribed maintenance medications (referring to full or partial agonists and antagonist medications such as naltrexone, buprenorphine, or methadone)
- *In a controlled environment:* when a person who previously met diagnostic criteria for an SUD is abstinent as a result of no longer having access to the substance when in an environment where access to the substance is restricted (e.g., correctional, detention, or residential rehabilitation programs)

Upon diagnosing an SUD, treatment providers assign patients to a given level of treatment intensity along the continuum of care, ranging from services offered at the primary care level to specialty services based on their treatment needs. The most widely used framework for such assessment utilizes the ASAM PPC-2R, which was one of the issues raised in the Forensic Dilemma at the start of this chapter. As in that example, these criteria may be relevant when a question arises as to whether the patient was given the proper treatment attention. The PPC-2R is a standardized approach to determine a person's SUD severity and characteristics with the treatment level they require (Mee-Lee and Shulman 2018). The PPC-2R examines every patient's treatment needs across the following six dimensions (each scored 0–4 based on the associated complication risks):

- Dimension 1: Intoxication and withdrawal potential
- Dimension 2: Biomedical conditions and complications
- Dimension 3: Emotional, behavioral, or cognitive complications
- Dimension 4: Readiness to change (transtheoretical model of change or stages of change)
- Dimension 5: Relapse or continued use potential
- Dimension 6: Recovery environment (including social, legal, vocational, educational, financial, or housing factors)

Treatment type needs for every dimension are determined and classified by level as follows:

- Level 0.5: Early intervention
- Level I: Outpatient treatment
- Level II.1: Intensive outpatient
- Level II.5: Partial hospitalization
- Level III.1: Clinically managed low-intensity residential services
- Level III.3: Clinically managed medium-intensity residential treatment
- Level III.5: Clinically managed high-intensity residential treatment
- Level III.7: Medically monitored intensive inpatient treatment
- Level IV: Medically managed intensive inpatient treatment

Subspecifiers are used, if applicable, to further specify treatment types as follows:

- D: Detoxification
- OMT: Opioid maintenance treatment
- BIO: Capable of managing complex medical comorbidity
- AOD: Alcohol or drug treatment only

- DDC: Dual diagnosis capable (the treatment facility is able to identify co-occurring psychiatric problems and refer to outside mental health treatment centers)
- DDE: Dual diagnosis enhanced capable (the treatment facility can manage patients with co-occurring psychiatric problems on-site)

# Dual Agency for Clinicians

Clinicians treating patients with SUDs may face challenges related to inherent dual agency. In this case, the clinician has a duty to treat the patient correctly but may also have an ethical pull, and sometimes obligation, to protect society as a whole from the behaviors of the patient.

Ethical principles guiding medical practice in any field include the following (Taylor 2013; Varkey 2021):

- Respecting and promoting the autonomy of competent patients to make their own decisions (in direct contrast with paternalism in medicine)
- Beneficence, or acting to maximize the welfare of a patient
- Justice, or treating patients equally
- Nonmaleficence, or the prevention of the intentional infliction of harm to patients

Physicians treating patients with SUDs sometimes encounter situations in which acting consistently with one medical ethical principle may violate another. Numerous examples of patient autonomy clashing with the principles of beneficence or nonmaleficence come to mind. Several theories of ethics are presented as a framework to resolve such ethical conflicts or moral dilemmas when they arise (Niveau and Welle 2018; Taylor 2013; Varkey 2021). These theories are as follows:

- *Principlism:* This approach examines moral dilemmas by identifying and focusing on common-ground moral principles shared among the four ethical tenets.
- *Deontological:* This approach prioritizes meeting moral obligations and duty. Simply said, it requires one (the physician, in this case) to "do the right thing."
- *Utilitarianism:* This approach pursues the goal of achieving the greatest amount of good for the greatest number of people.
- *Liberal individualism:* This approach prioritizes the patient's right to autonomy over all other ethical principles.
- *Virtue theory:* This approach requires an examination into the actor's intentions in their decision-making process, recognizing that deviating from the

rules or being subjected to the consequences may be overlooked as long as the individual was acting in good faith, showing good character and moral values.

- *Consequentialism:* This approach relates to assessing the moral worth of any given action undertaken by a physician based on the goodness (or alternatively badness) of its consequences. In other words, it is best described by the phrase, "the end justifies the means."
- *Dialectical principlism:* This approach requires balancing competing ethical principles to achieve an ethically sound direction (Weinstock 2015).

Moral dilemmas are common during the treatment of patients with SUDs. For example, does one discharge a patient with alcohol use disorder who is not taking their medications and driving after having consumed alcohol? Respecting the patient's autonomy would require the provider to continue treating the patient despite the individual's treatment noncompliance and the safety risks they pose, because the continued treatment relationship may offer further opportunities to support the patient and, ideally, usher the patient toward recovery in the future. On the other hand, that treatment may enable the patient's behaviors, in violation of the nonmaleficence principle. There may be issues involved with notification of public officials at departments of motor vehicles depending on the jurisdiction, or a consideration of when to breach confidentiality if the patient objects to discussion of the driving concerns with family. Similarly, should a physician prescribe a controlled substance to patients who may benefit from such medications but are at risk of misusing them? Prescribing the medication would prioritize beneficence toward the patient, whereas refusing to prescribe would prioritize nonmaleficence to others (and maybe the patient). A decision to move forward in one direction or another would require reasoning through theoretical choices and outcomes. Each of these areas may entail approaches to reasoning through decisions that could follow the ethical theories just described to resolve the conflict.

# Liability for Providers of SUD Treatment

Physicians treating any patient may be subject to professional liability as medical malpractice under federal and state tort laws if, as a direct result of substandard care provided, their patients suffer damages. Physicians who treat patients with SUDs are no exception to the duty to provide care as a reasonable practitioner. One common area of concern for physicians working with patients with SUDs is the liability risk associated with a patient's misuse of prescribed medications with addictive potential. Another relates to intentional or accidental overdose deaths from the use of prescribed medications such as opioids or benzodiazepines.

Patients should be able to provide informed consent to the treatments they receive. The three elements of the informed consent are as follows:

- *Information:* Patients should be informed of relevant information, including the risks, benefits, limitations of, and outcomes without treatment.
- *Competence:* Health care providers should assess and confirm their patient's medical decision-making capacity. A patient's capacity to provide informed consent should be unimpaired. Elements of medical decision-making capacity include the patient's ability to form and sustain a choice about their treatment, understand information presented, appreciate the nature of their situation, and manipulate information rationally (Appelbaum 2007).
- *Voluntariness:* Health care providers should assess and confirm that a patient's participation in treatment is voluntary and free of undue influence (unless they are court-ordered to receive treatment over objection) (Dennehy and White 2012; Sherman et al. 2021).

The following recommendations for licensed physicians may help minimize the liability risk when treating patients with SUDs:

1. Limit your medical practice to your scope of practice.
2. Ensure that you are licensed to practice medicine where the patient is located.
3. Have expertise in recognizing and diagnosing SUDs.
4. Possess sufficient skills and knowledge to provide a full range of treatment services for patients with SUD.
5. Be able to refer and support for additional SUD treatment interventions.
6. Recognize and manage drug or alcohol intoxication.
7. Recognize and manage drug or alcohol withdrawal.
8. Recognize and manage medical emergencies in the context of substance use (e.g., overdoses, high-risk withdrawal).
9. Do not overprescribe medications with addictive or diversion potential.
10. Conduct a physical examination when needed.
11. Obtain and document informed consent for treatment.
12. Obtain and follow up on necessary laboratory monitoring tests (including to assess the severity of the SUDs or monitor the tolerability of prescribed medications).
13. Keep accurate medical treatment records.
14. Take appropriate safeguards against diversion of prescribed medications.
15. Check the PDMP report when prescribing controlled substances and document the findings.
16. Coordinate and collaborate with other health care providers involved in the care of the patient if indicated.

17. Coordinate and collaborate with family members of patients if indicated (with patient's approval, unless there are authorized exceptions to requiring consent).
18. Educate the patient on their responsibility in the handling of prescribed controlled medications and safe disposing of unused portions.
19. Educate the patient upfront on the terms of discontinuing the prescribing of controlled substances, or the need to escalate the level of monitoring or care and maintain boundaries for violations of agreed-on rules.
20. Educate the patient about when a referral to more specialized services or higher levels of care might be necessary.
21. Monitor newer patients or higher-risk patients more closely, and prescribe smaller amounts of medications until enough clinical information is gathered and trust is established.
22. Ensure and respect patient confidentiality in treatment unless exceptions apply.

Ensuring and maintaining patient confidentiality is a core principle of medical practice in general, and it is particularly important when treating patients with SUDs. As noted earlier in this chapter, HIPAA set the first federal minimum privacy standards for patient health information. Beyond HIPAA, individual states may impose additional and stricter confidentiality and privilege standards. Privacy standards for substance use treatment (and release of records) are more stringent than those for medical or psychiatric care. They are established by the federal alcohol and drug abuse confidentiality regulations first enacted in 1972 and amended in 2020 as described in the earlier discussion of the CARES Act. Although maintaining patient confidentiality is an ethical duty of utmost import, it is far from absolute. Exceptions to absolute confidentiality include the need to ensure patient safety, the safety of identified third parties, and court-ordered disclosures. Patients should be informed of such limitations before initiating a treatment relationship.

*Telemedicine* refers to the provision of medical treatment (including for patients with SUDs) using video (or less frequently audio) conferencing. The practice of telemedicine has been increasing in popularity over the past couple of decades, but the COVID-19 pandemic accelerated its applicability tremendously (Fiacco et al. 2021; Tofighi et al. 2022). The use of telemedicine appears to be an effective means to deliver medical care that may offer equivalent outcomes to in-person care (Kermack et al. 2017; Shakir and Wakeman 2021). Health care providers using telemedicine to provide SUD care should ensure that they are using software and hardware that is consistent with the HIPAA standards for patient privacy. The prescribing of controlled substances using telemedicine is regulated by the Ryan Haight Online Pharmacy Consumer Protection Act (2008). The act requires prescribers to conduct an in-person medical evaluation at least once every 24 months if prescribing particular controlled substances (with some exceptions for medications, such as buprenorphine, made available during a declared public health emergency) (Implementation of the Ryan Haight Online Pharmacy Consumer Protection Act 2008). Given the evolving nature of these rules, it is important for practitioners to explore and follow the most recent expectations for the use of telemedicine for prescribing particular medications.

# Medical Licensure and Credentialing

Historically (until the beginning of the twentieth century), medicine was considered a self-regulated profession, with individual practitioners granted the responsibility for regulating and monitoring their own practice without any formal system to monitor the effectiveness and safety of said practice. Of course, practicing medicine is not a risk-free endeavor. Improper medical care can result in negative health outcomes for patients, including a risk of death. Thus, states and the federal government have enacted stringent regulations to ensure that individuals practicing medicine are qualified to do so, with the goal of protecting the public from poor medical care. The Tenth Amendment of the U.S. Constitution authorizes state governments to hold their own powers unless otherwise specified for the federal government, and one such power is that states protect the health, safety, and general welfare of individuals (unless superseded by federal authority).

All states, territories, and the District of Columbia have passed a medical practice act that defines and delineates the practice of medicine and delegates to state medical boards the authority to apply these standards and enforce the relevant laws. The Federation of State Medical Boards (FSMB) was formed in 1912 to represent the 71 state medical boards and provide unified guidance for their missions. In addition, a multitude of private and public agencies are tasked with examining, monitoring, and ensuring the qualifications of individuals practicing medicine.

There are multiple layers of qualifications that a physician must meet to practice medicine. In addition to attending medical school and receiving a Doctor of Medicine (M.D.) degree, an equivalent degree (e.g., Doctor of Osteopathic Medicine [D.O.]), or a foreign equivalent degree (e.g., Bachelor of Medicine, Bachelor of Surgery [M.B.B.S.]), physicians must pass qualifying certification examinations (the United States Medical Licensing Examinations administered by the FSMB), participate in postgraduate training (residencies, fellowship training, or both), acquire licenses to practice medicine in their respective states, and be credentialed by their local institutions. Licenses to practice medicine are administered by the various states' medical boards to individuals who meet specific qualifying training requirements and demonstrate their knowledge, skills, and abilities. State medical boards and credentialing boards at medical institutions are empowered to institute ongoing Continued Medical Education (CME) requirements to individual physicians to maintain their licensure and certifications.

Individual state medical boards are responsible for the following:

- Initial credentialing of physicians in accordance with the state's credentialing requirements
- Granting of licenses to practice medicine
- Establishment and implementation of a state's requirements for the maintenance of licensure
- Implementation of state regulations regarding medical licensure
- Review, investigation, and adjudication of complaints against individual licensed practitioners
- Disciplinary procedures to address poor medical practice, concerns related to an individual licensed practitioner's competence to practice, and other fraudulent, unprofessional, unethical, or unlawful behaviors
- Oversight of rehabilitation interventions for physicians when indicated

Additional certifications designed to assess and represent an individual physician's basic qualifications to practice medicine include board certifications by the National Board of Physicians and Surgeons and the American Board of Medical Specialties (through its subspecialty boards such as the American Board of Psychiatry and Neurology, which oversees addiction psychiatry board certifications; the American Board of Preventive Medicine, which oversees addiction medicine board certifications; or the American Board of Internal Medicine). Added qualifications embodied in some of these boards are viewed as optional but signify that a clinician has the requisite knowledge to practice safely. Furthermore, litigation for malpractice allows patients to pursue compensatory or punitive damages caused by negligent or deliberately harmful medical practice. All of these requirements provide checks and balances to protect the public and minimize the likelihood of receiving medical care that is incompetent, fraudulent, unprofessional, unethical, or unlawful.

Physician attributes sometimes addressed in malpractice suits are defined by the FSMB as follows (Federation of State Medical Boards 2015):

- *Competence:* possessing the requisite abilities and qualities (cognitive, noncognitive, and communicative) to perform effectively within the scope of the physician's practice while adhering to professional ethical standards
- *Dyscompetence:* failing to maintain acceptable standards of one or more areas of professional physician practice

- *Incompetence:* lacking the requisite abilities and qualities (cognitive, non-cognitive, and communicative) to perform effectively in the scope of the physician's practice
- *Impairment:* an inability to practice medicine with reasonable skill and safety due to the following:
  - mental, psychological, or psychiatric illness, disease, or deficit
  - physical illness or condition, including, but not limited to, those illnesses or conditions that would adversely affect cognitive, motor, or perceptive skills
  - habitual, excessive, or illegal use or abuse of drugs defined by law as controlled substances, illegal drugs, alcohol, or other impairing substances

It is important to note that in any employment matter, illness does not equate impairment, with the latter interfering with one's ability to engage safely in professional activities. The FSMB affirms that licensed health care professionals, state medical associations, hospitals, health care organizations, and other relevant bodies have a duty to report to the state medical board licensed physicians who may be compromised, incompetent to practice medicine, or suspected of unprofessional conduct. (SUD-related disability in the workplace is covered in more detail in Chapter 4.)

Upon determination that a physician is impaired, incompetent to practice medicine, or engaged in fraudulent, unprofessional, unethical, or unlawful behaviors, state medical boards may require a broad range of rehabilitative or disciplinary actions, including the following (Federation of State Medical Boards 2018):

- *Administrative action:* Certain nonpunitive actions that do not result in the modification or termination of a physician's license; these actions are generally administrative and may be issued for reasons such as failure to pay a licensing fee.
- *Fine:* In some cases, state boards may levy a monetary penalty against a physician.
- *CME requirements:* The physician is required to complete CME.
- *Conditions imposed:* The physician must fulfill certain conditions to avoid further sanction by the state board.
- *License denied:* The physician's application for a medical license or renewal of a current license is denied.
- *License restricted:* The physician's ability to practice medicine is limited (e.g., loss of prescribing privileges).
- *License revoked:* The physician's license is terminated; the individual can no longer practice medicine within the state or territory.

- *License surrendered:* The physician voluntarily surrenders their medical license, sometimes during the course of a disciplinary investigation.
- *License suspended:* The physician may not practice medicine for a specified period of time, perhaps due to disciplinary investigation or until other state board requirements are fulfilled.
- *Probation:* The physician's license is monitored by a state board for a specified period of time.
- *Reprimand:* The physician is issued a warning or letter of concern.

Physician health programs (PHPs) are peer-based monitoring, evaluation, and treatment-referral centers often governed by state laws and administered by collaborations between state medical societies, malpractice carriers, and state medical boards. Every state has a PHP that is independent of the state medical board and is typically administered by an independent agency or the state medical society to assess, monitor, provide oversight, and rehabilitate impaired physicians, as an alternative or a precursor to a referral to the state medical board. Individual practitioners may self-refer to the PHP (often to prevent or delay a referral to the state medical board), or they may be referred by health care organizations, medical schools, other practitioners, or law enforcement (Boyd and Knight 2012; Lenzer 2016).

Finally, grievances about medical care can be taken to court, either through a civil claim of a tort (wrongful action characterized as malpractice) or even a criminal matter pursuant to local and federal laws. These lawsuits offer an additional layer of recourse to address concerns over physicians who are impaired, incompetent to practice medicine, or engaged in fraudulent, unprofessional, unethical, or unlawful behaviors, separately from the administrative procedures described in this section.

It should be noted that there are also a number of nonphysician practitioners who work with individuals with SUDs in a treatment role. Each state can have different laws regarding what lies within a particular authorized scope of one's practice, and a full review of this topic is outside the scope of this book. Nevertheless, anyone working to treat or evaluate individuals with SUDs may also be subject to licensure complaints, civil liability, and criminal punishment depending on what might be happening in practice. Following basic standards of care, operating within the scope of one's license, and seeking supervision or referral for consultation can be remedies and actions to mitigate the risk associated with negative outcomes for both the patient and the practitioner.

# The Practice of Forensic Addiction Psychiatry

Forensic psychiatry is, broadly speaking, a psychiatric subspecialty involving the application of psychiatric knowledge to matters involving the legal regulation of psychiatric practice as well as the application of psychiatric knowledge to legal matters. As such, forensic psychiatrists receive additional training in the intersection between medicine and the law and serve as experts in addressing medical questions presented by legal professionals (e.g., lawyers or judges) or other third parties (e.g., employers, insurance companies, or licensing boards). These questions can arise from criminal, family, or civil matters. Forensic psychiatrists are also experts in the provision of care for individuals in the criminal legal system, including those in correctional settings. Given the relationship between SUDs and criminal matters (discussed in more detail in Chapter 8), it is unsurprising that forensic matters involving SUDs arise frequently in those contexts. Generally, evaluations that may benefit from a forensic and addiction psychiatrist may relate to criminal responsibility, civil medical malpractice litigation, and diversion courts (drug courts or driving while intoxicated courts), to name a few. Moreover, given SUD rates among incarcerated individuals, forensic addiction psychiatrists play a major role in delivering (and advocating for) evidence-based medical care for incarcerated patients with SUDs.

Forensic addiction psychiatrists may be invited to opine on relevant matters in written reports, as legal consultants, or as expert witnesses in court proceedings. In that capacity, the forensic addiction psychiatrist's role is distinct from that of a fact witness, with the latter testifying on their observations *without* an opinion. For example, an SUD treatment provider may be subpoenaed to produce medical records or testify on their knowledge of their patients as a fact witness or they may be asked to opine on a case; however, opinions offered as an expert are ill advised if one is in a treatment role, given ethical problems with those roles, with few exceptions (American Academy of Psychiatry and the Law 2005). Expert witnesses should strive to deliver expert opinions that are honest and objective, owing their fiduciary responsibility to the truth rather than to the evaluee or the retaining party. In contrast, a treating physician's fiduciary responsibility is to their patients.

A forensic evaluation differs markedly from a traditional doctor-patient treatment evaluation, most obviously in regard to confidentiality. Forensic addiction psychiatrists use the information they collect to deliver an opinion to a third party (typically the retaining party). So, it is important for the forensic psychiatrist to inform evaluees of the limits of confidentiality in forensic settings and to explain the differences between a forensic evaluation and a medical treatment evaluation. Given the import and implications of forensic evaluations, forensic addiction psychiatrists must abide by the ethics guidelines defined by the American Academy of Psychiatry and the Law (2005).

Although forensic addiction psychiatrists acting in forensic roles are not delivering clinical treatment, they are not necessarily shielded from scrutiny or even litigation. Forensic activities are generally covered separately in malpractice insurance, and professionals should review their coverage to that effect.

Substandard forensic evaluations can have grave and long-lasting consequences involving the freedom and livelihood of evaluees. Moreover, forensic psychiatric opinions are often delivered under oath and in an adversarial court process, which further increases scrutiny of the forensic services offered. Overall, it is important to rely on one's data and to offer opinions within the context of the data gathered, not based on personal views and biases. In other words, striving for objectivity and delivering opinions honestly are important elements in the preservation of the dignity and accuracy of forensic work.

# Conclusions

Clinicians should understand the legal structures in place for treating people with SUDs and the roles in which professionals can embark in forensic evaluations. As noted at the outset of this chapter, treatment of people with SUDs carries some risk but also has many rewards. In providing reasonable care, it is important to understand 1) how medications with addictive properties are regulated and 2) how current practices relate to the proper levels of care identified for patients with SUDs to help a practitioner prescribe appropriately and advocate for needed services. Understanding laws and limitations to reimbursement can help the practitioner avoid pitfalls and premature discharges of patients who may need more intensive services. In addition, practitioners must operate within the scope of their license, and regulatory bodies and licensing boards have established a variety of ways to help protect patients from harm. Finally, for practitioners operating in a forensic role, it is important to base opinions on data and consider all elements to strive for objectivity and minimize bias in evaluations to provide information and opinions in legal contexts.

## Key Points

- The Federal Register Schedule of Controlled Substances, which as of press time still lists cannabis as a Schedule I substance, could have legal ramifications for individuals who use cannabis and clinicians who recommend it.

- Prescribing rules for buprenorphine, although still governed by the Drug Addiction Treatment Act (2000), were loosened during the COVID-19 pandemic.

- Persons with substance use disorders (SUDs) are increasingly protected by statutes that require fair treatment by health insurance companies and the justice system.

- To serve their patients, clinicians should know the details of SUD nosology and the standards for insurance reimbursement for different levels of care.

- Clinicians should know the common areas of malpractice liability in working with patients with SUDs.

- Licensing bodies, board certification, and other outside influences help provide checks and balances aimed at safe patient care, and practitioners should be aware of the operation of these influences.

- Treatment and forensic practices differ in approach and ethical rules.

# References

Abraham AJ, Andrews CM, Grogan CM, et al: The Affordable Care Act transformation of substance use disorder treatment. Am J Public Health 107(1):31–32, 2017 27925819

American Academy of Psychiatry and the Law: Ethics guidelines for the practice of forensic psychiatry. May 2005. Available at: https://www.aapl.org/ethics.htm. Accessed November 13, 2018.

American Psychiatric Association: Substance-related and addictive disorders, in Diagnostic and Statistical Manual of Mental Disorders, 5th Edition. Arlington, VA, American Psychiatric Publishing, 2013, pp 543–665

American Society of Addiction Medicine: Treatment Criteria for Addictive, Substance-Related, and Co-Occurring Conditions, 3rd Edition. Rockville, MD, American Society of Addiction Medicine, 2013, p 153

Appelbaum PS: Clinical practice: assessment of patients' competence to consent to treatment. N Engl J Med 357(18):1834–1840, 2007 17978292

Boyd JW, Knight JR: Ethical and managerial considerations regarding state physician health programs. J Addict Med 6(4):243–246, 2012 23070127

Comprehensive Addiction and Recovery Act of 2016 (P.L. 114–198), 130 Stat. 695 (codified at 42 U.S.C. § 201 note)

Comprehensive Drug Abuse Prevention and Control Act of 1970 (P.L. 91–513), 84 Stat. 1236

Confidentiality of Substance Use Disorder Patient Records, 85 Fed. Reg. 42986, 43039 (Aug. 14, 2020) (to be codified at 42 C.F.R. pt. 2; SAMHSA-4162-20)

Confidentiality of Substance Use Disorder Patient Records, 87 Fed. Reg. 74216, 74286 (Dec. 2, 2022) (to be codified at 42 C.F.R. pt. 2 and at 45 C.F.R. pt. 164)

Coronavirus Aid, Relief, and Economic Security Act of 2020, S.3548, 116th Cong.

Croft B, Parish SL: Care integration in the Patient Protection and Affordable Care Act: implications for behavioral health. Adm Policy Ment Health 40(4):258–263, 2013 22371190

Dennehy L, White S: Consent, assent, and the importance of risk stratification. Br J Anaesth 109(1):40–46, 2012 22696558

Drug Addiction Treatment Act

Drug Enforcement Administration: 21 CFR Part 1308 Docket No. DEA-1362; A.G. Order No. 5931-2024. Schedules of Controlled Substances: Rescheduling of Marijuana. Available at: https://www.dea.gov/sites/default/files/2024-05/Scheduling%20NPRM%20508.pdf. Accessed May 25, 2024.

of 2000, H.R. 2634, 106th Cong.

Federation of State Medical Boards: Essentials of a state medical and osteopathic practice act. April 2015. Available at: https://www.fsmb.org/siteassets/advocacy/policies/essentials-of-a-state-medical-and-osteopathic-practice-act.pdf. Accessed October 30, 2023.

Federation of State Medical Boards: Guide to medical regulations in the United States. 2018. Available at: https://www.fsmb.org/u.s.-medical-regulatory-trends-and-actions/guide-to-medical-regulation-in-the-united-states/. Accessed October 30, 2023.

Fiacco L, Pearson BL, Jordan R: Telemedicine works for treating substance use disorder: the STAR clinic experience during COVID-19. J Subst Abuse Treat 125:108312, 2021 34016299

Implementation of the Ryan Haight Online Pharmacy Consumer Protection Act of 2008, 87 Fed. Reg. 74216 (Dec. 2, 2022) (to be codified at 42 C.F.R. pt. 2 and 45 C.F.R. pt. 164)

Kermack A, Flannery M, Tofighi B, et al: Buprenorphine prescribing practice trends and attitudes among New York providers. J Subst Abuse Treat 74:1–6, 2017 28132694

Lenzer J: Physician health programs under fire. BMJ 353:i3568, 2016 27364761

Mee-Lee D, Shulman GD: The ASAM criteria and matching patients to treatment, in The ASAM Principles of Addiction Medicine, 6th Edition. Edited by Miller S, Fiellin D, Rosenthal R, et al. Philadelphia, PA, Wolters Kluwer, 2018, pp 433–447

Mental Health Parity and Addiction Equity Act of 2008 (P.L. 110–343), 122 Stat. 3881 (codified as amended 42 U.S.C. § 201 note)

Niveau G, Welle I: Forensic psychiatry, one subspecialty with two ethics? A systematic review. BMC Med Ethics 19(1):25, 2018 29636102

Patient Protection and Affordable Care Act of 2010 (P.L. 111–148), 124 Stat. 119 (codified at 42 U.S.C. § 18001 note)

Shakir M, Wakeman S: Substance use disorder and telemedicine: opportunity and concern for the future. J Gen Intern Med 36(9):2823–2824, 2021 33078301

Sherman KA, Kilby CJ, Pehlivan M, et al: Adequacy of measures of informed consent in medical practice: a systematic review. PLoS One 16(5):e0251485, 2021 34043651

Spetz J, Hailer L, Gay C, et al: Changes in US clinician waivers to prescribe buprenorphine management for opioid use disorder during the COVID-19 pandemic and after relaxation of training requirements. JAMA Netw Open 5(5):e225996, 2022 35552728

Taylor RM: Ethical principles and concepts in medicine. Handb Clin Neurol 118:1–9, 2013 24182363

Tofighi B, McNeely J, Walzer D, et al: A telemedicine buprenorphine clinic to serve New York City: initial evaluation of the NYC public hospital system's initiative to expand treatment access during the COVID-19 pandemic. J Addict Med 16(1):e40–e43, 2022 33560696

Varkey B: Principles of clinical ethics and their application to practice. Med Princ Pract 30(1):17–28, 2021 32498071

Weinstock R: Dialectical principlism: an approach to finding the most ethical action. J Am Acad Psychiatry Law 43(1):10–20, 2015 25770274

Wen H, Druss BG, Cummings JR: Effect of Medicaid expansions on health insurance coverage and access to care among low-income adults with behavioral health conditions. Health Serv Res 50(6):1787–1809, 2015 26551430

# PART 2

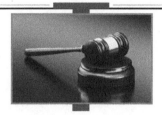

# CIVIL ISSUES

# CHAPTER 4

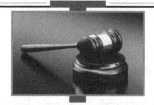

# EMPLOYMENT LAW AND ADDICTION

## Introduction

Most people with substance use disorders (SUDs) are gainfully employed and thus can be profoundly affected by the nuances of employment law. According to data gathered by the National Safety Council (2020), 1 of every 11 U.S. workers met criteria for an SUD in the past 12 months. Of all construction trade workers, 19% had an SUD, as did 16% of those in service occupations, 13.9% of transportation and material moving workers, 13.5% of installation and maintenance workers, and 13.4% of those in sales.

Clinicians and forensic examiners alike must know the basics of employment law, as it affects any patient or examinee who has a job, is applying for a job, or ever wants a job. Employment law influences the lives of substance users as they apply for jobs, if and when an accident or substance-related incident occurs, and if there is a threat of job termination because of substance use. Stigma and potential absences from work related to treatment for SUDs can also affect the employee. SUD-related disability is covered—in very specific and sometimes limited ways—by the Americans With Disabilities Act (1990) (ADA). Patients, their clinicians, and forensic mental health examiners should understand the variety of drug testing protocols for the workplace as well as the consequences of a positive test result showing recent substance use.

## FORENSIC DILEMMA

A 49-year-old male train conductor is alleged to have had alcohol on his breath at work. He is referred to the forensic evaluator with a phone call in which his supervisor asks, "Is he okay to come back to work?"

Consider the following:

1. What should the evaluator do first?
2. Whom should the evaluator interview?

During the interview, the train conductor acknowledges that there is a great deal of marital strife in his home, that a divorce is probably coming, and that he has been drinking a bit more than usual to prepare himself before he walks in the door after work. Although the conductor denies drinking on the job, he eventually says that he is probably drinking too much. The conductor asks, "Could you help me out, Doc, and refer me to someone who could help me beat this drinking thing?"

Consider the following:

3. What are the evaluator's legal obligations to the conductor? The employer?
4. How should the evaluator respond to the conductor's request for psychiatric and addiction treatment after the case has concluded?

The evaluator should first clarify the referral questions and obtain informed consent from the subject. The evaluator has an obligation to the employer who hired them to do the assessment; the evaluator also needs to know how to respond to the conductor, who is asking for some assistance with an apparent addiction problem. Unless there are extenuating circumstances (and even then, only after the conclusion of the evaluation process), the evaluator should not initiate treatment of the conductor: this would violate the boundary between forensic and clinical treatment (American Academy of Psychiatry and the Law 2005). It would be acceptable for the evaluator 1) to refer the conductor to treatment providers and 2) to explain to the conductor that the role of the evaluator cannot generally be mixed with the treatment role.

# Disability and SUDs

As with all forensic matters, it is very important for the clinician interacting with an employee involved with—or accused of being involved with—substances in the workplace to clarify the role of treating clinician versus forensic examiner. The clinician is obligated to provide accurate reports or information to whomever the patient indicates and, if in a treatment role, to provide appropriate care. The forensic examiner or workplace clinician is obligated to provide accurate information about the employee's substance use, any symptoms that meet actual diagnostic criteria, and present and future issues with the employee continuing in the workplace. Sometimes the forensic assessor must prognosticate about the likely downstream effects of substance use that might not be problematic at present. Often, a forensic assessor must explain laboratory testing in an understandable form to managers, attorneys, and human resources professionals who are tasked with protecting the workplace and other employees. All communications from the forensic assessor to others must comply with workplace contracts, union agreements, and relevant confidentiality law, including the Health Insurance Portability and Accountability Act of 1996 (HIPAA) and the more specific federal regulatory guidelines pertaining to SUDs and confidentiality (42 C.F.R. Part 2).

It is important to understand the terminology of disability assessment in the workplace. An *impairment* is best defined as a "significant deviation, loss, or loss of use of any body structure or function in an individual with a health condition, disorder, or disease" (Rondinelli 2008, p. 611). Impairment, of course, does not necessarily lead to or equate with *disability*, which is further defined as "activity limitations and/or participation restrictions in an individual with a health condition, disorder, or disease" (Rondinelli 2008, p. 611). A *limitation* is what the person cannot do, and a *restriction* is what the claimant-employee is medically advised not to do. Consider the following examples: A patient with a broken ankle may be able to bear weight but entirely unable to walk 10 miles, although the patient was advised by his physician not to bear weight on the affected limb at all. A person with opioid use disorder (OUD) may be restricted from working in a surgical operating room with access to a narcotics lockbox because his clinician has advised him to avoid that type of workplace. A person experiencing seizures and tremors related to alcohol use would have an impairment and would also—at least temporarily—be limited and restricted from working anywhere. By contrast, a person with anxiety following cocaine use might have a mood impairment but would not necessarily be limited or restricted from working in most environments.

# AMERICANS WITH DISABILITIES ACT

The ADA of 1990, which was further amended in 2008, was designed to protect individuals with a disability, as defined in the law, from discrimination in multiple domains, including employment discrimination (Americans With Disabilities Act 1990). People with drug- or alcohol-related diagnoses are protected by the ADA in some very specific instances, although these protections are increasingly narrowed by court rulings (Westreich 2002). Interestingly, alcohol problems are addressed quite differently from drug problems in the ADA. The ADA covers only a person who is not "currently" using drugs, whereas no such limitation exists in the alcohol portions of the act (U.S. Commission on Civil Rights 2024). Any individual with an employment issue related to substance use should consult an attorney familiar with the ADA, state and local statutes, and the practical workings of the U.S. Equal Employment Opportunity Commission.

For any protected condition under the ADA, including addiction to drugs or alcohol, a disability or impairment as defined earlier in this chapter (not merely a diagnosis) must exist. Situations that would not qualify for protections under the ADA include those in which the person has only a history of impairment or when the person does not have a qualifying disability. At times, diagnostic records can help or confuse the picture, because a person may have received a misdiagnosis or may have been treated assuming that they have a disability when they do not.

Although the ADA aims to provide a structure that is nationwide and under statutory protection to eliminate discrimination against people with disabilities, including drug and alcohol users, the ADA does not treat drug use disorders like other diseases and disabilities. The law carves out exceptions under the safe harbor provisions of the act, such that an individual using illicit drugs would be excluded from the definition of disability. Therefore, an individual with an alcohol use disorder has different protections than someone with an OUD. Although some states have legalized marijuana use, the federal government has not, so marijuana use would still be considered use of illegal substances in the ADA regardless of the state.

Having a potentially disabling condition does not equate with disability, according to the ADA. The ADA sets out specific provisions for limitations on areas of impairment that are required to be met for an individual to qualify as having a disability. These include impairments in "major life activities," such as caring for oneself, performing manual tasks, seeing, hearing, eating, sleeping, walking, standing, lifting, bending, speaking, and reproductive functions, among others (see Table 4–1).

Case law has both broadened and whittled down the actual protections available to drug and alcohol users under the ADA, although some substantive protections remain in place. To understand case law in context, it is also important to realize that if an employee comes to work intoxicated or experiencing withdrawal, their protections under the ADA would potentially be limited. The ADA's overarching "direct threat exception" means that if the individual poses a direct threat to the safety of themselves or others related to their disability, the person will not qualify for aspects of the ADA including accommodations or even job protection. It is also critical to understand that there can be other

**Table 4–1.** Major life activities and bodily functions under the Americans With Disabilities Act

| Major life activities | Major bodily functions |
|---|---|
| Caring for oneself | Functions of the immune system |
| Performing manual tasks | Normal cell growth |
| Seeing and hearing | Digestive system, bowel, and bladder |
| Eating | Neurological system |
| Sleeping | Respiratory system |
| Walking | Circulatory system |
| Speaking | |
| Learning | |
| Concentrating | |
| Working | |
| Communicating | |

*Source.* Office of Federal Contractor Compliance Programs: ADA Amendments Act of 2008 Frequently Asked Questions. U.S. Department of Labor, 2009. Available at: https://www.dol.gov/agencies/ofccp/faqs/americans-with-disabilities-act-amendments. Accessed November 2, 2023.

forces at play in the employment context beyond the ADA. For example, even if an individual has an SUD that qualifies as a disability under the ADA, there are still no allowances for violation of specific workplace rules, and the ADA does not supersede the Drug-Free Workplace Requirements of Federal Contractors (1988) or statutes established by the U.S. Department of Transportation (DOT), the U.S. Department of Defense (DOD), or the Nuclear Regulatory Commission (NRC).

The ADA does not specify what constitutes current drug use, although definition of the term *current* is very much debatable. In *Shaffer v. Preston Memorial Hospital* (1997), one appeals court judge defined the term broadly in finding that nurse-anesthetist Deborah Shaffer, who was denied a return to her position although she successfully completed a 21-day inpatient treatment program for fentanyl addiction, did not deserve ADA protection because her drug use was "current." In its ruling, the court articulated the following:

> Contrary to Shaffer's assertion, the ordinary meaning of the phrase "currently using drugs" does not require that a drug user have a heroin syringe in his arm or a marijuana bong to his mouth at the exact moment contemplated. Instead, in this context the plain meaning of currently is broader. (*Shaffer v. Preston Memorial Hospital* 1997)

In this matter, the court may well have been influenced by records in evidence showing that Shaffer had experienced a relapse to opioid use while working at a different hospital after completing her rehabilitation program.

So, what does it mean to be covered by the ADA? To be covered by the ADA, an individual is entitled to be free from discrimination but also may be entitled to accommodations, assuming that with those accommodations they can perform the essential functions of their job. If the individual is unable to perform the essential functions of their job with or without accommodations, an employer is not obligated to keep them on the payroll. Accommodations, however, allow a worker with a disability to maintain employment without discrimination. For example, an employee who uses a wheelchair may be perfectly capable of working if the job entails getting to the office and sitting at a desk. The employer's accommodations may include ramps and a desk with height adjustment.

For individuals with an SUD-related disability, ADA entitlements apply to those who have not endangered anyone in the workplace and must take time off from work for treatment or require other reasonable accommodations. Examples of reasonable accommodations might include allowing time off to pick up a daily methadone prescription, changing work assignments to relieve an employee of relapse-provocative duties, if possible, or temporarily reassigning the patient to a non-safety-sensitive position while they complete treatment. So, in some circumstances, the ADA can be quite helpful to the person who is employed while dealing with addiction. An employer is also protected from having to make accommodations that would be unreasonable.

## EMPLOYER OR PRIVATE DISABILITY POLICIES

As opposed to the ADA, which usually provides some job protection for people with SUDs, employer-funded or private disability insurance policies may or may not cover SUDs, depending on how the policy is written. Short-term disability policies provide coverage for living expenses for 3–6 months if the covered individual is disabled from work because of a chronic condition, illness, or injury. Most short-term disability policies cover SUDs: *own occupation policies* would pay out if the individual is prevented by their SUD from doing their specific work, whereas *any occupation policies* would pay out only if the individual cannot work in any position. Long-term disability policies (usually written for 6 months to 2 years of disability) are less likely to cover SUDs, although some do. It should also be noted that many long-term disability policies would provide lifetime coverage for physical health conditions (including neurocognitive conditions induced by alcohol, for example) but not for primary SUDs. Parity laws are concerned with health insurance coverage, whereas disability policies are not required to have parity with coverage arrangements.

Disability evaluations for SUDs have enormous import for the examinee and for the financial coffers of the insurance company. For disability policies (which are becoming less common) in which the subject of the assessment is covered for drug or alcohol use, the forensic examiner will need at least a rudimentary knowledge of the policy language to answer the relevant questions. Often, the ultimate issues in the disability evaluations center around 1) present impairment, which disability policies usually cover; and 2) potential relapse, which the policies often do not cover.

The philosophical underpinnings of modern concepts of addiction often underlie disability insurance disputes. Addictive disorders are often viewed as "soft" disabilities, in that the insurer may limit claim approvals. Typical arguments might be that a chronic SUD may have been a preexisting condition and therefore excluded from payment, that the claimant is choosing to use addictive substances, or that the claimant is simply noncompliant with treatment if a relapse occurs. This putative choice to use, or noncompliance with treatment, can be used as evidence that the claimant is not even attempting to mitigate the circumstances of the condition, thereby invalidating the disability insurance policy. Similarly, disability insurers can argue that disability insurance pays out only for actual occurrences rather than something that might occur, such as a relapse to substance use. The addicted person in stable (or even not-so-stable) recovery is left to argue that although they are well now, a relapse is so likely that a real disability exists.

One relevant legal case, *Colby v. Union Security Insurance Co.* (2013), addressed whether the risk of relapse should itself be considered a disability. Julie Colby, M.D., an anesthesiologist in a busy Massachusetts practice, was found "asleep or unconscious" on a hospital table and had a positive drug screen for fentanyl. Soon after this event, Colby took a leave of absence from her job and entered addiction treatment at Talbott Recovery Campus in Atlanta, Georgia, in a program specifically designed for physicians. She received a diagnosis of opioid dependence, dysthymia, and obsessive-compulsive traits, in addition to degenerative disc disease that had caused back pain that had led to her initial opioid use. Although Colby's insurance company paid disability benefits for the 12 days she was at Talbott, the company refused to pay any further costs, noting that "risk for relapse is not the same as a current disability" (*Colby v. Union Security Insurance Co.*2013). A trial court ruled that this denial of benefits, based on the grounds that the "[long-term disability plan] does not cover future risk generally or treats physical and psychological future risks differently, absent language allowing these distinctions, is arbitrary and capricious" (*Colby v. Union Security Insurance Co.* 2013). In essence, the insurance company was told that the summary denial of benefits was unfair, and it had to pay the benefits. The insurance company still refused to pay the benefits and appealed, arguing that a risk of relapse does not amount to a current disability under the plan and would not prevent the plaintiff from working in her occupation. The First U.S. Circuit Court of Appeals in Boston found for Dr. Colby, citing examples of non-addiction-related relapses that are, in fact, covered by disability insurers as a framework for their decision. Examples included a case involving an orthopedic surgeon at risk of heart attack or an air traffic controller at risk of seizures provoked by blinking runway lights. Although informative as a Circuit Court of Appeals case, and given that private disability insurance companies can write policies that cover multiple jurisdictions, this case decision did not lead to binding change. Thus, it is important for evaluees and patients to understand that private disability insurance for SUDs is still an area in which coverage, especially long term, may be limited.

# SOCIAL SECURITY ADMINISTRATION DISABILITY PROGRAMS

The Social Security Administration (SSA) administers the Social Security Disability Insurance (SSDI) and the Supplemental Security Income (SSI) programs, which provide financial assistance to people with disabilities. The SSDI pays benefits for those who have contributed a certain amount through Social Security taxes on their earnings, whereas the SSI provides benefits for adults and children with limited income and resources.

Federal benefits for addictive disorders are managed under the SSDI program, and they have a specific set of rules administered by the SSA. Ultimate determinations are made by SSA administrative law judges and claims examiners. Although earlier iterations of the SSDI program provided disability payments for addiction alone, the rules were changed on March 29, 1996 (Contract With America Advancement Act 1996), to deny new disability payments for addiction unless the disability would continue even if the applicant stopped using drugs: a judicial determination is made as to whether the addiction is a material factor to the disability. The evaluation criteria were explained as follows:

> [W]e will evaluate which of your current physical and mental limitations, upon which we based our current disability determination, would remain if you stopped using drugs or alcohol and then determine whether any or all of your remaining limitations would be disabling.
> (i) If we determine that your remaining limitations would not be disabling, we will find that your drug addiction or alcoholism is a contributing factor material to the determination of disability.
> (ii) If we determine that your remaining limitations are disabling, you are disabled independent of your drug addiction or alcoholism and we will find that your drug addiction or alcoholism is not a contributing factor material to the determination of disability." (20 C.F.R. Ch. III [4–1–10 Edition] § 404.1535)

SSDI and SSI recipients who received benefits by virtue of an addictive disorder were studied in advance of the 1996 changes and, in the language of the regulations, more than half were addicted to alcohol only, 16% were addicted to drugs, and 27% were addicted to both (Waid and Barber 2001). Of those studied, 79% received SSI benefits, their average age was 43 years, and the majority

(73%) were male. Approximately 40% identified as Black, although Black people made up only 28% of the entire SSI population who were blind or had a disability as of June 1996.

Since 1996, applicants for SSDI benefits for addiction must show 1) that disability would exist even after the drug or alcohol use stopped and 2) that the remaining disability is severe enough to constitute a true disability. Common examples of this include liver pathology, which continues after the person stops drinking, or alcohol-related neurocognitive decline that continues after alcohol use is stopped. Although there is no absolute requirement that the drug and alcohol use cease before benefits are awarded, the applicant must make the theoretical argument about what the disabilities would be in the event that drug or alcohol use stopped. In general, applicants are viewed more favorably in circumstances when they have, in fact, stopped using drugs or alcohol. Individuals who are granted disability payments for addiction based on the assumption that they will still be disabled if they stopped their use may be assigned a representative payee who can receive the benefits to "help create a stable living environment for the beneficiary and ensure that the basic current needs of food, shelter, clothing, and medical care are met" (Social Security Administration 2021).

Treating physicians are often asked to write reports for SSDI on the work they believe their patient can and cannot do because of the impairment. In the case of SUDs, this determination may be subjective. However, the SSA gives preference for a treating clinician to first evaluate the patient (Social Security Administration 2021). The presence of a co-occurring psychiatric disorder, or a related medical problem, may be highly relevant and should be included in this type of report. Although these types of requests for impairment reports are common in clinical practice, clinicians should be sure to discuss them in detail with their patients and obtain informed consent for doing them and sending them to a government agency. Potential for disruption of the clinical treatment exists, because the obligation to write a truthful report may conflict with the desire to render whatever assistance the patient requests. Clinicians should be mindful of pressures to misrepresent opinions (Christopher et al. 2011). Also, it is important that treating clinicians work with their patients to complete the paperwork rather than refer them elsewhere, because the risk of a patient with a disability not getting SSI or SSDI when it is needed is also part of the balance in patient care.

In addition to the role of treating clinicians in providing reports, physicians may choose to do consultative examinations for individuals referred to them through the SSA. These consultative examinations are essentially independent medical examinations for the SSA. In addition, the SSA requires continuing disability reviews for individuals who have been granted disability payments, and these reviews can occur every 6 months or up to every 7 years when no medical improvement is expected. Although forensic experience and credentials are not required, these consultative examinations and continuing disability reviews are distinct from clinical treatment and essentially operate as forensic assessments meant to be presented as objective opinions and as evidence used in SSA administrative law hearings before an administrative law judge (Social Security Administration 2001).

# Workplace Drug and Alcohol Testing and Monitoring

Although forensic drug and alcohol testing should always be rigorous and thoughtfully executed (see Chapter 5), the occupational aspects of this type of testing require specific protocols, in anticipation of legal and procedural challenges to the testing itself. Employers have a legitimate interest in preserving a safe and collegial workplace, whereas employees have a legitimate interest in behaving as they please outside of the workplace. Although the changing legal status of cannabis in the United States, along with the recent postpandemic difficulty in hiring and retaining employees, has roiled the drug testing world, many aspects of drug testing remain unchanged. Different professions may use different drug testing services and protocols.

As an example, DOT testing is one of the most stable occupational drug and alcohol testing structures in the United States and has changed little in the last 10 years. It remains a gold standard for clear requirements for testing, an insistence on chain-of-custody protocols, and a clear set of procedures and consequences in response to a nonnegative test result. DOT testing, as required by federal law (Omnibus Transportation Employee Testing Act 1991), seeks to ensure that commercial transportation employees in safety-sensitive positions are free of intoxicating substances while on the job. These regulations cover commercial transportation employees in all transportation industries, including trucking, aviation, and bus transportation. The following transportation workers are covered by DOT rules (Federal Motor Carrier Safety Administration 2021a):

- Anyone employing drivers with a commercial driver's license to operate commercial motor vehicles on public roads
- Drivers with a commercial driver's license who operate commercial motor vehicles on public roads
- Interstate motor carriers
- Intrastate motor carriers
- Federal, state, and local governments
- Civic organizations (e.g., transport of veterans with disabilities, Boy Scouts or Girl Scouts)
- Faith-based organizations

Transportation workers in these categories can expect to be tested for drugs and alcohol in preemployment tests, in reasonable-suspicion tests, in return-to-duty tests, and in follow-up tests (U.S. Department of Transportation 2016). These required tests are carefully delineated because they may be contested in employment actions when a transportation worker feels they have been tested unfairly. For instance, the rules of random testing, while both unannounced and sometimes done at home or off duty, are clearly defined. For the notified employee, a late arrival to the testing site for a drug test is equivalent to having a positive test result. However, random *alcohol* testing may only occur when the driver is on duty or immediately before or after that duty.

The consequences of a positive drug test, an alcohol concentration of at least 0.02 mg/dL, or a refusal to test are immediate removal from the roadways. (Note that the legal limit for alcohol is substantially lower for a commercial driver as opposed to a private driver.) DOT regulations then require evaluation and treatment by a government-certified substance abuse professional who can eventually produce a return-to-duty document. However, the driver must have a negative test result before they return to work; during the first year back at work, they must show at least six unannounced, directly observed urine toxicology results under the auspices of the substance abuse professional. The substance abuse professional may recommend continuing testing for up to 5 years after the return to work, in addition to whatever random testing is already occurring.

As of December 2021, official DOT guidance described the drugs tested in DOT protocols as marijuana, cocaine, opiates (opium and codeine derivatives), amphetamines and methamphetamines, and phencyclidine (Federal Motor Carrier Safety Administration 2021b). Importantly, this DOT guidance specifically allows additional drug testing under the company's own policy, allows the use of nonurine specimens, and contemplates employment consequences different from those described in the official DOT program. Businesses outside of the transportation industry may—and often do—construct drug and alcohol testing programs different from the standard DOT policy.

Of course, non-DOT testing programs are similarly important to the well-being of employee and employer alike. Agencies such as the DOD, the NRC, and the Federal Bureau of Investigation have distinct testing programs, and private corporations often develop their own programs, usually based on a combination of the employer's specific needs and the Drug-Free Federal Workplace Act (Drug-Free Federal Workplace 1988; Drug-Free Workplace Requirements of Federal Contractors 1988). In general, these policies are acceptable as long as they are nondiscriminatory, although they are always susceptible to challenge in court. A guidance document from the Substance Abuse and Mental Health Services Administration (2021) on developing workplace drug and alcohol testing programs specifies the most relevant questions for each program:

1. Who receives testing?
2. When are the drug tests given?
3. Who conducts the testing?
4. What substances are tested for?
5. Who pays for the drug testing?
6. What steps are taken to ensure the accuracy of the drug tests?
7. What are the legal rights of employees who receive a positive test result?

These questions address the fundamental fairness of the testing program and are often interrogated in hearings during a labor dispute. Successful employment drug and alcohol testing programs provide comprehensive and well-thought-out responses to these questions in written materials available to the managers responsible for administering the program and to the employees whose well-being depends on a fair, effective, and nondiscriminatory testing program.

Importantly, different testing methodologies have different pros and cons. Forensic testing is discussed in depth in Chapter 5, but several specific issues essential for employment-related drug testing are described here. The time frame of substance use and the resultant effects are quite important in the employment sphere. Cannabis is the most troublesome, because a positive urine drug screen can occur weeks to months after use, and the presence of $\Delta$-9-tetra-hydrocannabinol (THC) in the employee's body denotes little about the employee's level of intoxication. Similarly, a positive breathalyzer breath alcohol level can occur many hours after the last ingestion of alcohol, necessitating that employers set a reasonable accepted breath alcohol level for the particular workplace. Given the often-fraught nature of labor relations, drug policies must contemplate all possible sources of unfairness toward covered employees and must, of course, protect the dignity of those employees, even when drug testing is mandatory. Sometimes in employment situations, employees may prefer a blood test to a urine test because they need not use the bathroom in a semipublic manner, and the observation of a blood test is naturally less intrusive compared with a urine test. In addition, the cost of a drug or alcohol test is often directly related to its accuracy and vulnerability in a courtroom or hearing room. Businesses must decide on the type and frequency of testing based on their relationship with labor, the relevant rules in place, the costs, and the likelihood and seriousness of legal challenges by employees.

## Safety-Sensitive Positions

The notion of safety-sensitive positions—usually those for which drug and alcohol testing will be required—is central to testing protocols in various industries. A person's right to avoid unreasonable search and seizure under the Fourth Amendment is in tension with the necessity for avoiding harm caused by intoxicated employees. Many testing protocols, and many court cases, turn on exactly how this tension should be resolved. Defining which job positions are safety sensitive can be difficult in all but the most obvious circumstances. Federal agencies have led the way in defining safety-sensitive roles and, for federal employees, consider all those employed in "law enforcement, national security, the protection of life and property, health or safety, or other functions requiring a high degree of public trust" (Drug-Free Workplace 1988) to be in safety-sensitive positions and therefore subject to mandatory drug testing. These agencies include the DOT, the DOD, and the NRC. Federal agencies such as the Federal Aviation Administration (FAA) can also have their own regulations pertaining to certain sensitive positions (14 C.F.R.).

Transportation industries share several core requirements for designating safety-sensitive employees at specific points in their employment. As summarized earlier in this section, employees being hired for safety-sensitive positions must be drug tested in the pre-employment phase and if there is any reasonable cause or suspicion that they are under the influence of alcohol or drugs at work. In addition, tests must be done immediately after an employee is involved in an accident and before the employee is able to return to work following a testing violation (Substance Abuse and Mental Health Services Administration 2020).

In *Skinner v. Railway Labor Executives' Association* (1989), an important U.S. Supreme Court review of this question, the Federal Railroad Administration promulgated a set of rules requiring postaccident drug tests for all employees involved in accidents as well as for employees who broke safety rules. A group of railway trade unions sued, claiming that these rules would constitute an unreasonable search under the Fourth Amendment. The U.S. Supreme Court ruled the testing permissible for employees in safety-sensitive positions, with Justice Anthony Kennedy writing for the majority:

> [T]he Government interest in testing without a showing of individualized suspicion is compelling. Employees subject to the test discharge duties fraught with such risks of injury to others that even a momentary lapse of attention can have disastrous consequences based on the interests of the general public.... While no procedure can identify all impaired employees with ease and perfect accuracy, the Federal Railroad Administration regulations supply an effective means of deterring employees engaged in safety-sensitive tasks from using controlled substances or alcohol in the first place. (*Skinner v. Railway Labor Executives' Association* 1989)

*National Treasury Employees Union v. Von Raab* (1989) is another important case that explored the safety-sensitive nature of various roles. The U.S. Customs Service proposed mandatory drug testing for all of its employees who were directly involved in drug interdiction, who were required to carry firearms, or who handled classified intelligence materials. A suit by the federal employees' union and one of its officials asserted that the testing requirements were so broad as to constitute a violation of the Fourth Amendment. Again, the U.S. Supreme Court agreed with the testing requirement (for those interdicting drugs and carrying weapons), although it did not opine on whether handling classified information should be considered a safety-sensitive position.

# Impaired Professionals (Physicians, Attorneys, and Pilots)

Although many jobs have safety designations, there are also professions where public trust is paramount. Thus, several professions have high-profile and intentionally well-publicized protocols for assuring the public that their members are unimpaired by drugs or alcohol (Ross 2003). Physicians, attorneys, and pilots are examples of professions that have well-defined programs for monitoring drug- or alcohol-induced impairment, likely stemming from the public nature of their work, certain potential safety considerations for some of them, and the well-publicized results of on-the-job failure for each. The following section describes a few of these professions and some of the employment and fitness-for-duty nuances related to impairment and SUDs. Of course, professionals may commit misconduct that has nothing to do with SUDs. This chapter focuses solely on SUD-related impairments and employment and licensing matters that arise as a result of substance use that affects work.

## PHYSICIANS

Substance use, unsurprisingly, is the most common cause of impairment among physicians (Austin et al. 2021; Cottler et al. 2013). Substance use may be a marker for, or an exacerbating factor of, physician burnout and may also correlate with physicians' relatively easy access to medications. Although physicians with SUDs may experience the usually expected damage to their physical and emotional health, relationships, and general well-being, their occupational function may be unaffected or at least unchallenged, given the depth of expertise and overlearned nature of the work. Some specific work-related symptoms of SUDs among physicians are as follows (Ross 2003):

- Late to appointments; increased absences; unknown whereabouts
- Unusual rounding times, either very early or very late
- Increase in patient complaints
- Increased secrecy

- Decrease in quality of care; careless medical decisions
- Incorrect charting or writing of prescriptions
- Decrease in productivity or efficiency
- Increased conflicts with colleagues
- Increased irritability and aggression
- Smell of alcohol; overt intoxication; needle marks

If these symptoms impair physicians' ability to provide treatment, they have an ethical obligation to discontinue practice if they cannot provide safe care and to seek treatment. Similarly, colleagues of an impaired physician have an ethical—and often legal, depending on the state—obligation to protect patients by making reports to licensing boards to determine whether the impaired physician should cease practice. Most states have a medical licensing board that is mandated 1) to provide licensure to physicians and other professionals but also 2) to protect the public from any impaired professionals or professionals whose actions are unsafe or harming patients. Practitioners should be familiar with the requirements in their state regarding reporting of suspected impaired physician colleagues.

Physicians reported to their medical board may immediately lose their license, because an investigation is done to determine whether there is an actual impairment. Most states also have physician-centered groups or physician health plans, often run by the state medical society, that assist physicians who may be impaired. Usually, these physician-focused groups do not report a physician to the state medical board unless the physician is actually impaired in practicing medicine but declines to cease practicing. Although different states have different regulations, usually the treating physician of an impaired (or potentially impaired) physician is not obligated to report the impaired physician (over objection) to authorities. For instance, the New York State statute on contacting the licensing agency, the Office of Professional Medical Conduct (OPMC), reads as follows:

> All licensed health professionals, including physicians, physician assistants, and specialist assistants, are required by state law to report colleagues whom they suspect may be guilty of misconduct. Failure to report suspected instances of misconduct is, in itself, misconduct. If you believe a colleague's actions may constitute misconduct, contact OPMC.... If the colleague is affiliated with a hospital, a report can be made to the facility's professional practices committee, which must then inform OPMC.... *However, this requirement does not apply if compliance would violate a physician-patient relationship.* (New York State Department of Health 2016; emphasis added)

When the treating physician is managing a clinical or forensic case involving an addicted physician whose patient care appears to be substandard, the best option is often physician self-report. However, if the apparently impaired physician declines to self-report, the treating physician should consult with colleagues and an attorney knowledgeable about local statutes to determine the best course. Managing the care or monitoring of a physician impaired by an SUD is an important, albeit often difficult, part of addiction treatment: the goal is to rehabilitate the impaired physician with the expectation of a return to medical practice, so long as safe patient care can be ensured (Candilis et al. 2019). Issues of countertransference and the boundaries between clinician and mandated reporter roles often arise in this type of work, and they are best managed with careful attention and consultations with colleagues and knowledgeable risk management staff.

## ATTORNEYS

Attorneys also have a special, and much scrutinized, place in the public eye, and pressures associated with their roles can be a breeding ground for self-soothing behaviors such as addictive substance use. In a 2016 study of 12,825 licensed and employed attorneys in 19 states, researchers gathered self-reported data about their mental health and alcohol and drug use and found that more than 20% reported "hazardous, harmful, and potentially alcohol dependent drinking" (Krill et al. 2016). Using Alcohol Use Disorders Identification Test (AUDIT) scores, researchers found that attorneys were more likely to have positive screening results for alcohol-related problems if they were male, were relatively young, or had been working in the field for a relatively short duration.

Recent research suggests that perhaps these gender patterns are changing. In a 2021 study of 2,863 California attorneys surveyed randomly, 25% of female attorneys had considered leaving the profession because of mental health concerns, compared with 17% of male attorneys. Researchers found that 60% of female attorneys and 46% of male attorneys met AUDIT-Concise (AUDIT-C) criteria for risky drinking, and 34% of female attorneys and 25% of male attorneys met AUDIT-C criteria for hazardous drinking; both differences were statistically significant (Anker and Krill 2021).

The legal profession has taken steps toward treating addiction as a chronic, relapsing condition rather than as a moral failing, and treatment programs and protective agencies have focused on helping attorneys impaired by addiction to return to work and daily life. As with physicians impaired by addiction, impaired attorneys now have access to supportive programs focused on their particular stressors and professional obligations. Each state has a lawyer assistance program that can be easily accessed for confidential support and service referrals (American Bar Association 2022). These programs have well-codified procedures to assist the attorney and the public.

# PILOTS

The issuance of medical certification for professional and amateur pilots, as well as air traffic control professionals, is governed largely by FAA rules. There are three classes of medical certification: transport pilot (first class), commercial pilot (second class), and private pilot (third class). Pilots fall into a category of personnel who are under special scrutiny, for obvious reasons. They undergo regular physical examinations and performance evaluations, and they may be subject to random drug and alcohol testing related to employment or other factors. When addiction or even substance use in the cockpit comes to light, especially for commercial pilots, public outrage necessitates enforcement of strict rules and a demonstration to the flying public that those rules are followed (e.g., ABC News 2001).

There is no leeway in FAA rules about alcohol or drug use—both commercial and private pilots are proscribed from ingesting any alcohol in the 8 hours before flying (the bottle-to-throttle rule), may not be under the influence of alcohol, may not have a blood alcohol level of 0.04 mg/dL or greater when they fly, and may not fly "while using any drug that affects the person's faculties in any way contrary to safety" (14 C.F.R. Part 91.17 [2011]). Official guidance to pilots from the FAA is even stricter: it suggests waiting 24 hours after the last alcohol use before flying and notes that cold showers, black coffee consumption, and 100% oxygen do not improve sobriety (Federal Aviation Administration 2023). Pilots are also warned to consider the possibility of a hangover even if 8 hours have passed.

In a review of 1,042 aviation accidents between 2013 and 2017 in which the pilot was killed, the National Transportation Safety Board (2020) found urine toxicology results showing substance use in 952 cases (91%). Approximately one-third of the pilots were commercial pilots, with the rest being cargo, private, student, sport, or unlicensed pilots. Of the pilots' postmortem results, 266 (28%) had a positive result for at least one potentially impairing drug, 94 (10%) had a positive result for at least one controlled substance, and 47 (5%) had a positive result for an illicit drug (mostly THC). Sedating histamines, such as diphenhydramine (Benadryl and others), were found in 11.9% of samples, and sedating pain relievers (mostly opioids) were found in 5.3% of samples. Alcohol was not tested for, and the study could not measure actual impairment; no group of pilots without aviation accidents was included for comparison. Most concerning to the National Transportation Safety Board was a disturbing trend: the marked increase during the years 1990–2017 in all categories of potentially sedating drugs found in the body of pilots involved in fatal aviation accidents. As noted in Figure 4–1, findings for benzodiazepines tripled, and those for sedating antihistamines and illicit drugs doubled.

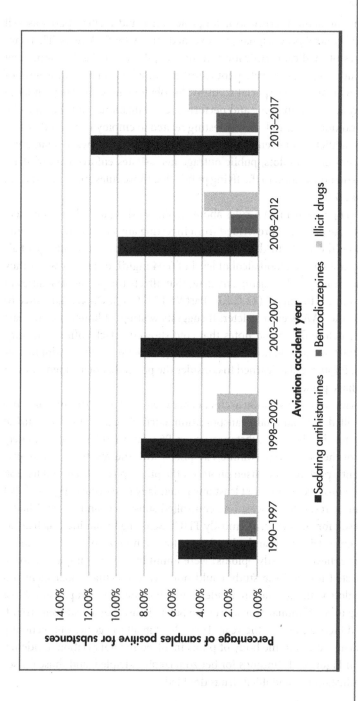

**Figure 4–1. National Transportation Safety Board Safety Research Report, 2013–2017.**

*Source.* National Transportation Safety Board: 2013–2017 Update to Drug Use Trends in Aviation. Safety Research Report, February 13, 2020. Available at: https://www.ntsb.gov/safety/safety-studies/Documents/SS2001.pdf. Accessed December 18, 2021.

In response to data implicating medications in some airplane crashes, the FAA tried to educate all pilots about the regulations that govern pilots' clearance to fly with a medical deficiency (14 C.F.R. § 61.53 [2004]). In addition, the FAA enhanced its educational efforts about over-the-counter medications in a publication intended for all licensed pilots (Federal Aviation Administration 2019).

In addition to the aviation industry's strict rules about on-the-job impairment for pilots, a collaborative program called the Human Intervention Motivational Study (HIMS) is specifically designed to assist commercial pilots find help for addiction and, in some circumstances, return to the cockpit (Human Intervention Motivational Study 2021). As with most such effective programs, HIMS is a collaboration of employees (in this case, pilots), along with company executives and health care professionals. FAA oversight of the program allows for effective integration of treatment protocols with the potential for regaining licensure and returning to work as a pilot. In addition, efforts have been made for pilot peer assistance programs so that pilots can provide mutual support (Pinsky et al. 2020). Individuals identified to have substance use issues can be part of a monitoring program, again similar to those of other professions. Treating psychiatrists working with pilots should be mindful of the public safety risks and their potential duty to disclose such risks, and they should work with their patients in support of self-disclosure when feasible (Pinsky et al. 2020).

# Elite Sport and Athletics

The assessment, monitoring, and treatment of substance use in elite sport—including at the Olympic, National Collegiate Athletic Association (NCAA), and professional levels—has taken on great importance in the United States. Publicity about substance use by elite athletes, the acquiescence of some team personnel, and the downstream consequences of that substance use have led to ongoing public scrutiny. In fact, monitoring these athletes for substance use protects their health and safety and directs those to treatment who may need it. Maintaining a level playing field for all competitors necessitates prohibition of performance-enhancing drugs and agreement on which drugs classify as such. Athletes are role models for young people, and society has a legitimate interest in providing healthy and life-affirming examples. Finally, because advertisers and fans will not want to be associated with a drug-infested industry, the business necessities of modern sport require effective and transparent policies.

Some athletes use anabolic androgenic steroids, human growth hormone, and numerous other prescription medications and illicit substances to improve their abilities and, in essence, cheat their way to better performance. The biological risks of anabolic androgenic steroid use include hormonal abnormalities, musculoskeletal damage, and profound mood alterations, among others. In addition, these substances are prime examples of the damage that illicit drug use by athletes can inflict: the majority of anabolic androgenic steroid users are not elite athletes but young people emulating their heroes, either for athletic performance or merely for physical appearance (U.S. Food and Drug Administration 2017). This copycat use of anabolic androgenic steroids causes immeasurable damage to younger users, who often double, triple, or quadruple the dosages used by their heroes. One study reported that 5.9% of middle school and high school students have used anabolic androgenic steroids at least once (Eisenberg et al. 2012).

In some circumstances, the elite athlete may have a legitimate medical need for a banned substance. For instance, an Olympic athlete with asthma may be treated with albuterol (Ventolin and others), which is on the banned list for Olympic athletes, or a professional baseball player may be prescribed amphetamine/dextroamphetamine (Adderall). Sport officials can issue a therapeutic use exemption (TUE), giving the athlete permission to use a necessary medication even if it is on the banned list for the sport. These TUEs must be granted judiciously to permit needed medical treatment while still preserving a fair competitive balance for all athletes on the field. For instance, although the NCAA does not consider TUEs for cannabinoids, it will consider exemptions for athletes who are prescribed anabolic androgenic steroids, stimulants, $\beta$-blockers, diuretic medications, $\beta_2$ agonists, peptide hormones, and in specific situations, narcotic medications (National Collegiate Athletic Association 2021). The athlete must demonstrate to an NCAA medical panel that their physician has recommended the banned medication and that no alternative medication exists; the athlete then must maintain on-campus medical records.

Although some substances (e.g., amphetamines) occupy the middle ground between performance-enhancing use and addiction, pure addiction occurs in the population of elite athletes who, despite their superlative athletic skills, remain vulnerable to the peer pressure, self-medication, trauma response, and genetic loading that drive addiction for the rest of the population. Sports injuries treated with opioid narcotics may generate an addictive response, leaving the athlete susceptible to a narcotic addiction long after the injury has healed. Although use of stimulants such as cocaine or sedatives such as heroin is not consistent with stellar athletic performance, addicted athletes may be able to hide their addiction for substantial periods of time, absent regular, random drug testing.

Alcohol and cannabis, although legal for use by adults in many jurisdictions, present substantial problems for elite athletes and their employers. Although alcohol is legal and relatively unstigmatized, alcohol use by athletes has surely caused enormous losses in performance as well as the usual relationship, mental health, and educational deficits that most alcohol users experience.

Given the increasing decriminalization of cannabis, athletes must now judge the substance's effect on their functioning, absent any legal or occupational bar to its use. Cannabis is discussed further in the next section.

# Cannabis: A Special Case

Cannabis is the most commonly used drug by the workforce (Quest Diagnostics 2021). Over the last 20 years, the status of cannabis has morphed from being bundled with other so-called drugs of abuse into a separate and less-stigmatized category, and today cannabis use in some jurisdictions may not be used to deny or terminate employment (Quest Diagnostics 2021). As of February 2022, however, cannabis remained classified as a Schedule I substance, one of many "drugs with no currently accepted medical use and a high potential for abuse" (Drug Enforcement Administration 2024). This remaining federal hard line against cannabis has, quite naturally, sown confusion among stakeholders affected by state laws that permit medical or recreational cannabis use, remove criminal penalties, and, in some cases, protect employees from adverse job actions solely for their use of cannabis.

As of 2022, 37 states and the District of Columbia allow medicinal cannabis, and 18 states and the District of Columbia have legalized recreational cannabis (National Conference of State Legislatures 2022). Therefore, employers and employees face myriad legal, business, and practical challenges. Most important are the numerous thorny ethical and public policy questions that face our nation given this evolving landscape, especially the tension between the public policy good and the individual harm that many see associated with marijuana decriminalization and legalization, and the constraints on civil liberties implied in the prohibition of a widely used and admired substance.

Employees question whether medicinal marijuana prescribed (or at least recommended) by a licensed physician will be exempted from usual drug testing protocols. Employers must manage a rapidly changing set of legal obligations concerning safety-sensitive positions, potential ADA lawsuits, confidentiality, and the notoriously long-lasting THC molecule in drug tests. Relatively sparse data exist on workplace accidents or lost productivity associated with cannabis, the effects of instituting drug testing programs for cannabis, and the cost/benefit ratios of these testing and treatment programs.

Most importantly, employers must grapple with the rapidly changing case law and societal perception regarding cannabis, along with the discordance between federal law and state laws regarding its legalization. Only data-based and collaborative discussions about the issue will promote the most effective and legally defensible policies regarding cannabis in the workplace.

From an employment regulatory and legal standpoint, the tide may be shifting to the benefit of cannabis-using employees, given the evolving views toward legalizing cannabis use. Twenty U.S. states now protect the employment rights of cannabis users, to varying degrees. These protections span legislation that requires that a positive test itself cannot, under the law, mean that an employee is actually impaired, enforces some protections for the employee with a valid medical marijuana card, or simply bars any discrimination against employees who have a positive test for, or use, cannabis of any sort (California NORML 2021). New York City specifically bans preemployment drug testing, but the statute exempts a long list of safety-sensitive (and politically sensitive) positions, such as police officers and positions requiring construction safety training, involving the care of children or medical patients, operating under federal contracts or grants, requiring testing as part of a collective bargaining agreement, or involving DOT-required testing (Chodoff et al. 2019). Nevada (Nevada Assembly 2019) and New Jersey (Diana and Riccobono 2021) similarly prohibit denying employment solely on the basis of a preemployment drug test positive for THC, although both states similarly exempt employers with safety-sensitive positions from following this rule.

Trial and appeal judges must apply the relevant law to the actual cases that come into their courtrooms. At the same time, they must ensure that employers obey a rapidly changing set of legal obligations concerning safety-sensitive positions, potential ADA-based lawsuits, and confidentiality.

In *Ross v. RagingWire Telecommunications* (2008), the California Supreme Court found that employers need not accommodate an employee's medicinal cannabis use irrespective of the Compassionate Use Act (1996), which provides that people using cannabis under the care of a physician are not subject to criminal prosecution by the state. The court commented that the Compassionate Use Act does not grant cannabis the same status as legal prescription drugs, and it noted that cannabis remains illegal under federal law and therefore cannot be "completely legalize[d] for medical purposes" (*Ross v. RagingWire Telecommunications* 2008). This case showed typical judicial reasoning of the time, which differentiated medical cannabis from FDA-approved medication, and granted precedence to federal law over state law.

By contrast, in the Arizona case *Whitmire v. Wal-Mart Stores Inc.* (2019), a medical-cannabis-using employee prevailed against her employer. Walmart was found to have discriminated against Carol Whitmire, who had a valid Arizona medical cannabis card for treatment of sleep problems. After a minor workplace injury, Whitmire was seen in a medical clinic and given a urine drug screen, which revealed a THC level greater than 1,000 ng/cc. Walmart alleged that Whitmire's "positive drug test result for marijuana indicated that she was impaired by marijuana during her shift that same day" (*Whitmire v. Wal-Mart Stores Inc.* 2019).

Whitmire was eventually terminated on the basis of the positive drug test result. She filed suit, alleging that she had been discriminated against in violation of state antidiscrimination laws. The court agreed, reasoning that "without any evidence that Plaintiff used, possessed, or was impaired by marijuana at work,…it is clear that Defendant discriminated against Plaintiff…by suspending and then terminating Plaintiff solely based on her positive drug test" (*Whitmire v. Wal-Mart Stores Inc.* 2019). The relatively high level of THC went unaddressed as a potential contributor to workplace impairment.

The evolving federal and state law postures toward workplace-related cannabis matters, combined with the scattershot case law on the subject, necessitate management by the clinicians and labor attorneys who respond to cannabis use and testing in the workplace. It has been recommended that workplace cannabis policy be carefully designed to include a clear mission and set of expectations, a defensible testing protocol, offers of clinical assistance to employees who need it, defined consequences for positive THC test results, and a policy that allows eligible employees to return to work (Hazle et al. 2020). Furthermore, workplace assessments should examine as separate issues use and impairment due to that use. This type of intentional workplace cannabis focus, designed with the collaborative effort of addiction professionals, human resources specialists, and labor attorneys, will produce the most workable cannabis policy and evaluation practices for all parties involved.

# Fitness-for-Duty Evaluations and Independent Medical Examinations for Disability

Forensic (i.e., nonclinical) psychiatric assessments are often requested for the substance-using employee who wants to return or decline to return to work or is considered "unfit" to return to work. These examinations and their reports should include information from collateral informants, any relevant medical records, and forensic protocol substance testing.

A psychiatric fitness-for-duty evaluation is usually requested by the employer to get a concrete response as to whether the psychiatrically ill or substance-using employee is fit for duty. The not-so-subtle subtext is the employer's desire to make certain that no harm comes to the impaired employee, other employees, customers, or the business itself. The forensic examiner must provide a well-substantiated opinion regarding the employee's fitness to return to work. Sometimes this is obvious, such as in the case of an individual with severe alcohol use disorder who drinks before driving a school bus. More often, the employer relies on the examiner's evaluation as to the correct diagnosis, disease course and likely prognosis, an understanding of the job obligations, any relevant contract issues, and opinion in a report that will be defensible under cross-examination later. The forensic report should include a directed mental status examination, a review of the available medical documents, discussions with collateral informants, and conversations with the treating clinicians. It is important 1) to clarify who will have access to the information obtained and the report and 2) to ensure that the employee is notified of any limits of confidentiality.

An independent medical examination (IME) in the employment context, which can encompass disability and fitness-for-duty evaluation (Anker and Krill 2021), necessitates a complete evaluation of the employee or subject, including all of the elements involved in an IME. The IME report should directly answer the employer's specific questions so that the best possible psychiatric outcome occurs. Typical questions for a substance-related IME are as follows:

1. Does the patient have the capacity to return to their previous position?
2. Will the patient experience relapse if they return to their previous position?
3. Are there any "reasonable accommodations" that would allow the patient to return to their previous position?
4. Are there other job positions that would protect the patient's sobriety?

These are difficult questions, and complete answers may be impossible. The American Academy of Psychiatry and the Law has issued a practice resource for evaluations in employment contexts that is a very useful compendium of information, including numerous caveats and clinical points for consideration (Anker and Krill 2021). Of course, no assessor can determine what will happen in the future, but it is possible to make reasonable prognoses based on the employee's symptom picture, diagnosis, and treatment plan. The reasonable accommodations question in the context of SUDs is usually answered by defining whether needed work changes to allow for attendance at treatment or recommended work changes would support the employee's sobriety and success in the workplace.

# Conclusions

In the occupational setting, the emergence of SUDs often signals the need for the individual to access treatment. In some work contexts, an employee who has an SUD or a positive test result for substance use will require monitoring, and the employee's ongoing ability to function in the workplace can depend on these interventions. In considering occupational and employment issues involving SUDs, the legal and regulatory landscape can be complex and involves a balance between the rights of individuals and their employers. Legal protections exist for both.

# Key Points

- Most people with substance use disorders (SUDs) are gainfully employed.
- People with SUDs are typically protected—in very specific circumstances—by the Americans With Disabilities Act.
- High-profile job positions—like pilot or physician—often have specific protocols for management of SUDs before a return to work.
- The extra scrutiny of elite athletes must translate into transparent and fair workplace programs that address both performance-enhancing drugs and addictive drugs.
- Because they may determine an examinee's ability to remain employed, independent medical examination reports and those written to help assess fitness for duty must be accurate, fair, and as well documented as possible.

# References

ABC News: Pilot fired for failing alcohol breath tests. January 22, 2001. Available at: https://abcnews.go.com/US/story?id=94332andpage=1. Accessed November 2, 2023.

American Academy of Psychiatry and the Law: Ethics Guidelines for the Practice of Forensic Psychiatry. Washington, DC, U.S. Department of Transportation, May 2005. Available at: https://www.aapl.org/ethics.htm. Accessed January 27, 2022.

American Bar Association: Directory of Lawyer Assistance Programs. Available at: https://www.americanbar.org/groups/lawyer_assistance/resources/lap_ programs_by_state/. Accessed February 4, 2022.

Americans With Disabilities Act of 1990 (P.L. 101–336), 104 Stat. 328 (codified as amended at 42 U.S.C. §§ 12101–12213 [2008])

Anfang SA, Gold LH, Meyer DJ: AAPL practice resource for the forensic evaluation of psychiatric disability. J Am Acad Psychiatry Law 46(1):102, 2018 29618542

Anker J, Krill PR: Stress, drink, leave: an examination of gender-specific risk factors for mental health problems and attrition among licensed attorneys. PLoS One 16(5):e020563, 2021 33979350

Austin EE, Do V, Nullwala R, et al: Systematic review of the factors and the key indicators that identify doctors at risk of complaints, malpractice claims or impaired performance. BMJ Open 11(8):e050377, 2021 34429317

California NORML: State and city laws protecting marijuana users' employment rights. 2021. Available at: https://www.canorml.org/employment/state-laws-protecting-medical-marijuana-patients-employment-rights/. Accessed February 27, 2021.

Candilis PJ, Kim DT, Sulmasy LS, et al: Physician impairment and rehabilitation: reintegration into medical practice while ensuring patient safety: a position paper from the American College of Physicians. Ann Intern Med 170(12):871–879, 2019 31158847

Chodoff LL, Humma TL, Peerce MJ, et al: New York City adopts law prohibiting pre-employment testing for marijuana. National Law Review, May 10, 2019. Available at: https://www.natlawreview.com/article/new-york-city-adopts-law-prohibiting-pre-employment-testing-marijuana. Accessed November 5, 2023.

Christopher PP, Arikan R, Pinals DA, et al: Evaluating psychiatric disability: differences by forensic expertise. J Am Acad Psychiatry Law 39(2):183–188, 2011 21653261

Colby v Union Security Insurance Co., 705 F.3d 58 (1st Cir. 2013)

Compassionate Use Act of 1996, Calf. Health and Saf. Code § 11362.5

Contract With America Advancement Act of 1996, H.R. 3136, 104th Cong.

Cottler LB, Ajinkya S, Merlo LJ, et al: Lifetime psychiatric and substance use disorders among impaired physicians in a physician's health program: comparison to a general treatment population. J Addict Med 7(2):108–112, 2013 23412081

Diana M, Riccobono MJ: Recreational marijuana is legal in New Jersey: what employers need to know. National Law Review, February 23, 2021. Available at: https://www.natlawreview.com/article/recreational-marijuana-legal-new-jersey-what-employers-need-to-know. Accessed November 5, 2023.

Drug-Free Federal Workplace, Executive Order No.12564, 3 C.F.R. 224 (1988)

Drug-Free Workplace Requirements of Federal Contractors of 1988 (P.L. 100–690), 41 U.S.C. § 701, §§ 5152–5158, 102 Stat. 4304

Eisenberg ME, Wall M, Neumark-Sztainer D: Muscle-enhancing behaviors among adolescent girls and boys. Pediatrics 130(6):1019–1026, 2012 23166333

Federal Aviation Administration: What over-the-counter (OTC) medications can I take and still be safe to fly? November 11, 2019. Available at: https://www.faa.gov/sites/faa.gov/files/licenses_certificates/medical_certification/medications/OTCMedicationsforPilots.pdf. Accessed November 2, 2023.

Federal Aviation Administration: Alcohol and flying: a deadly combination. Available at: https://www.faa.gov/pilots/safety/pilotsafetybrochures/media/alcohol.pdf. Accessed November 2, 2023.

Federal Motor Carrier Safety Administration: Drug and Alcohol Testing Program. Washington, DC, U.S. Department of Transportation. Available at: https://www.fmcsa.dot.gov/regulations/drug-alcohol-testing-program. Accessed December 9, 2021a.

Federal Motor Carrier Safety Administration: Which Substances Are Tested? What CDL Drivers Need to Know. Washington, DC, U.S. Department of Transportation. Available at: https://www.fmcsa.dot.gov/regulations/drug-alcohol-testing/which-substances-are-tested. Accessed July 22, 2021b.

Hazle MC, Hill KP, Westreich LM: Workplace cannabis policies: a moving target. Cannabis Cannabinoid Res 7(1):16–23, 2020 33998870

Human Intervention Motivational Study: What is HIMS? Available at: https://himsprogram.com/about-hims. Accessed December 19, 2021.

Krill PR, Johnson R, Albert L: The prevalence of substance use and other mental health concerns among American attorneys. J Addict Med 10(1):46–52, 2016 26825268

National Collegiate Athletic Association: Medical exceptions procedures. June 29, 2021. Available at: https://www.ncaa.org/sport-science-institute/medical-exceptions-procedures. Accessed on December 19, 2021.

National Conference of State Legislatures: State medical cannabis laws. 2022. Available at: https://www.ncsl.org/research/health/state-medical-marijuana-laws.aspx. Accessed June 2, 2022.

National Safety Council: Substance use disorder by occupation. 2020. Available at: https://www.nsc.org/getmedia/9dc908e1–041a-41c5-a607-c4cef2390973/ substance-use-disorders-by-occupation.pdf. Accessed November 5, 2020.

National Transportation Safety Board: Safety Research Report: 2013–2017 Update to Drug Use Trends in Aviation (NTSB/SS-20/01). 2020. Available at: https:// www.ntsb.gov/safety/safety-studies/Documents/SS2001.pdf. Accessed November 2, 2023.

National Treasury Employees Union v Von Raab, 489 U.S. 656 (1989)

Nevada Assembly, Bill No. 132, 80th Legislative Session (2019)

New York State Department of Health: Understanding New York's Medical Conduct Program: physician discipline. March 2016. Available at: https:// www.health.ny.gov/publications/1445. Accessed December 18, 2021.

Office of Federal Contractor Compliance Programs: ADA Amendments Act of 2008 Frequently Asked Questions. Washington, DC, U.S. Department of Labor, 2009. Available at: https://www.dol.gov/agencies/ofccp/faqs/americans-with-disabilities-act-amendments. Accessed November 2, 2023.

Omnibus Transportation Employee Testing Act of 1991 (P.L. 102–143), 105 Stat. 917 (codified as amended in scattered sections of 49 U.S.C.)

Pinsky HM, Guina J, Berry M, et al: Psychiatry and fitness to fly after Germanwings. J Am Acad Psychiatry Law 48(1):65–76, 2020 31753966

Quest Diagnostics: Marijuana workplace drug test positivity continues double-digit increases to keep overall drug positivity rates at historically high levels. May 26, 2021. Available at: https://www.prnewswire.com/news-releases/marijuana-workforce-drug-test-positivity-continues-double-digit-increases-to-keep-overall-drug-positivity-rates-at-historically-high-levels-finds-latest-quest-diagnostics-drug-testing-index-analysis-301299762.html. Accessed February 5, 2022.

Rondinelli RD: Guides to the Evaluation of Permanent Impairment, 6th Edition. Chicago, IL, American Medical Association, 2008, p 611

Ross S: Identifying an impaired physician. Virtual Mentor 5(12):420–422, 2003 23267571

Ross v RagingWire Telecommunications, 174 P.3d 200 (Cal. 2008)

Shaffer v Preston Memorial Hospital, 107 F.3d. 274 (4th Cir. 1997)

Skinner v Railway Labor Executives' Association, 489 U.S. 602 (1989)

Social Security Administration: Disability evaluation under Social Security. 2001. Available at: https://www.ssa.gov/disability/professionals/bluebook/. Accessed November 5, 2023.

Social Security Administration: Guide for Organizational Representative Payees. 2021. Available at: https://www.ssa.gov/payee/NewGuide/toc.htm. Accessed June 12, 2024.

Substance Abuse and Mental Health Services Administration: Considerations for Safety- and Security-Sensitive Industries. Rockville, MD, Substance Abuse and Mental Health Administration. Available at: https://www.samhsa.gov/workplace/legal/ federal-laws/safety-security-sensitive. Accessed June 28, 2020.

Substance Abuse and Mental Health Services Administration: Drug Testing Resources. Rockville, MD, Substance Abuse and Mental Health Services Administration. Available at: https://www.samhsa.gov/workplace/resources/drug-testing. Accessed October 14, 2021.

U.S. Commission on Civil Rights: Sharing the Dream: Is the ADA Accommodating All? n.d. Available at: https://www.usccr.gov/files/pubs/ada/ch4.htm. Accessed May 4, 2024.

U.S. Department of Transportation: Federal Drug and Alcohol Testing Regulations (FM-SCA-E-06–003). September 2016. Available at: https://www.fmcsa.dot.gov/sites/fmcsa.dot.gov/files/docs/Drug%20and%20Alcohol%20Brochure%20for%20Drivers.pdf. Accessed November 1, 2023.

U.S. Drug Enforcement Administration: Drug Scheduling. n.d. Available at: https://www.dea.gov/drug-information/drug-scheduling. Accessed May 4, 2024.

U.S. Food and Drug Administration: Teens and steroids: a dangerous combo. December 4, 2017. Available at: https://www.consumermedsafety.org/safety-articles/teens-and-steroids-a-dangerous-combo#:~:text=Watch%20for%20signs%20of%20steroid,and%20Drug%20Administration%20(FDA). Accessed November 2, 2023.

Waid D, Barber SL: Follow-up of former drug addict and alcoholic beneficiaries. Research and Statistics Note No 2001–02, October 2001. Available at: www.ssa.gov/policy/docs/rsnotes/rsn2001–02.html. Accessed February 5, 2022.

Westreich LM: Addiction and the Americans With Disabilities Act. J Am Acad Psychiatry Law 30(3):355–363, 2002 12380414

Whitmire v Wal-Mart Stores Inc., 359 F. Supp. 3d 761 (D. Ariz. 2019)

# CHAPTER 5

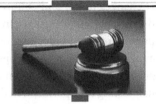

# DRUG AND ALCOHOL TESTING IN THE LEGAL SPHERE

## Introduction

Forensic drug and alcohol testing can be broadly defined as any specimen testing conducted for legal or regulatory decision-making, separate and apart from treatment purposes. Forensic testing is done with the understanding that the results might be scrutinized and even challenged in a courtroom or other legal arenas. Thus, testing is conducted with procedures in place to minimize the possibility of test inaccuracy, including evasion and tampering. These procedures include a chain-of-custody protocol to guarantee the provenance of the sample, both screening and more sophisticated confirmatory laboratory testing, and a split-sample protocol to allow for a confirmation test based on the laboratory protocol in case the first test result is contested. Although the clini-

The authors thank J. D. Matheus, M.A., for his review of this chapter.

cian treating an individual with a positive result can simply ask the patient for another test or collect other clinical information to confirm or negate the result, these remedies are often unavailable in the legal realm. Because the testee's job, future employability, personal reputation, or even liberty may rely on the results of a drug or alcohol test, that test must be accurate, the test must be consented to by the testee or mandated through a legally authorized process (e.g., court order), and the test result must be delivered in a timely manner.

Overall, rates of positive forensic drug test results tend to track the rates in clinical testing and reflect changes in law and culture more generally. For instance, when cannabis is decriminalized or legalized in a particular jurisdiction, any increased use in the population would result in increased positive rates for both clinical tests and forensic tests. One major supplier of forensic drug and alcohol tests, Quest Diagnostics, monitors changes in positivity rates in the forensic (mostly occupational) testing they perform. In their sample of more than 7 million occupational drug tests, rates of positive tests in the U.S. workforce have generally decreased over the past 5 years except for results for cannabis, which increased from 3.1% of general workforce positive test results in 2019 to 3.6% in 2020 (Quest Diagnostics 2021). There was a similar increase in positive cannabis test results in postaccident testing, with a jump from 2.4% in 2012 to 6.4% in 2020. Regarding attempts to evade occupational drug tests (which Quest designates as nonnegative tests), Quest found in 2020 that 0.009% of their tests had an acid-base abnormality indicating tampering, 0.012% of the samples had been substituted for a fluid not obtained from the testee, and 0.17% were ruled invalid for other reasons. Between 2016 and 2020, positive drug test rates (including marijuana) rose from 4.7% to 6.2%; in the construction industry, positive drug test rates remained stable at 4.0% in 2016 and 4.1% in 2020.

## FORENSIC DILEMMA

A 29-year-old woman who works filling boxes at a large e-commerce retail store is called in for a random urine drug screen (UDS). She is given a urine container and directed to a private bathroom. After 10 minutes, she emerges and tells the collector that she has never been able to urinate while "under pressure" and asks to be allowed to return to work. Although the employee complies with the tester's request that she try for a little longer, she emerges from the bathroom without the requisite urine after 10 additional minutes. At that point, the collector directs her to drink three 12-oz bottles of water, which she does. After waiting 30 minutes, the employee produces urine with a specific gravity of 1.0020, too dilute for the testing protocol.

Consider the following:

1. How should the tester respond to the employee's representation that she is unable to produce urine for the test?

2. How should the tester respond to the employee's production of dilute urine?

   Although the employee eventually produces a nondilute specimen, 10 days later the result is positive for benzoylecgonine—a metabolite of cocaine. The employee insists that this is impossible because she has never used cocaine in her life, and she now recalls that the tester put "a white powder" into her urine sample, which she (the employee) thinks might have been cocaine.

3. What are the next steps?
4. Can the employee's accusation be correct?

   The first positive result was confirmed in a second test because the entire urine sample was split into A and B samples, as is usually done in forensic drug and alcohol testing. However, the employee continues to assert that she has never used cocaine, and the case eventually goes before a due process hearing with a representative each from the employer and the employee's union. After the hearing, the employee is required to 1) attend treatment arranged by the company's employee assistance program and 2) undergo random drug testing.

5. What are possible explanations for this result? What are the implications if any of these explanations are accurate?
6. Should ongoing testing of this employee include other drugs of abuse?
7. Are there any clinical implications of this positive drug test result?

It is common for testees to find it difficult to produce a required urine sample, even when production is not directly observed. This difficulty should be addressed compassionately with encouragement, and eventually 40 oz of water should be provided to help with urine production. If the testee is unable to produce urine after 3 hours, their condition can be defined as paruresis or shy bladder (Knowles and Skues 2016; Swotinsky 2015). Although paruresis is usually considered an anxiety-related condition, a clinical evaluation by a urologist is indicated; in some U.S. Department of Transportation (DOT) protocols, this can exempt the employee from further urine testing (Federal Motor Carrier Safety Administration 2015). If the employee delivers too-dilute urine by the testing program criteria, options are to wait for another specimen or to excuse the testee until the next day. (These options should be clearly spelled out in the testing protocol.)

If the testee disputes a positive confirmation result, the B sample should be tested to rule out any laboratory error. If the B sample is positive for the same substance and the testee wishes to continue disputing the result, a hearing or trial usually is held with experts for both the testee and the laboratory testifying about the results. (The specifics on the hearing depend on whether a union represents the employee and on employment law in the relevant jurisdiction.) A DNA test of skin cells found in the urine and the testee's own DNA can further connect the urine sample to the testee. Cocaine introduced into a urine container would be unmetabolized and therefore would not show a benzoylecgonine result: the result would simply be "cocaine." It is possible for a testee to use a banned substance inadvertently through a contaminated drug or unknowing ingestion: most forensic drug policies have a policy of terminal responsibility, in which the testee is responsible for whatever is in their body. Given the substantial risk of cross-addiction, clinical considerations militate for broad testing in any person who has a positive drug test. However, labor unions and employee representatives often prevent this type of suspicionless drug testing, arguing that it is an unreasonable intrusion on the employee. If a forensic drug test result is positive, this can push the testee toward receiving needed clinical assistance, in addition to facing any legal implications that result.

## Collection and Specimen Handling Protocols

The collection and handling of forensic drug and alcohol specimens is extremely important to test integrity. These tests are often challenged in court, so the beginning steps in the analysis must be beyond reproach—even minor deviations from the protocol can result in legal roadblocks to any actual use of the results. First, the testing protocol must be clear and demonstrably fair to the party being tested. For instance, preemployment drug testing, along with the consequences of a positive test result, must be clearly designated. In many, although not all, jurisdictions, a preemployment drug test (but not alcohol) is not considered a medical test under the Americans With Disabilities Act and may therefore be used to deny employment to an applicant (Americans With Disabilities Act National Network 2022). Forensic tests, which are random, must be truly and demonstrably random to counter any allegation of discrimination or unfairness in the testing regimen. Postaccident or for-cause testing should be done only after an event has occurred that is clearly defined in the drug testing protocol (Swotinsky 2015). Prescheduled or periodic forensic testing, although usually of little utility, must be clearly defined in the testing protocol.

Once a test has been scheduled, collection procedures for the specimen are the next step that must be carefully delineated and executed. The specimen donor's identity must be established and verified, usually with government- or employer-issued photo identification. Guidelines specifically warn against accepting any nonphoto identification or any identification from a coworker or another donor (Substance Abuse and Mental Health Services Administration 2014). Testers must maintain strict security at the testing site, use tamper-proof specimen containers and seals, and deploy any mandated on-site checks such as temperature strips, specific gravity readings, or adulterant checks. For urine samples, the testing protocol must clearly define whether an observer collection is necessary: observers are always of the same gender as the donor, but these protocols will likely require updating as issues related to transgender employees begin to be recognized. Although ensuring the source of blood samples, hair samples, and saliva samples is less cumbersome than it is for urine samples, collectors must stay vigilant for any anomalies in the process because any test may be challenged if there is even the appearance of carelessness.

Chain-of-custody forms (CCFs), both paper and electronic, are designed to establish that the sample came from the donor, was transported in a timely manner to the laboratory, and was evaluated and then reported in a manner satisfactory to any observer. (Federal CCFs are used in DOT testing and are the gold standard, but non-DOT forensic testers may construct their own forms.) Failure by the donor, collector, transporter, or laboratory technician to sign and date the CCF can become a serious problem in proving the veracity of the test. Although minor errors can sometime be corrected, the CCF can have five fatal flaws that render the sample unusable in all circumstances, as noted in Table 5–1 (U.S. Department of Transportation 2017).

After the CCF is completed properly, the specimen must be packaged and transported in a manner precisely laid out in the particular testing policy. Even the perception of careless handling, in the absence of any actual deviation from the rules, can lead to a successful appeal of a positive drug test result. In one celebrated case, the collector appropriately packaged and transported the sample but kept it in his personal refrigerator for 48 hours before shipping it. An oversight panel negated the eventual positive results, although it acknowledged that the collector did not breach the written protocol in any way (Belson and Schmidt 2012).

# Laboratory Analysis

Many creative nonlaboratory devices are often used in criminal and civil forensic matters to monitor individuals who must remain abstinent from drugs, alcohol, or both. Internet-connected breathalyzers (e.g., Soberlink) can be programmed to remind the user to take a breathalyzer test several times per day. These test results are then reported to whomever the user has designated, often an attorney, an ex-spouse, or a clinical monitor. Difficulties with these systems often relate to problems with internet connectivity, occasional failure of the device itself, and poor planning as to when the tests should be done. Addiction experts, rather than attorneys or parties to a particular legal or employment matter at hand, are best situated to recommend a breathalyzer testing regimen. Similarly, breathalyzer systems connected to the car's ignition can prevent a person with elevated breath alcohol from operating a motor vehicle. Sweat-patch testing for drugs is available but can be monitored only after the sweat patch has been removed.

**Table 5–1.**   Potential issues that can invalidate drug testing

1. No form with the sample

2. No specimen included with the form

3. No printed collector name and signature

4. Two separate collections for one chain-of-custody form

5. Specimen and chain-of-custody form identification numbers do not match

# OVERVIEW OF TESTING AND TEST RESULTS ACROSS SPECIMENS

Testees often want to know how long a particular substance will be detectable in their body after the last use. As noted earlier in this chapter, the answer depends on many variables: the particular substance, the tissue being tested, the level of detection (LOD) set by the laboratory, the screening and confirmation methods used, and the physiological characteristics of the testee. Individuals being tested sometimes assume that all drug tests are the same and reassure themselves by taking an over-the-counter urine dipstick test before showing up for a more sophisticated workplace test the next day, with disastrous results. Generally speaking, breath, blood, and oral fluids contain substances for the shortest period of time, urine and sweat for a moderate amount of time, and hair for the longest time (Swotinsky 2015).

The chart of UDS detection times in Table 5–2 should be used only as a general guideline rather than a standard for testees concerned about their results. This section provides more information about testing across laboratory procedures and substance types.

# TYPES OF TOXICOLOGY TESTING

Laboratory analyses of forensic drug and alcohol tests are arranged for maximum possible accuracy and reproducibility. Because these results will likely be subjected to legal scrutiny, the testing procedures and documentation of those procedures must be well considered and up to state-of-the-art specifications for drug and alcohol testing. Although point-of-contact tests such as urine dipstick and saliva tests are perfectly reasonable as clinical tools and can yield benefit for their immediate results, they are rarely sufficiently structured to be permissible, or at least convincing, in a legal venue. Rather, documented screening and confirmation tests done in a laboratory credentialed by the National Laboratory Certification Program (RTI International 2021) by appropriately certified personnel are the gold standard in any legal setting.

**Table 5–2.**    Approximate detectability of drugs and alcohol in urine
drug screens

| Drug | Detection time |
|---|---|
| Alcohol | 7–12 hours |
| Amphetamine | 2–4 days |
| Benzodiazepines | |
|    Short acting | 3 days |
|    Long acting | 3 weeks |
| Chlorodehydromethyltestosterone (Turinabol) | 18 months |
| Cocaine metabolite (benzoylecgonine) | 2–4 days |
| Marijuana (cannabinoids) | |
|    Single use | 3 days |
|    Daily use | 10–15 days |
|    Heavy, long-term use | ≥30 days |
| Opioids | |
|    Morphine | 2–3 days |
|    Hydrocodone | 24 hours |
|    Heroin metabolite 6-monoacetylmorphine | <1 day |
|    Oxycodone | 3 days |
| Phencyclidine | 8 days |
| Stanozolol (Winstrol) | 4 months |
| Testosterone suspension | 7 days |

*Source.*    Adapted from DieOff.org 2019; Mayo Clinic Laboratories 2021; Swotinsky 2015.

Screening tests, usually semiquantitative immunoassay tests, are often the first pass at a specimen because they are relatively inexpensive and provide quick results, thereby allowing the laboratory to focus on any nonnegative test results with more sophisticated analysis. The initial screening immunoassay tests have varying levels of cross-reactivity with molecules similar to the drug being tested for, and the definition of a positive screening test result is set by the laboratory (which designates a particular LOD). The LOD, which may vary in different laboratories or testing regimens, often explains why the exact same sample may be listed as positive in one laboratory but negative in another. For instance, a commonly used forensic screening LOD for Δ-9-tetrahydrocannabinol (THC) is 50 ng/mL, with 15 ng/mL being used as the confirmatory cutoff (Kulig 2017; Onondaga County Medical Examiner 2021).

Once a screening test shows a positive result, confirmatory testing begins. As should be expected, these confirmatory tests are more accurate, take longer to perform, and are more expensive. Laboratories often use gas chromatography and mass spectroscopy (GC/MS) techniques to separate the specific molecule being tested for and compare it to chemical analogs (Sparkman et al. 2011).

As noted, various body tissues and fluids can be subjected to forensic drug and alcohol testing. Urine is most commonly used because it is noninvasive to collect (at least physically) and has the advantage of the kidneys' concentrating effects on various substances. Blood can also be tested for drugs and alcohol, and breath testing for alcohol is straightforward and simple to administer. Both blood and breath testing are helpful because they are difficult to evade. Hair has the advantage of aggregating substances over the length of time that the hair shaft grows, and reliable testing can often be done that looks back 90 days or more. Importantly, however, hair often does not reveal recent use. Point-of-contact saliva and fingernail tests are increasingly used in both clinical and forensic environments.

## ALCOHOL USE BIOMARKERS

Alcohol use confirmatory tests that can pass muster in forensic-level analyses include tests of the alcohol metabolites ethyl glucuronide and ethyl sulfate. These metabolites can last as long as 80 hours in the urine, as opposed to the much shorter time that alcohol itself can be found in the urine or via breathalyzer or blood tests (Jatlow et al. 2014). Another highly specific alcohol biomarker, phosphatidyl ethanol, is formed from phosphatidylcholine by the enzyme phospholipase D in the presence of ethanol and can be detected for up to 12 days after alcohol ingestion (Andresen-Streichert et al. 2018). Phosphatidyl ethanol quantitative levels are also found to correlate with the severity of alcohol use.

## TESTING FOR PERFORMANCE-ENHANCING DRUGS

In the world of performance-enhancing drugs, the lists of potentially enhancing drugs are so long that testing for each one specifically would be impractical and cost prohibitive. For example, the list of anabolic androgenic steroids banned for Olympic athletes (World Anti-Doping Agency 2022) includes 62 named substances and ends with the phrase "and other substances with a similar chemical structure or similar biological effect(s)." An evaluation of the athlete's urinary testosterone/epitestosterone ratio, however, can provide a proxy evaluation as to whether the athlete has ingested any exogenous anabolic androgenic steroids. For other commonly used performance-enhancing drugs (e.g., erythropoietin, peptide hormones, and growth factors), specific tests must be done.

# TOXICOLOGY TESTING VALIDITY ASSESSMENTS

*Validity checks* are methods that specimen collectors and laboratory personnel can use to ensure that the particular tissue sample (whether urine, blood, or hair) actually comes from the testee and is unadulterated by substances or conditions that would cause a false-negative result. For urine testing, most forensic laboratories will validate only a sample with urine creatinine ≥20 mg/dL, specific gravity between 1.005 and 1.030, pH between 4.5 and 8.0, and a temperature (just after voiding) of no different than 2 degrees from body temperature. Laboratories usually check for the presence of adulterants such as glutaraldehyde, phenazopyridine (Pyridium), or nitrites (American Society of Addiction Medicine 2017a). For blood and hair samples received in the laboratory, reliance on the CCF is usually more important than any validity checks.

As noted earlier in this chapter, results of forensic drug tests must be carefully reported. The tester must ensure 1) that only individuals with appropriate access to the results get them and 2) that the results themselves are absolutely accurate and beyond reproach. If there has been uncertainty in the testing process itself at any point, the details must be reported along with the results. Many testing facilities use a reporting protocol that is common in DOT-regulated testing (Swotinsky 2015). *Negative results*, of course, are samples that do not contain the particular drug, substance, or metabolites for which the test was conducted; *positive results* denote a sample that contained the tested-for drug, substance, or metabolite at a level above the specified LOD. Urine test results reported as *invalid* have oxidant, pH, creatinine, or specific gravity readings outside of the usual physiological levels, although the levels are not so abnormal that the test can be definitively ruled *adulterated*. Invalid hair test results may occur when hair has been chemically treated (e.g., through bleach and other products), because these chemicals can leave a residue on the outside of the hair shafts or chemically affect the presence of metabolites, which may invalidate the hair shaft testing. For any testing, an invalid test result does not equate with a positive or negative result and is its own finding, so there should be no suppositions of recent drug use associated with invalid tests. Adulterated urine samples are those that do not comport with physiological norms, such as those with a pH <3 or ≥11, or that contain apparent adulterants at far above the level possibly found in human urine. Adulterated samples imply an act of changing the sample but do not impute reasoning for doing so. Dilute urine samples are those with a creatinine level of 2–20 mg/dL and a specific gravity of 1.0010–1.0030, and testees with results in this category are usually retested. As noted in the Forensic Dilemma at the beginning of this chapter, a dilute sample may involve deliberate shifting of fluid balance, but it may or may not be the result of a desire to hide the truth about recent drug consumption. *Substituted samples* are those with creatinine and specific gravity both outside the normal physiological range. *Rejected for testing* denotes a sample that had to be rejected by the laboratory because of a fatal flaw in the CCF or testing process: this flaw is described with the test report. These latter two categories again may or may not mean activity on the testee's part to subvert the test result, because a sample can be substituted in error or rejected because of accidental mishandling by the laboratory. At the same time, these various types of results may warrant further scrutiny and discussion with the testee.

Alcohol tests can sometimes have false-positive results after ingestion of nonbeverage alcohol. For example, breathalyzer testing performed very soon after mouthwash use is a common problem, as are very low ethyl glucuronide and ethyl sulfate results after the application of perfume or cologne. Although there have been numerous claims of mistaken positive cocaine results after the testee handles cocaine-laden dollar bills or has sexual relations involving the application of cocaine to mucous membranes, there is sparse scientific evidence for positive test results from either situation (Dasgupta 2019). These claims must be carefully investigated on a case-by-case basis.

Some common causes for false-positive results in screening tests include poppy seeds from dietary sources giving a positive result for codeine and morphine. However, any level higher than 2,000 ng/mL is almost certainly not the result of poppy seed ingestion (American Society of Addiction Medicine 2017b). Also, a test of the same sample for 6-monoacetylmorphine can distinguish heroin from ingestion of poppy seeds. People subject to random testing (e.g., pilots, people on parole) should avoid poppy seeds to prevent questioning about positive results. The antidepressant sertraline cross-reacts with some benzodiazepine assays, and bupropion and pseudoephedrine can be mistaken for the amphetamine/methamphetamine mixture in amphetamine and dextroamphetamine (Adderall) and other prescribed stimulant medications. The dextromethorphan in over-the-counter cough suppressants can be read as phencyclidine (PCP) by some screening tests.

Table 5–3 illustrates some common substances that can result in false-positive toxicology test results.

# DOT Protocols for Forensic Drug and Alcohol Testing

Different venues for forensic drug and alcohol testing require specific protocols for collections, laboratory assessment, and delivery of results. These protocols are based on the relevant law, risk to the public, the likelihood of legal challenge, and not insignificantly, the cost to the entity ordering the tests. Highway safety, which is important to nearly every person in the United States, is managed by the DOT, which has implemented model (although hardly infallible) rules and

**Table 5–3.** Common substances that can appear as a false positive in drug tests

| Drug tested | Actual substance that can appear as a false-positive result |
| --- | --- |
| Amphetamines | Labetalol, ranitidine, bupropion, pseudoephedrine, ephedrine, amantadine, desipramine, selegiline, trazodone, methylphenidate, Vicks inhalers |
| Barbiturates | Phenytoin, nonsteroidal anti-inflammatory drugs |
| Benzodiazepines | Sertraline |
| Marijuana | Proton pump inhibitors, dronabinol, nonsteroidal anti-inflammatory drugs |
| Opiates | Ofloxacin, rifampicin, poppy seeds (papaverine), fluoroquinolone |
| Phencyclidine | Venlafaxine, dextromethorphan, ketamine |

regulations to ensure that commercial drivers are free of any influence of drugs and alcohol. These regulations for the physical qualifications and examinations of commercial drivers are established by the Code of Federal Regulations (49 C.F.R. § 391.41 Physical Qualification for Drivers [1970]) and various guidelines promulgated by the Federal Motor Carrier Safety Administration (including its *Medical Examiner's Handbook*, Federal Motor Carrier Safety Administration 2024). In addition to disqualifying potential commercial drivers who have impaired movement of their extremities, uncontrolled diabetes, epilepsy, or any other medical condition likely to interfere with their ability to operate a motor vehicle, federal regulations disqualify driver candidates who use federal Schedule I substances, amphetamines, narcotics, habit-forming drugs, or any other drugs or substances (including over-the-counter medications and supplements) that might affect the driver's ability to function. The DOT tests for the following substances: marijuana, cocaine, amphetamines, phencyclidine, and opiates (including hydrocodone, hydromorphone, oxymorphone, and oxycodone).

Federal regulations require that commercial drivers have "no current diagnosis of alcoholism." A driver may be allowed to use a banned substance if it is prescribed by a licensed medical practitioner who "is familiar with the driver's medical history and assigned duties; and has advised the driver that the prescribed substance or drug will not adversely affect the driver's ability to safely operate a commercial motor vehicle" (49 C.F.R. 391.41[b][12][i][ii][A][B] Physical Qualification for Drivers [1970]).

Medical examiners are directed to carefully review their examinee's responses to questions about drug or alcohol use. Specifically, examiners should ask how often alcohol is used, ask about any habit-forming drugs, and refer examinees for a more in-depth evaluation if they appear to need one. The use of standardized questionnaires, like the Alcohol Use Disorders Identification Test (AUDIT), the CAGE (Cut Down, Annoyed, Guilty, and Eye-Opener) Assessment, and the T-ACE (Tolerance, Annoyed, Cut Down, Eye-Opener) Screening Tool, is recommended to minimize subjectivity of the examination (keeping in mind that these instruments may not have been validated in forensic settings). Under DOT rules, drug testing is required before granting a commercial driver's license (CDL), although alcohol testing is not required. However, the employer may ask the driver to complete an alcohol test before performing a safety-sensitive function and may make a job offer contingent on passing an alcohol test. Postaccident testing is mandatory after all fatal crashes and if the driver receives a moving traffic violation. Even in the absence of an accident or a traffic ticket, reasonable-suspicion tests are conducted when a supervisor sees behavior suggestive of drug or alcohol misuse. Random testing is allowed, as is return-to-duty testing for drivers who have violated the prohibited drug or alcohol standards and have undergone treatment.

In these changing times of cannabis decriminalization, the DOT has maintained its strict stance on cannabis, even regarding the use of medical marijuana. Relying on the federal government's continued scheduling of marijuana as a Schedule I substance, given its role of "assur[ing] the traveling public that our transportation system is the safest it can be," and in response to U.S. Department of Justice advice to federal prosecutors under the Obama administration to avoid prosecution of marijuana-related criminal cases, the DOT put out a guidance on October 22, 2009 (which is still in effect) as follows:

> We want to make it perfectly clear that the DOJ guidelines will have no bearing on the Department of Transportation's regulated drug testing program. We will not change our regulated drug testing program based upon these guidelines to Federal prosecutors.
>
> The Department of Transportation's Drug and Alcohol Testing Regulation—49 C.F.R. Part 40, at 40.151(e)—does not authorize "medical marijuana" under a state law to be a valid medical explanation for a transportation employee's positive drug test result.... [M]edical Review Officers will *not* verify a drug test as negative based upon information that a physician recommended that the employee use "medical marijuana." Please note that marijuana remains a drug listed in Schedule I of the Controlled Substances Act. It remains unacceptable for any safety-sensitive employee subject to drug testing under the Department of Transportation's drug testing regulations to use marijuana. (Swart 2009; emphasis in original)

Even if cannabis is reassigned to Schedule III of the Controlled Substances Act, individuals tested by DOT and those doing the testing would be well advised to avoid making any changes until there is explicit guidance from DOT on the subject of cannabis. It is not entirely clear whether the prescribed medical use of methadone or buprenorphine would disqualify a driver from having a CDL. Although both agents could reasonably be described as habit forming, an examining physician might just as reasonably find that these medications do not "adversely affect the driver's ability to safely operate a commercial motor vehicle," thereby allowing a CDL driver to work even with the prescription of these two medications.

# Forensic Drug and Alcohol Testing in the Criminal Legal System

Although substance use can affect individuals in court in a variety of contexts (e.g., child welfare, parental custody, housing tenancy) as described elsewhere in this book, the following section discusses substance use testing in criminal legal contexts. The criminal system has obvious needs for drug and alcohol testing, not only for ensuring that jails and prisons are free of illicit substances but also in evaluating and monitoring parole and probation participants to make certain that they are complying with mandates to remain drug and alcohol free. In one data set from the Bureau of Justice Statistics (2021b), 47% of federal prisoners were mandated for drug trafficking or possession, as were 15% of state prisoners. While incarcerated, 25% of federal prisoners were mandated to have drug testing, as were 12% of state prisoners.

There is no question that U.S. prisons and jails have significant numbers of people with addiction problems (see Chapter 10 for more information). For instance, 1.7% of state prisoner deaths in 2008 were attributable to drug and alcohol intoxication; this percentage slowly rose over the ensuing years to rates of 5.1% in 2017, 6.0% in 2018, and 6.6% in 2019, with the increase almost certainly attributable to illicit fentanyl within carceral settings (Bureau of Justice Statistics 2021a). The California penal system, which was placed under federal receivership in 2005 and therefore kept more specific records of all substance-related deaths, reported that in 2019, 38 deaths were attributable to single opioids, 9 to amphetamine, 8 to amphetamine plus opiates, 4 to mixed opiates, 3 to opioids plus alcohol, 1 to opioids plus nortriptyline, and 1 to a calcium channel blocker (Imai 2021).

The medical treatment of substance use disorders (SUDs) within the criminal legal system is, of course, a necessary component for decreasing the death toll. Accurate drug and alcohol testing in the general criminal legal population (not just decedents) is necessary to assess the problem's magnitude. This testing should take place at a variety of junctures within criminal case processing and incarceration (Swotinsky 2015), including 1) at criminal sentencing and bail-setting, to allow for periodic drug testing of convicted felons who need it; and

2) during jail or prison terms, to direct treatment resources to those who need them and to maintain drug- and alcohol-free facilities. Finally, accurate testing is needed to monitor parolees and probationers for adherence to any legal requirements for abstinence and to direct them to treatment once identified.

Accurate testing is tremendously important in the criminal justice system, given the consequences for a prison inmate or parolee found to have a positive result. Forensic methods should always be used in these settings. Yet even with rigorous protocols in place, erroneous results can occur, leading to unfair sanctions and widespread disaffection with the testing protocols themselves (Requarth and Joseph 2019). The specific types of testing done in the criminal system are dictated by the specific circumstances of the testing protocol as well as the costs involved. To screen large populations for drug or alcohol use, random UDSs are typically used. In parole or probation scenarios, in which the testee is not incarcerated for all or most of the time, random drug screens can also be done, but portable technology like internet-connected breathalyzers (Soberlink, SCRAM, and others) or wearable sweat-assessment technology (PharmChek and others) is increasingly used and can provide greater accuracy through more immediate testing and facilitate testing for both the testee and the system reviewing the results.

Dedicated drug courts, described in Chapter 9, rely on their drug testing protocols to support the combined role of justice and health care defined by the term *therapeutic jurisprudence*. Judicial decisions about how to respond to a positive drug or alcohol test result often rely on recommendations from the court's substance abuse professionals, who must interpret the test in scientific and clinical terms. The dual role of the drug tests—both punitive and therapeutic—necessitates a transparent and intentionally designed program that fulfills both roles as effectively as possible. Given that drug courts must use the drug and alcohol testing available to them, often without the benefit of sophisticated toxicological guidance on the testing, it is important that these courts use qualitative UDSs rather than rely on quantitative reports that appear to (but do not really) quantify the amount or pattern of the substance use (Cary 2004).

Drug testing in an effective drug court can have profound meaning for the offender, whether the test is positive or negative. For the offender who has never had a supportive experience in a courtroom, having a series of negative test results and being supported and congratulated on those results from the bench can provide effective motivation for sobriety going forward. In addition, a positive drug test result met with understanding, concern, and enhanced therapeutic maneuvers from the court team can provide a reparative experience for the drug court client. However, drug courts can and usually do reserve the right to sanction individuals who have multiple positive drug and alcohol test results, because these sanctions are a legitimate and sometimes necessary function of the court.

# Forensic Drug and Alcohol Testing in Child Custody Disputes

As with the justice system in general, child custody disputes often contain components of drug and alcohol testing, with important consequences for the testee. Although the legal focus in these matters is on the well-being of the minor child, keeping children in contact with their parents is always an important, if secondary, component of this judicial decision. In one survey of divorcing couples (Amato and Previti 2003), 11% of respondents listed alcohol or drug use as an important reason for their marriage's failure, outdone only by infidelity (21.6%) and incompatibility (19.2%). In addition, parental alcohol or drug use as an identified condition necessitating removal of a child from a home has been increasing (National Center on Substance Abuse and Child Welfare 2021a) (see also Chapter 6 for more information about legal issues related to substance use and pregnancy and family matters generally).

Government guidance on the use of drug and alcohol testing in child welfare situations (National Center on Substance Abuse and Child Welfare 2021b) focuses on some highly relevant points for evaluators. First, drug testing should be only one aspect of the decision to determine case planning and removal of a child, because a drug test alone cannot ascertain whether the individual being tested has an SUD, nor can it determine whether the individual is a fit parent, even with an SUD. Although a series of tests can define a pattern of use or denial about the severity of use, the results alone cannot define whether there is a safety risk to a child related to a parent's ingestion of a particular substance. Evaluators should 1) look to test results as only one aspect of the data, 2) consider standardized screening assessments, and 3) use behavioral observations as well as information from collateral informants. In some instances, drug testing can function as a motivating tool for some parents to engage with their treatment and therefore become more effective parents. However, forensic evaluators and treating clinicians must look at testing for different purposes, even though in some cases drug testing can be a part of motivational enhancement tools aimed to support the well-being of children and families.

The practical aspects of evaluating substance use in the context of child custody disputes necessitates protecting the child's best interests, maximizing parenting time for the parents involved, and presenting information as needed for court processes that is both accurate and acceptable in legal contexts (Westreich 2017). Custody disputes are, by nature, adversarial, and individuals accusing a subject of having an addiction problem must be interviewed. However, the findings from such interviews should be carefully examined for evidence of misrepresentation or exaggeration, conscious or otherwise.

If in the context of child custody a court determines that a monitoring program should be instituted for one parent or both, such a program should be designed 1) with the specific problematic substances in mind and 2) with any information about likely contexts for substance use that might endanger a child. For instance, the parent who has driven while intoxicated might be provided with an ignition lock system (Intoxalock and others), which allows the car to operate only when the driver provides a breath sample negative for alcohol. Monitoring programs should be designed for the problem at hand: some are designed to quickly identify drug or alcohol use while the parent has custody of the child. In these types of regimens, there must be a mechanism to immediately remove the child from the intoxicated parent's care. This removal can be arranged via a monitor (available 24/7) who contacts the attorneys involved, or the other spouse, in the event of a positive test result. In some cases, there may be more concern over a long period of time, such as with a parent who has acknowledged or been accused of occasional cocaine use. Because this is different from the acute issues of the intoxicated driving example, it is often recommended to perform routine drug testing over time. For example, random UDSs and quarterly hair drug screens for cocaine and metabolites might be in order, coupled with an action plan for any positive results. Table 5–4 presents a summary of various testing methods often used in child custody disputes, along with their advantages and disadvantages.

Any person involved in a child custody dispute in which there have been allegations of drug or alcohol problems should contact an attorney familiar with the law in that jurisdiction. Especially around the issue of drug or alcohol testing, for the reasons noted earlier in this chapter, a knowledgeable attorney will advocate for the best possible outcome for both the child and the parents, always understanding that the court's primary concern will be the well-being of the child. Multiple law firms offer internet-based guidance along with contact information, and this is often where prospective clients turn for legal resources.

# Forensic Drug and Alcohol Testing in the Clinical Sphere

## SCREENING DURING TREATMENT WITH OPIOID MEDICATIONS FOR PAIN

Starting in the 2000s, as the rapid growth of opioid use disorder (OUD) stemming from prescription opioids became apparent, calls for drug testing as a matter of course during treatment with opioids came to the fore (National Academy of Medicine 2017). As one component of standard-of-care pain management treatment, regular UDSs were recommended for the patient being pre-

**Table 5–4.**    Drug and alcohol testing in a child custody dispute
testing method

| Technology | Pros | Cons |
|---|---|---|
| Urine drug screens | Widely available<br>Not physically invasive | Relatively easily evaded<br>Observation is awkward |
| Ethyl glucuronide/ethyl sulfate (metabolites of alcohol) | Can detect use over 3 days | False-positive results at low levels |
| Remote alcohol breathalyzer testing | Can be scheduled or random | Intrusive: testee must always be alert for a random test |
| Hair testing | Can detect a wide range of drugs<br>Can detect use over 90 days | Scientific data are sparse although improving |
| Point-of-service testing (saliva, breath, sweat) | Immediate results | Expensive to get a tester to the testee quickly |
| Ignition lock | Can prevent drunk driving | Does not monitor testee when they are not driving |

scribed opioid medications. Although it is slightly counterintuitive (i.e., the patient is supposed to have opioids in their urine), clinicians find the results valuable in identifying patients who are illicitly taking other opioids or sedative medications or who are obtaining opioid prescriptions for the express purpose of selling them to others. Simple in-office UDS procedures are best in pain management and primary care clinics, as part of the assessment routine for patients seen in the clinic. By using noninvasive, relatively less intrusive, and inexpensive technology, clinicians can sort out the few patients who are potentially feigning their symptoms and gathering prescriptions for later profit or endangering themselves by taking other sedative medications. Given the legally fraught situation of opioid prescription, the testing should be considered forensic for the benefit of both the patient and the prescribing clinician.

# SCREENING DURING TREATMENT WITH MEDICATIONS FOR OPIOID USE DISORDER

For individuals who become addicted to opioid medications, whether via prescription of opioids for pain management or otherwise, medications for OUD (MOUD) are the standard-of-care treatments even if there remains a dearth of active prescribers for MOUD. For patients taking buprenorphine (Suboxone and others), methadone, or naltrexone (Vivitrol), regular UDSs are highly recommended. In addition to ascertaining that the patient is taking (rather than selling) the daily dose of buprenorphine, the clinician can know whether the patient is taking other, potentially sedating and therefore dangerous medications. Some buprenorphine-treated patients may unintentionally ingest drugs such as fentanyl or PCP, because illicit drugs often contain substances of unknown provenance, and various drugs can even be sprinkled on an otherwise harmless-appearing marijuana joint. Because all patients receiving MOUD should be screened, UDSs are the test of choice: clinicians should choose an unobserved protocol in most cases, but they should switch to an observed protocol if sample tampering is suspected. The following guidance from the Substance Abuse and Mental Health Services Administration nicely delineates the rationale for ordering UDSs as well as deciding between unobserved and observed protocols:

> Conduct random urine tests that include a wide spectrum of opioids—including morphine, oxycodone, and buprenorphine—and periodically include buprenorphine metabolites. This will help monitor response to treatment and determine whether patients are taking at least some of their prescribed buprenorphine.
> Use **unobserved** specimen collection to preserve patient privacy and dignity:
>> Do not let patients bring backpacks, jackets, or other items into the bathroom.
>> Do not let others enter bathrooms with patients.
>> Temperature test the urine sample.
> Use **observed** specimen collection (obtained by a staff member of the same gender) or oral fluid testing if there is reason to suspect tampering or falsification.
> Contact patients at random; ask them to bring in their medication within a reasonable period (24 to 48 hours) to count the tablets/films to ensure that all medication is accounted for.
> Provide a limited number of days of medication per prescription without refills (e.g., several days or 1 week per prescription) until the patient has demonstrated stability and lowered diversion risk. (Substance Abuse and Mental Health Services Administration 2021; emphasis in original)

# SCREENING IN DRUG TREATMENT PROGRAMS, ELITE SPORTS, AND DURING PREGNANCY

In addition to the clearly forensic environments of drug and alcohol testing in highway safety, criminal justice, and pain management scenarios, some testing environments demonstrate a tension between a clear clinical mission and a forensic component to that mission. For instance, drug treatment programs, elite sport drug testing, and pregnancy drug testing may have clinical goals as well as a mandate for reporting the findings to officials for formal case processing. Although clinical treatment may be the goal of a particular test facility, the program may assign consequences (e.g., discharge from the program) for a positive test result. The individual patient usually experiences this type of consequence as unhelpful, but one rationale given is that the program may need to protect other clients from a patient chronically experiencing relapse. This is an evolving area of debate in practice, because removal from treatment also has significant potential downstream consequences. In some instances, regulatory authorities and third-party payers are developing "no eject and no reject" policies to handle these matters to maximize continuity of care.

In mixed forensic and clinical scenarios, it is equally important that the testee be made aware of any consequences from a positive test result. Although it can be tempting to use the less complicated and less expensive clinical testing protocols in these situations, the potential for negative consequences for the testee necessitates a full forensic protocol. Practically speaking, this protocol often uses a document signed by the testee, acknowledging the test protocol and the potential consequences of a positive result. Such a document both 1) ensures that the testee is aware of the full meaning of the test and 2) protects the testing agency from accusations that the sanctions imposed after a positive result are arbitrary, egregious, or otherwise unfair. Although observed collection protocols are sometimes contemplated for highway safety and child custody testing, these protocols should at least be considered in these mixed scenarios, given the high likelihood of eventual legal challenge.

# Methods Used to Evade a Forensic Drug or Alcohol Test

As noted earlier in this chapter, test results can be difficult to ascertain owing to cross-reactivity of substances or because they can be tampered with or evaded. Although detection determinations may be illuminating for these circumstances, it is also useful to understand from a legal perspective how test results can be modified by the testee. Testees may attempt to intentionally evade the testing in a variety of creative mechanical and chemical ways. Sending another person to the testing site should be defended against by most careful identification processes, as should the provision of a sample from another person. Simply diluting a positive specimen by ingesting large amounts of any liquid is a common and generally unsuccessful strategy, given now-standard specific gravity checks. Supplying another person's urine for the testing is another common strategy, often foiled by a simple temperature check. Companies sell receptacles that can be taped to the lower abdomen and filled with drug-negative urine, thereby providing a sample at near-body-temperature (e.g., Whizzinator). Even more sophisticated strategies, such as catheterizing oneself with negative urine, are sometimes used by health care professionals desperate to avoid a positive test. External adulteration of urine samples with bleach or toilet water is sometimes attempted. Agents that supposedly eliminate toxins (sold as Urineluck,

Quick Fix Plus, and Klear) can be purchased online, although they are usually quickly identified in forensic testing.

Jurisdictions differ on the legality of evading a drug test, although most ban the sale or use of adulterants or other instruments to fake a drug test. For example, Texas defines falsifying a drug test as a misdemeanor; the statute reads as follows:

(a) A person commits an offense if the person knowingly or intentionally uses or possesses with intent to use any substance or device designed to falsify drug test results.
(b) A person commits an offense if the person knowingly or intentionally delivers, possesses with intent to deliver, or manufactures with intent to deliver a substance or device designed to falsify drug test results. (Texas Health and Safety Code § 481.133 1991)

Individuals involved with forensic drug and alcohol testing should be methodical with their testing procedures and detail oriented in their provision of the results of those drug tests. The seriousness of the mission requires a level of thoughtfulness, completeness, and skepticism even beyond that necessitated by clinical tests. However, collectors and testers should remain respectful toward the testee, and they should avoid letting any stereotypes about drug or alcohol users contaminate the specimen collection process. On a practical level, some tampering is difficult to detect. For example, it is impossible to ban drinking copious quantities of water that result in the dilution of one's own body fluid. Also, suspicions can certainly turn out to be inaccurate at times. Collectors and testers must remain professional in all of their interactions, even with the person intentionally evading a drug test. In addition to the simple common decency reflected in this professionalism, inappropriate actions or comments toward the testee could influence the outcome of any subsequent litigation.

# Expert Testimony

In the oft-litigated world of drug and alcohol testing, expert witness testimony is commonly necessary to explicate the nuances of the testing report (e.g., NMS Labs 2024). *Fact witnesses*, usually toxicologists, are called to court to explain laboratory procedures, including the laboratory's standard operating procedure, the analytical processes used, the calculation and review of analytical results, chain-of-custody documentation, the details of sample storage, and the accreditations and licensing of laboratory personnel. *Expert witnesses* may offer opinions on the fact testimony itself and may interpret the results according to their own education, training, and experience.

The *litigation package* used in court or hearing rooms regarding a contested result often spans hundreds of pages. These packets include, at a minimum, the test results, completed chain-of-custody documentation, the collection instructions, documentation of the screening test results, the confirmation test documents, and copies of the licensures and registrations for all relevant equipment and personnel in the laboratory. These litigation packages are usually the central documents in any case in which the laboratory procedures are questioned by the recipient of a positive drug test result, and the results of this litigation often bear directly on the employability of the testee or have other implications, depending on the test's context. In addition, of course, incorrect or sloppy procedures on the part of a laboratory can negate the results in question and damage the laboratory's reputation.

In one such case (*Landon v. Kroll Laboratory Specialists, Inc.* 2011), a forensic testing laboratory reported that a probationer's saliva sample was positive for THC, although the testee had a blood test the same day that was negative for THC. In addition to some problems with the saliva collection device and procedures, documents revealed that the laboratory used an immunoassay test with a screening cutoff of 1.0 ng/mL, despite the manufacturer's recommendation to use a cutoff of 3.0 ng/mL, and that no GC/MS confirmation test was ever ordered or completed. The court noted the seriousness of a probation drug test, given that the potential consequence of the test was incarceration of the individual. In reversing the results, the court noted that "we hold that a drug testing laboratory may be held liable in tort to the subject of a drug test for failing to use reasonable care under the circumstances." (Landon v Kroll Laboratory Specialists, Inc. 2013)

# Medical Review Officers

*Medical review officers* (MROs) organize and oversee forensic testing regimens and are prepared to manage the types of testing anomalies mentioned in this chapter. Introduced by statute into the U.S. transportation system in 1988, the MRO is essentially a liaison between the clinical world and the laboratory world, tasked with overseeing the testing procedures to yield outcomes that are fair and reasonable. A federal regulation describes the obligations for MROs (49 C.F.R. Part 40 Subpart G, Medical Review Officers and the Verification Process). Although by law an MRO must oversee DOT testing, MROs are also often employed to manage non-DOT-regulated testing. MROs must be licensed physicians who are knowledgeable about addiction and capable of interpreting laboratory test results related to SUDs. MROs are knowledgeable about specimen collection procedures, chain-of-custody reporting, the interpretation of drug and validity test results, and the role of MROs within the testing procedure. In addition to this technical knowledge, the MRO is usually tasked with managing any interactions between the program, the testee, and any treating clinicians involved in a particular situation.

A major training organization for MROs requires that MROs have the following (Hartenbaum et al. 2003):

- Knowledge and clinical training in SUDs involving controlled substances, including detailed knowledge of alternative medical explanations for laboratory-confirmed drug test results
- Knowledge of issues relating to adulterated and substituted specimens and possible medical causes of an invalid result
- Knowledge of the Procedures for Transportation Workplace Drug and Alcohol Testing Programs, the DOT MRO Guidelines, and DOT agency rules applicable for any employer for which the MRO provides services
- Knowledge of the pharmacology of "drugs of abuse"
- Knowledge of accepted pharmacological treatment and standard prescribing practices for specific disease processes
- Authorization to prescribe controlled substances consistent with U.S. Drug Enforcement Administration rules and regulations
- Knowledge of ethical considerations in workplace drug testing programs
- Knowledge of laboratory testing methodology and quality control
- Knowledge of laws and regulations related to the use of illicit and licit substances
- Knowledge of chemical dependence and addiction behavior

A variety of training courses exist for MROs, all of which are available to licensed physicians (American College of Occupational and Environmental Medicine 2024; American Osteopathic College of Occupational and Preventive Medicine 2024).

## Conclusions

Drug and alcohol testing in forensic contexts must be ordered carefully, managed with chain-of-custody methods, and assessed using laboratory methods that are demonstrably accurate and reproducible. Given the serious consequences that can flow from a test result found to be positive or adulterated in some way, fundamental fairness demands these rigorous collection and assessment techniques. The inevitable legal challenges to these tests should be met with professional responses and litigation packages that accurately represent the science of the testing protocol and the degree of certainty about the test result that can be inferred by that science.

# Key Points

- Forensic drug and alcohol testing often cannot be repeated to find a more accurate answer.

- Paruresis (shy bladder) is most commonly a manifestation of anxiety rather than a physiological abnormality.

- Under the Americans With Disabilities Act, a preemployment drug test is not considered a medical test.

- Screening drug tests usually use immunoassays, whereas confirmation tests usually use gas chromatography/mass spectroscopy.

- Positive drug and alcohol test results alone do not denote impairment or a diagnosis of a substance use disorder.

# References

Amato P, Previti D: People's reasons for divorcing: gender, social class, the life course, and adjustment. J Fam Issues 24(5):602–626, 2003

American College of Occupational and Environmental Medicine: Learning: MRO resources. Available at: https://acoem.org/Learning/MRO-Resources. Accessed April 14, 2024.

American Osteopathic College of Occupational and Preventive Medicine: About AOCOPM. Available at: https://www.aocopm.org/. Accessed April 14, 2024.

American Society of Addiction Medicine: Appropriate Use of Drug Testing in Clinical Addiction Medicine: Consensus Statement. Rockville, MD, American Society of Addiction Medicine, 2017a. Available at: https://sitefinitystorage.blob.core.windows.net/sitefinity-production-blobs/docs/default-source/guidelines/the-asam-appropriate-use-of-drug-testing-in-clinical-addiction-medicine-full-document.pdf?sfvrsn=700a7bc2_0. Accessed January 2, 2021.

American Society of Addiction Medicine: Drug Testing Pocket Guide. Rockville, MD, American Society of Addiction Medicine, 2017b. Available at: http://eguideline.guidelinecentral.com/i/840070-drug-testing-pocket-guide/. Accessed January 2, 2022.

Americans With Disabilities Act National Network: Is testing for the illegal use of drugs permissible under the ADA? Available at: https://adata.org/faq/testing-illegal-use-drugs-permissible-under-ada#:~:text=A%20test%20for%20the%20illegal, prohibit%2C%20or%20authorize%20drug%20tests. Accessed November 19, 2022.

Andresen-Streichert H, Müller A, Glahn A, et al: Alcohol biomarkers in clinical and forensic contexts. Dtsch Arztebl Int 115(18):309–315, 2018 29807559

Belson K, Schmidt MS: Braun wins appeal on positive drug test and avoids suspension. The New York Times, February 23, 2012. Available at: https://www.nytimes.com/2012/02/24/sports/baseball/braun-wins-appeal-on-positive-drug-test-and-will-avoid-suspension.html. Accessed February 6, 2022.

Bureau of Justice Statistics: Mortality in State and Federal Prisons, 2001–2019: Statistical Tables. Washington, DC, U.S. Department of Justice, 2021a. Available at: https://bjs.ojp.gov/library/publications/mortality-state-and-federal-prisons-2001–2019-statistical-tables. Accessed December 28, 2021.

Bureau of Justice Statistics: Profile of Prison Inmates, 2016. Washington, DC, U.S. Department of Justice, December 2021b. Available at: https://bjs.ojp.gov/library/publications/profile-prison-inmates-2016. Accessed February 7, 2022.

Cary PL: Urine Drug Concentrations: The Scientific Rationale for Eliminating Use of Drug Test Levels in Drug Court Proceedings. Alexandria, VA, National Drug Court Institute, 2004. Available at: https://www.ndci.org/wp-content/uploads/Urine_Drug_Concentrations.pdf. Accessed February 6, 2022.

Dasgupta A: Miscellaneous issues: paper money contaminated with cocaine and other drugs, cocaine containing herbal teas, passive exposure to marijuana, ingestion of hemp oil, and occupational exposure to controlled substances, in Critical Issues in Alcohol and Drugs of Abuse Testing, 2nd Edition. New York, Elsevier, 2019, pp 463–476

DieOff.org: How long do steroids stay in your system? November 9, 2019. Available at: https://www.dieoff.org/how-long-do-steroids-stay-in-your-system. Accessed January 16, 2022.

Federal Motor Carrier Safety Administration: Shy Bladder. Washington, DC, U.S. Department of Transportation, May 20, 2015. Available at: https://www.fmcsa.dot.gov/regulations/drug-alcohol-testing/shy-bladder. Accessed February 7, 2022.

Federal Motor Carrier Safety Administration: Medical Examiner's Handbook. Washington, DC, U.S. Department of Transportation, 2024

Hartenbaum NP, Martin DW; American College of Occupational and Environmental Medicine: Qualifications of medical review officers (MROs) in regulated and non-regulated drug testing. J Occup Environ Med 45(1):102–103, 2003 12553185

Imai K: Analysis of 2019 Inmate Death Reviews in the California Correctional Healthcare System. Sacramento, CA, California Correctional Health Care Services, 2021. Available at: https://cchcs.ca.gov/wp-content/uploads/sites/60/MS/2019-Inmate-Death-Reviews.pdf. Accessed December 28, 2021.

Jatlow PI, Agro A, Wu R, et al: Ethyl glucuronide and ethyl sulfate assays in clinical trials, interpretation, and limitations: results of a dose ranging alcohol challenge study and 2 clinical trials. Alcohol (Hanover) 38(7):2056–2065, 2014 24773137

Knowles SR, Skues J: Development and validation of the Shy Bladder and Bowel Scale (SBSS). Cogn Behav Ther 45(4):324–338, 2016 27216857

Kulig K: Interpretation of workplace tests for cannabinoids. J Med Toxicol 13(1):106–110, 2017 27686239

Landon v Kroll Laboratory Specialists, Inc., 91 A.D.3d 79, 934 N.Y.S.2d 183, 2011 N.Y. Slip Op. 8567 (2011)

Landon v Kroll Laboratory Specialists, Inc., 934 N.Y.S.2d 183 (N.Y. App. Div. 2d Dept. 2011), aff'd, 999 N.E.2d 1121 (N.Y. 2013)

Mayo Clinic Laboratories: Opiates: interpretation. Available at: https://www.mayocliniclabs.com/test-catalog/drug-book/specific-drug-groups/opiates#. Accessed January 5, 2021.

National Academy of Medicine: First, Do No Harm: Marshaling Clinician Leadership to Counter the Opioid Epidemic. Washington, DC, National Academy of Medicine, 2017. Available at: https://nam.edu/wp-content/uploads/2017/09/First-Do-No-Harm-Marshaling-Clinician-Leadership-to-Counter-the-Opioid-Epidemic.pdf. Accessed February 6, 2022.

National Center on Substance Abuse and Child Welfare: Child Welfare and Alcohol and Drug Use Statistics. Rockville, MD, Substance Abuse and Mental Health Services Administration, 2021a. Available at: https://ncsacw.samhsa.gov/research/child-welfare-and-treatment-statistics.aspx. Accessed December 29, 2021.

National Center on Substance Abuse and Child Welfare: Drug Testing for Parents Involved in Child Welfare: Three Key Practice Points. Rockville, MD, Substance Abuse and Mental Health Services Administration, 2021b. Available at: https://ncsacw.samhsa.gov/files/drug-testing-brief-2-508.pdf. Accessed December 29, 2021.

NMS Labs: Court testimony and deposition services. 2024. Available at: https://www.nmslabs.com/expert-services/service-offerings/court-testimony-and-deposition-services. Accessed April 14, 2024.

Onondaga County Medical Examiner: Forensic Toxicology Scope of Testing and Detection Limits. Syracuse, NY, Onondaga County Health Department Center for Forensic Services, 2021. Available at: http://www.ongov.net/health/meo/documents/toxicologytesting.pdf. Accessed January 5, 2022.

Quest Diagnostics: Marijuana workplace drug test positivity continues double-digit increases to keep overall drug positivity rates at historically high levels. May 26, 2021. Available at: https://newsroom.questdiagnostics.com/2021-05-26-Marijuana-Workforce-Drug-Test-Positivity-Continues-Double-Digit-Increases-to-Keep-Overall-Drug-Positivity-Rates-at-Historically-High-Levels,-Finds-Latest-Quest-Diagnostics-Drug-Testing-Index-TM-Analysis#:~:text=SECAU-CUS%2C%20N.J.%2C%20May%2026%2C,world's%20leading%20provider%20of%20diagnostic. Accessed February 5, 2022.

Requarth T, Joseph G: Leaked documents say roughly 2,000 NY prisoners affected by erroneous drug tests. Gothamist, November 21, 2019. Available at: https://gothamist.com/news/leaked-documents-say-roughly 2000-ny-prisoners-affected-by-erroneous-drug-tests. Accessed February 6, 2022.

RTI International: National Laboratory Certification Program. Available at: https://www.rti.org/impact/national-laboratory-certification-program-nlcp. Accessed December 31, 2021.

Sparkman OD, Penton Z, Kitson F: Gas Chromatography and Mass Spectroscopy: A Practical Guide, 2nd Edition. Cambridge, MA, Academic Press, 2011

Substance Abuse and Mental Health Services Administration: Urine Specimen Collection Handbook for Federal Agency Workplace Drug Testing Programs. Rockville, MD, Substance Abuse and Mental Health Services Administration, 2014. Available at: https://www.samhsa.gov/sites/default/files/specimen-collection-handbook-2014.pdf. Accessed December 30, 2021.

Substance Abuse and Mental Health Services Administration: Medications for Opioid Use Disorder. Treatment Improvement Protocol, TIP 63 (Publ No PEP21–02–01–0002). Rockville, MD, U.S. Department of Health and Human Services, 2021. Available at: https://store.samhsa.gov/sites/default/files/SAMHSA_Digital_Download/PEP21–02–01–002.pdf. Accessed February 6, 2022.

Swart J: DOT Office of Drug and Alcohol Policy and Compliance Notice. Washington, DC, U.S. Department of Transportation, 2009. Available at: https://www.transportation.gov/sites/dot.gov/files/images/ODAPC%20Medical%20Marijuana%20Notice.pdf. Accessed December 27, 2021.

Swotinsky RB: The Medical Review Officer's Manual: MROCC's Guide to Testing, 5th Edition. Beverly Farms, MA, OEM Press, 2015

Texas Health and Safety Code § 481.133—Offense: Falsification of Drug Test Results (1991)

U.S. Department of Transportation, Rule 49 C.F.R. Part 40 § 40.199 (2017)

Westreich LM: Evaluating and monitoring drug and alcohol use during child custody disputes. Curr Psychiatr 16(4): 2017

World Anti-Doping Agency: World Anti-Doping Code: International Standard Prohibited List, 2022. 2022. Available at: https://www.wada-ama.org/sites/default/files/resources/files/2022list_final_en.pdf. Accessed November 6, 2023.

# CHAPTER 6

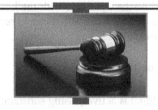

# ADDICTIONS IN PREGNANCY, FAMILY, AND DIVORCE

## Introduction

Substance use disorders (SUDs) and related laws can affect family systems dramatically. Pregnant women with SUDs face unique challenges, such as barriers to accessing care and, in some jurisdictions, risks of punitive actions such as prosecution if substance use harms the fetus or child. Child welfare removal of children from their home of origin and placement into foster care are increasingly related to SUDs among parents. Substance use among youth can have negative effects on school performance and heightens risks for juvenile justice entanglements. Laws for educational supports that protect children with disabilities may have limits for youth engaging in active substance use, especially if they are using illegal drugs. SUD treatment consent requirements vary by age across states; whether parental figures have the right to information about such treatment also varies across states. This chapter outlines many interactions between substance use and related legal and regulatory issues for pregnant women, youth, and family systems across a variety of contexts.

---

## FORENSIC DILEMMA

A 32-year-old woman with alcohol use disorder, opioid use disorder (OUD), and PTSD discovers that she is 12 weeks pregnant. She regularly used substances before and after she conceived. Now she desires to cut back her use because she is motivated to deliver a healthy baby and raise the child on her own. She has a history of taking medications for addiction treatment but did not remain in care after initial months of stability. Four years earlier, she delivered a baby with neonatal abstinence syndrome. The child has spent time in foster care, but she is hoping to have the child returned to her custody. The woman is living with a friend while the child lives with the biological paternal grandmother. She has had no direct contact with the child recently, and she comes to a clinician's office for treatment.

Several immediate questions emerge:

1. Given that this individual is actively using substances while pregnant, do the mandated reporting laws require the clinician to report it to children's services?
2. What do the laws and policies support with regard to returning a child to a mother with addiction and a history of custody loss?

Depending on the state in which the woman lives, there may be a mandate to report her substance use even before the baby is born. Practitioners should be familiar with the state requirements in their regions. If the baby is born with substance use issues, such as neonatal abstinence syndrome or fetal alcohol syndrome, typically a mandated report to child welfare would occur. Some states will then pursue linkages to treatment, but others may move to prosecute the mother if the baby is harmed by the substance use. Racial and ethnic disparities worsen negative outcomes, by increasing the risk of child removal and prosecution stemming from legal sanctions. Many of these outcomes are also tied to other socioeconomic disparities and social determinants of health. If the child is removed from the mother's custody, efforts will be made to determine whether the mother can improve with treatment. Time standards must be followed that may lead to termination of parental rights if the mother continues to demonstrate an inability to safely care for the child. Therefore, it is critically important that treatment be offered for both mother and child to try to keep the family together as much as possible without compromising safety. A father may face related challenges if he has an SUD that prevents safe parenting.

# Addiction in Pregnancy and Breastfeeding and the Rights of Fetuses, Infants, and Young Children

Addiction in pregnancy is a growing area of concern, particularly as highlighted by the opioid epidemic. The number of women with opioid-related diagnoses at the time of delivery increased by 131% between 2010 and 2017 (Hirai et al. 2021). According to a 2019 CDC survey, approximately 7% of women reported taking prescription opioid pain relievers during pregnancy, and 20% self-reported misuse of these prescriptions (Ko et al. 2020). Although data from another study by Desai et al. (2014) are somewhat older, they are noteworthy in that almost a quarter of women enrolled in Medicaid across 46 states filled an opioid prescription during pregnancy in 2007. Rates of neonatal abstinence syndrome were highest in states with the highest rates of opioid prescribing (Patrick et al. 2015). Substance use has been associated with increased maternal mortality, although the reasons for this are multifactorial and are attributable to limited access to and use of prenatal and pediatric health care and to social determinants related to nutrition, housing, and environment (Wolfe et al. 2005).

With emerging data highlighting the multiple issues pertaining to substance use and pregnancy, the American College of Obstetricians and Gynecologists (ACOG) recommends early universal screening, brief intervention, and referrals to treatment to improve outcomes for both infants and mothers. ACOG advises that such screening should be part of routine care and recognizes that waiting until a mother shows poor prenatal care or poor follow-up with prenatal services would be too late, missing opportunities for earlier course correction in the trajectory of the lives of the child and mother. ACOG further advises that breastfeeding should be encouraged for women receiving appropriate and stable medications for addiction, such as opioid agonists, if they are not concomitantly using illicit drugs and as long as other illnesses are not creating contraindications or other cautionary directions for breastfeeding. ACOG further suggests that breastfeeding should be halted if women experience a substance use relapse (American College of Obstetricians and Gynecologists 2017). Although the clinical issues surrounding pregnant and parenting women with SUDs are critical to address, this chapter highlights legal issues pertaining to these situations.

# Legal Rights for Mother and Unborn Child

Legal concerns over the rights of infants and unborn babies of pregnant mothers with SUDs and other conditions have a long and complex history. Boudreaux and Thompson (2015) provided an excellent overview in which they explained how, over the course of history, rights between mother and unborn child have typically rested on legal decision-makers balancing the various factors and interests involved for both (Epstein 1995). This type of balance has been codified in statutes for some issues and resolved through litigation in others.

Over centuries, legal commentary has focused on the well-being of the unborn child from the moment of conception (Boudreaux and Thompson 2015). Two distinct cases along these lines are of note. In *Dietrich v. Inhabitants of*

*Northampton* (1884), the Massachusetts Supreme Judicial Court held that a fetus was not owed a separate duty, because it was part of the mother. In contrast, in *Bonbrest v. Kotz* (1946), the court viewed a fetus as a "distinct" individual when it was viewed as "viable."

These issues evoke current controversies related to when a fetus is viable and the legal issues that flow from viability. Federal laws and legal cases come into play that examine these issues. *Roe v. Wade* (1973) is the landmark U.S. Supreme Court decision in which first-trimester abortions were legalized, with the court finding that any restrictions to their legalization conflicted with a mother's right to privacy protected under the Fourteenth Amendment. In rendering its decision, the court balanced multiple interests, including the state's interest in protecting women and protecting prenatal life. Thus, under this ruling, the court determined that the right to abortion can exist but only up until a fetus reaches independent viability (Boudreaux and Thompson 2015). *Roe* established a Fourteenth Amendment constitutional protection based ultimately on what the U.S. Supreme Court of the time viewed as a woman's right to privacy and, thus, a right to terminate a pregnancy. For nearly 50 years, this case was the law of the land.

With its ruling in *Dobbs v. Jackson Women's Health Organization* (2022), the U.S. Supreme Court overturned *Roe* in June 2022. The court determined that there is no constitutional "right to abortion" and that instead this issue could be determined on a state-by-state basis and required a balancing test, which could allow consideration of the potential viability of younger fetuses with medical advances. The case centered around a Mississippi law, the Gestational Age Act, which was passed in 2018 and banned abortion after the first 15 weeks of pregnancy unless there was a medical emergency or severe fetal abnormality but did not provide exceptions for rape- or incest-related pregnancies. Later, an even more restrictive antiabortion bill was passed that prohibited abortion in Mississippi at the time of a fetal heartbeat (usually beginning at 6 weeks of pregnancy). Since the *Dobbs* decision, there have been legislative efforts across states to either ban or broaden abortion laws. These legal shifts are important to track within one's state, as they can help practitioners understand some of the issues that might come into play regarding an unborn child, a wish for an abortion, and a mother's active substance use.

Federal statutes also guide the balancing test when issues such as pregnancy and unborn babies, in particular, come to the attention of decision-makers and lawmakers. The federal Unborn Victims of Violence Act (2004) recognizes an embryo or fetus still in utero as a potentially separate entity and legal victim of certain crimes of violence. This act provides language that allows for conduct to be punished when such conduct causes the separate death or specific serious bodily injury to a child in utero (Unborn Victims of Violence Act 2004). This law was enacted in response to the case of Scott Peterson, who was convicted of murdering his wife, Laci, and their unborn child (Boudreaux and Thompson 2015).

As of May 1, 2018, 38 states had fetal homicide laws that protect fetuses by giving them victim rights when killed by violent acts against pregnant mothers, according to the National Conference of State Legislatures. In addition, at least 29 state laws protect the fetus from conception to birth (Boudreaux and Thompson 2015).

Separate from the violent acts of others on pregnant women, laws have also considered situations in which women engage in conduct that can be harmful to their unborn child (separate from abortion). Conceptually similar to considering what might ensue from general harm to an unborn fetus, several states have enacted laws relevant to substance use by pregnant women. According to research by the Guttmacher Institute, an organization that analyzes policy developments in this area, laws range in type and scope. For example, some states consider substance use during pregnancy as child abuse, whereas other states mandate that health care professionals report substance use by pregnant mothers (without necessarily defining it automatically as child abuse) (Guttmacher Institute 2024). The distinctions between what happens when a call is made to child welfare, depending on state law and policy, may be very broad: these include 1) whether the response would automatically invoke referrals to substance use treatment or other supports; 2) whether the conduct would be fully referred to as child abuse, and thus lead to a more direct child welfare case flow that could potentially lead to child removal; and 3) whether the response to the report would simply be a notation in a children's protective services file that could be used later as evidence of abuse if other problems surfaced for the mother and children.

Some states allow for the civil commitment of pregnant women specifically for substance use. States have also enacted laws that help support drug treatment targeted to pregnant women. At the same time, several states invoke various child welfare laws for pregnant women using substances. A brief overview of these laws and policies is presented in Table 6–1. According to one study examining policies in eight states, more punitive policies were associated with greater odds of babies born with neonatal abstinence syndrome; however, this association did not hold true for states with policies that simply require reporting (Faherty et al. 2019).

Case law in this area is also noteworthy. *Johnson v. State* (1992) was an early Florida case in which the prosecution prevailed in convicting a pregnant woman for prenatal harm to a fetus. The defendant was sentenced to drug rehabilitation and probation after she was found guilty of "gestational substance abuse," related to the idea that the substances were passed to the fetus through the umbilical cord. Although this was a landmark type of case for conviction, the Florida Supreme Court ultimately overturned the conviction on the follow-

**Table 6–1.**   State laws regarding substance use and pregnancy

| Focus area | Number of states |
| --- | --- |
| Substance use during pregnancy viewed as child abuse | 12+DC |
| Health care professionals required to report suspected prenatal drug use | 7+DC |
| Substance use during pregnancy viewed as grounds for civil commitment | 3 |
| Funded or creation of drug treatment programs for pregnant women | 25 |

*Source.*   Guttmacher Institute 2024.

ing technical grounds: 1) the underlying Florida statute was not applicable in this case; and 2) passing substances from mother to unborn child was seemingly not specifically delineated in the statute, making it more of a health issue than a criminal child abuse issue contemplated in the statute. Alabama and South Carolina, however, have upheld, via state supreme court rulings, convictions for criminal child abuse for substance use in pregnancy (Guttmacher Institute 2024). In a South Carolina case,P a 23-year-old African American woman who gave birth to a stillborn baby was convicted of homicide for alleged cocaine use that caused the fetus's death. In an Alabama case, a pregnant mother with methamphetamines in her system was charged criminally after giving birth prematurely to an infant who did not survive (Boudreaux and Thompson 2015). In yet another example, a Mississippi county prosecuted 20 cases over 4 years (Liu and Hensley 2019), relying on a felony child abuse law that addressed poisoning as child abuse.

In *Beltran v. Strachota et al.* (2014), Beltran was court ordered into substance use treatment for much of her pregnancy after she stopped taking prescribed Suboxone while pregnant. She sued, claiming that she was denied due process of law, guaranteed by the Fifth and Fourteenth Amendments, in response to how her situation was managed under Wisconsin Act 292 of 1997 (which was referred to colloquially as the Cocaine Mom Law; DeVille and Kopelman 1999). This law allowed the Wisconsin courts to have jurisdiction over fertilized eggs, embryos, fetuses, and pregnant women when they severely lacked self-control over their use of substances and the unborn or newborn baby was determined to be at substantial risk as a result (Boudreaux and Thompson 2015). Although some states have made drug use during pregnancy potentially criminal, others have relied on mechanisms that invoke child protection laws. These child protection laws were built with a protective stance but are themselves complicated in terms of substance use and parenting, and some can lead full circle to child removal and even prosecution, as discussed in the following sections.

# Child Custody Disputes

Approximately one in eight children lives with at least one parent with an SUD (Brice and Generes 2022). When such substance use negatively affects an individual's ability to parent and keep the child safe, the child can be removed from parent custody. (Drug and alcohol testing in the context of child custody matters is addressed further in Chapter 5.) The child welfare system is one avenue for this to occur, but divorce is another. In a divorce context, a court of law would review a particular case and make a determination of what placement would serve the best interests of the child (the origins of this standard are described next). The following terminology in custody and divorce proceedings is important to understand (Brice and Generes 2022):

- *Legal custody* is the legal authority to be responsible for making decisions for the minor child, with decisions ranging from medical care and school issues to other areas of decision-making.
- *Physical custody* refers to who has physical oversight of the child where the child is residing.
- *Joint custody* refers to a legal assignment of shared decision-making for the child.
- *Joint physical custody* refers to situations typically involving when a child spends time within each parent's home.
- *Sole custody* refers to situations when only one parent retains either physical custody or decision-making authority through legal custody.

Some states have shifted from using the terms *custody* and *visitation* to *parenting time* and *parental responsibilities* (Gjelten 2023). These terms must be distinguished from *parental rights*, which are those rights that any parent would have for their child as the child's legal custodians. Parental rights are the ultimate right of responsibility for a child; loss of parental rights is permanent, and these rights can be lost only through voluntary abdication or a court intervention and decision.

Two landmark U.S. Supreme Court cases related to child custody are worth noting and understanding in terms of standards on which certain custody and parental rights decisions are made. In *Santosky v. Kramer* (1982), a case was brought against the parents of three minor children in New York, where the state law permitted termination of parental rights after proof by a fair preponderance of the evidence that it was justified. The case was appealed to the U.S.

Supreme Court. The court found that natural parents have a constitutional right to due process and that there is a fundamental liberty interest in the care and custody of their children protected by the Fourth Amendment. To provide fair procedures when a state moves to terminate parental rights, there is a balancing of three factors that must be considered: private interests, risk of error, and the government interest supporting the state's need to occasionally terminate such fundamental rights of a parent. As such, the court found that a New York statute that relied on a "fair preponderance of the evidence" violated the due process clause of the Fourteenth Amendment.

To understand this case, it is important to note that there are three general standards of proof for the fact finder at trial to judge and weigh the evidence: 1) preponderance of the evidence (the lowest standard), 2) clear and convincing evidence (a midlevel standard), and 3) evidence that is beyond a reasonable doubt (the highest standard where liberty is at stake). Given the total and permanent nature of termination of parental rights and the threatened loss to the familial bond that becomes irrevocable, the U.S. Supreme Court found that on one hand, the fair preponderance of the evidence standard that New York was using was too lenient to balance the risk of an erroneous finding; on the other hand, the risk to the child that might ensue by not terminating parental rights was potentially too high to make the points of concern too difficult to prove. Thus, the court found that the standard of proof that balances the parental rights, the fiscal and administrative interests in the costs of these proceedings, and the government's interest in supporting the welfare of the child requires at least the elevated clear and convincing evidence standard. The court's ruling meant that across the country, state laws can support a higher standard of beyond a reasonable doubt, but not a lower standard of proof of preponderance of the evidence, to determine whether to terminate parental rights.

Removal from custody is increasingly associated with parental substance use (see Figure 6–1). Although such removal is not the same as termination of parental rights, it is a first step to that final legal decision. In understanding how the courts will determine whether to terminate parental rights, it is also important to note that risk factors for termination of parental rights among parents who have substance use challenges have been identified. This means that together, SUDs can increase the risk of removal of the child from custody and can compound the risk for termination of parental rights. Of course, children must live in safe environments and society must protect them. However, removal of children from biological families comes at costs in different ways, and the ideal situation would be to develop means to prevent removals and keep children safe and families intact. Thus, working to treat substance use among parents should be a primary prevention effort on many levels. Risks for termination of parental rights for parents with substance use challenges include having younger children, parental incarceration, lack of treatment progress, co-occurring mental

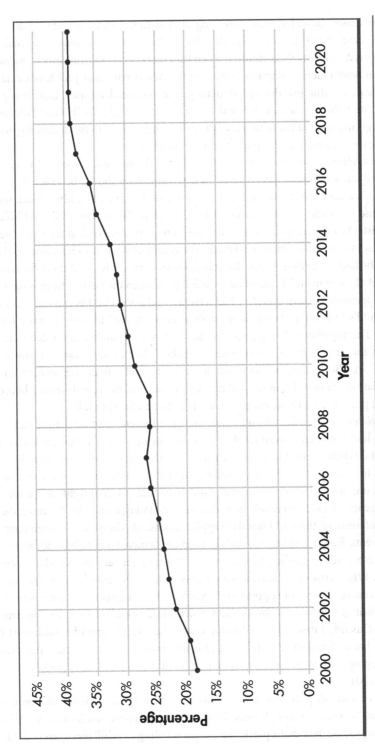

**Figure 6–1.** The percentage of children in out-of-home care with parental alcohol or other drug abuse as a condition associated with removal has steadily increased from 18.5% in 2000 to 39.1% in 2021.

*Note.* Estimates based on all children in out-of-home care at some point during the fiscal year.

*Source.* National Center on Substance Abuse and Child Welfare 2023.

health issues, homelessness, parenting skill deficits, and domestic violence (Hong et al. 2014). A review reported that mothers who used substances had a greater risk of losing their children when they had criminal justice involvement, mental health factors, ongoing substance use of a particularly problematic nature (e.g., cocaine use during pregnancy, intravenous drug use), lack of supports, or failure to attain prenatal care (Canfield et al. 2017). Generally, in making custody determinations, courts will examine the parent's failure to provide a safe and nurturing environment for the child.

In a related case, *Painter v. Bannister* (1966), the appellate court in Iowa examined what standard was required to determine who should be granted custody of a minor child. Harold Painter was married with two children when his wife and one child died in a motor vehicle accident. His in-laws (Mr. and Mrs. Bannister) took care of the surviving child while Painter tried to recover from his loss. After a time, Painter asked for the return of his son to his custody. By then, he had remarried. When the grandparents refused, he sued them for custody. Although the trial court first awarded custody to the father, the grandparents appealed, arguing that they had a right to raise the child because it was in the child's best interests for them, with a more "stable" lifestyle, to raise the child. The appellate court applied the "best interests" standard and ruled in favor of the grandparents. They noted that the father's home was "unconventional, arty, Bohemian" and although it was likely intellectually stimulating, the appellate court found that the stability and security of the grandparents' home would provide a better developmental environment for the child.

*Painter* has been criticized because the grandparents had no natural rights, and it had not been proven by clear and convincing evidence that the father's parental rights needed to be terminated. Whether this case would have been found for the grandparents if the suing parent at the time had been the mother is also unknown. However, one could speculate that paternal rights at the time the case was decided were not viewed as they are today. Generally, however, the best-interests-of-the-child standard applies to custody decisions between natural parents. Recent legal trends offer grandparents increasing rights within state laws, especially regarding visitation and at times related to custody (Justia 2022). When custody is at issue for parents with SUDs, grandparents may become central figures of support and may have legal rights for various actions with their grandchildren. In addition, federal legislation, such as the Uniform Child-Custody Jurisdiction and Enforcement Act (1997), provides guidance to states that adopted their own laws and is designed to deter interstate parental kidnapping and promote uniform management of custody and visitation cases (Hoff 2001).

In custody disputes involving a parent with an SUD, evidence of ongoing use may be sought through periodic drug testing. These results may then be used to provide data that a particular parent is failing to fulfill their parental duties. Judges can also impose conditions on parents, such as avoiding use of substances immediately before or during visits or requiring supervised visitation only (Gjelten 2023). Drug or alcohol use itself may not result in a loss of custody but can point to concerns. Behaviors that create unsafe situations, such as arrests for driving under the influence or evidence of child neglect, would be more likely to result in a loss of custody. Parental fitness examinations and evaluations of parents facing termination of parental rights proceedings are complex, given that they involve both functional areas and an understanding of how functioning intersects with contextual factors (Azar et al. 1998). Forensic psychiatrists embarking on conducting these examinations need to understand the local laws, the standards used by judges in that jurisdiction, and other factors (Azar et al. 1998). Child psychiatry and children's mental health expertise are also important in many cases involving custody evaluations that examine, for example, child-parent bonding and child development issues.

# Child Welfare Systems and Considerations of Child Abuse and Neglect

Child protection in the United States has a long and complex history. Myers (2008) described three major phases of its evolution, beginning in colonial times when child protection was not structured but laws allowed for child removal when parents did not "train" their children properly. The laws then evolved from the late 1870s to the mid-1960s, when organized child protection grew through nongovernmental societies established for the welfare of children. Myers (2008) noted a third modern era when government protections and systems grew in each state starting in 1962. By way of background, in the 1960s, there was a significant rise in attention to child abuse. Pediatric radiologist C. Henry Kempe, M.D., coined the term *battered-child syndrome* after viewing x-rays of classic injuries sustained related to physical abuse of children (Kempe et al. 1985). Medical interest in child abuse was growing before that and was discussed in the academic literature. For example, Caffey (1946) reported on a case involving a child with multiple fractures and a subdural hematoma. In *Landeros v. Flood* (1976), the California Supreme Court found that physicians should be able to suspect and diagnose child abuse and then should be required to report it to proper authorities. Thus, the 1960s and 1970s saw an increase in the identification and reporting of child abuse through medical professionals.

The wave that began in 1962 stemmed from federal activity in this space, in parallel to the growing interest in child abuse identification by medical professionals. In 1962, Congress amended the Social Security Act, codifying child protective services as part of all child welfare and requiring states to develop children's protection services (Myers 2008). The amendment also provided Title IV-E funding to states for their child welfare services. State legislation requirements for child abuse reporting (influenced by Kempe and others) came into being around the same time, and they were first passed in 1963 but authorized as law in all states by 1967. With child abuse reporting on the rise, the child welfare system of protection developed.

Child welfare systems developed across two major components: 1) to receive reports of abuse and investigate them and 2) to protect children from abuse, even if it meant removal from their home. Foster care became the answer to those removals. Although emphasis is always on individuals of natural biological relation taking care of children in need, non-kinship-based foster services have also developed.

With the development of child protection services came tensions in terms of keeping children in their natural environments while shoring up those environments by giving parents the tools they need to do better versus removing children from unsafe situations. Specific tensions in regard to *removal* (taking a child from their natural supports), *preservation* (keeping a child within a family to keep the family whole), and *reunification* (bringing removed children back to their natural supports), as well as pressures to establish adoption as *permanency* to foster child stability, all contribute to the pushes and pulls tugging at children in child welfare services. States are frequently sued for leaning too far in one direction or another, often after a reunification decision or failure to remove a child goes awry with a highly publicized poor outcome for a child.

In the landmark case of *DeShaney v. Winnebago* (1989), the U.S. Supreme Court ruled that it is not a violation of the Fourteenth Amendment when a state does not intervene from protecting people from actions of private parties, even if the private parties affect an individual's safety. In that case, a child was suspected to have been seriously physically abused by his father, and the social services agency did not remove the child from the father's custody. The child eventually experienced serious brain injury. The social services agency was sued under a 42 U.S.C. § 1983 civil rights claim, arguing that the child's liberty interest in bodily integrity and substantive Fourteenth Amendment due process rights had been violated when they did not intervene to protect him. The court, however, held that the state was not in violation because there was no constitutional requirement to prevent violence from a private actor, making a distinction between what happens in a private home versus a state-sponsored institution.

Child abuse protection issues and child welfare system laws are often highly relevant in the context of SUDs. According to national data, cases of child removals from homes due to alcohol or drug abuse have risen markedly, from 18.5% in 2000 to 39.1% in 2021 (National Center on Substance Abuse and Child Welfare 2023) (see Figure 6-1). Although prevalence rates vary across studies (Seay 2015), it is estimated that 50%–80% of parents in the child welfare system have substance use problems. Families with caregiver substance use face numerous challenges in child welfare, from investigation to removal and reunification, and they have a range of other complicated outcomes (Canfield et al. 2017; Marsh and Smith 2011).

There is growing interest in and focus on helping to enhance the potential for children to remain in their natural environments with the proper supports. One review, for example, highlighted innovative interventions that use trauma-informed addiction treatments to help improve outcomes for families (Bosk et al. 2019). One of the challenges in providing integrated services, however, relates to the different structures of the child welfare system and public substance use services, with some authors suggesting that a more integrated approach is needed to better serve families (Marsh and Smith 2011).

Federal legislation is also relevant beyond child abuse and children's protective services. The Child Abuse Prevention and Treatment Act (1974) requires states to have procedures and policies for the protection of suspected child abuse and neglect. This act requires states to have policies and procedures that include referral to child protection and other services when babies are born with evidence of being affected by substance use (e.g., neonatal abstinence syndrome or fetal alcohol syndrome). Thus, when babies are born with these circumstances, mandated reporting becomes the rule. As noted earlier in this chapter and reviewed here briefly, the issue is more complicated and more varied when a pregnant woman is using substances, because the landscape of mandated reporting in those circumstances varies from state to state, as shown in a survey by Jarlenski and colleagues (2017). In that survey, 20 states had laws requiring health care providers to report perinatal substance use to children's protection services, and 4 states had laws requiring such reporting only when there was belief that there was actual child maltreatment. Thirteen states with reporting laws had provisions that promoted SUD treatment. Thus, for the clinical case described in the Forensic Dilemma at the start of this chapter, it is important to consider the laws in one's particular state. Practitioners should explore whether mandated reporting would also include laws offering protections and referrals to treatment or would be more punitive in nature. Mandated reporting would obviously not be optional, but in terms of treatment alliance and patient care, it might help to understand the implications of such a report.

Given the high prevalence of substance use among families involved in child welfare services, it is also helpful to understand some additional areas of law related to removal of children from their home. The Adoption and Safe Families Act (1997) was passed by Congress to help facilitate better approaches to parental substance use for those involved in child welfare services. The act was seen as a major change in child protection policy when it was passed. Part of the Adoption and Safe Families Act came about because children were held in foster care for long periods in order for parents to prove that the environment was safe enough for reunification; this limbo period then precluded the children from being assigned permanent placements (also known as *permanency determinations*). The law then required custodial decisions to be made more quickly, to get to the goals of adoption permanency or reunification. If the parental environment was determined to be unsafe, the move toward termination of parental rights would need to ensue. Some have noted how the Adoption and Safe Families Act philosophy promoted child permanency (identification of a permanent home for the child) over biological family preservation and facilitation of parental rehabilitation (Marsh and Smith 2011). The law has specific provisions that allow agencies to forgo "reasonable efforts" to prevent removal under certain circumstances, and they must file termination of parental rights petitions if a child has been in foster care for 15 of the most recent 22 months. Furthermore, states are given financial incentives for successful adoptions, with greater financial incentives when the adoption is of a child with special needs (Public Broadcasting Service 2003).

Another important factor regarding child welfare practices is the systemic racial and ethnic disproportionality of child removals and other disparities across the child welfare system. Removal rates of Native American children have been very high historically. As a result, the Indian Child Welfare Act (1978) was passed with a number of provisions, including that Native American child welfare court proceedings were heard whenever possible in tribal courts, that tribes had a right to intervene in state court proceedings, that there were more specific guidelines for reunification and placement of Native American children, and that grants would be made available to assist with related child welfare services (Child Welfare Information Gateway 2023). Additionally, African American families are overrepresented in reports of suspected maltreatment: they are subjected to child protective service investigations at rates higher than other families, and their children have a higher likelihood of being removed from home (Child Welfare Information Gateway 2021). There has been increasing attention to these issues, and evidence is emerging in regard to interventions to improve child welfare outcomes that can help preserve Black families when SUDs are involved (Huebner et al. 2021). Recognizing that the risk of disparities in SUDs themselves disproportionately criminalizes Black individuals (see Chapter 10), it is all the more important to evaluate disparities in child welfare and how families may be disproportionately affected toward prosecution for "child abuse" related to SUDs, in lieu of remedies that direct parents toward treatment that could help facilitate safe reunification.

At the state level, several efforts have been made to improve outcomes for families when a caregiver is using substances. In 2018, the child welfare code in Kentucky was amended to factor in parental drug use during pregnancy, requiring a mother with a child born with neonatal abstinence syndrome to enroll in a drug treatment program within 90 days and to keep appointments for postnatal care or risk petitions for termination of parental rights (Coleman 2019). Although these efforts are framed as a way to encourage treatment, the risks to the family of nonadherence are high. Other states have developed interventions aimed to reduce the effects of substance use in pregnant women on themselves and their children. In Texas, the Pregnant and Parenting Intervention provides a multitude of resources, ranging from case management to education and support for families struggling with substance use (Texas Health and Human Services Commission 2023). A Montana law was passed that protects pregnant women by offering "safe harbor from prosecution" when they seek addiction treatment (Coleman 2019; Safe Harbor Act 2019).

Medications for addiction treatment have been recognized federally as important and allowable treatments for parents. For example, the Office of Civil Rights reached a voluntary resolution in West Virginia in an investigation of the state children's services agency. A couple was denied custody of their niece because one of them was prescribed Suboxone and had a history of OUD. The couple filed a complaint, claiming that the denial was a violation of both the Americans With Disabilities Act (1990; ADA) and the Rehabilitation Act (1973) (Legal Action Center 2022). The agreement mandated revised policies and staff training about the medications as proper treatments. The U.S. Department of Justice sent letters clarifying that courts prohibiting medication-assisted treatment as a condition of child custody or visitation were possibly engaging in practices that were in violation of the ADA (Legal Action Center 2019). Although these examples of rights-driven policy advances are promising, scholars have noted several remaining gaps regarding prevention and expansion of treatment opportunities and access for women with SUDs, particularly OUD, surrounding their reproductive years (Saunders et al. 2018). As more research emerges on the importance of treating and examining SUDs across a generation and on providing whole-family care, such laws and policies may become more common.

# Special Issues in Pregnancy and Addiction: Delivery, Shackles, and Correctional Practice

SUDs among pregnant individuals raise many hurdles, not the least of which is access to treatment. Even if treatment is available, pregnant women's fears that their substance use will be detected and that they will be prosecuted or face termination of parental rights become barriers to care (Stone 2015). Although many state policies are evolving to align with the disease model of addiction (as noted throughout this chapter and book), state policy views toward pregnant women with addiction remain punitive in many places (Coleman 2019; Davis 2020). Physician attitudes have also been studied, with research showing that just over half of physicians support mandated reporting of substance use during pregnancy as child abuse but also support treatment over criminalization (Abel and Kruger 2002).

On the provider side, turning away pregnant women with SUDs from care may occur for many reasons. Some states have passed laws that forbid certain substance use treatment providers from declining care to individuals because they are pregnant. Unfortunately, one study (Davis et al. 2022) showed that such laws did not yield better outcomes for pregnant patients in accessing SUD care. Davis et al. (2022) suggested that states should consider expanding such laws to all treatment providers and monitoring compliance with these provisions. SUD providers should be aware of whether such laws exist in their state and, regardless, should not decline care to individuals just because they are pregnant, although they may benefit from clinical consultation with an obstetrician or gynecologist and SUD expert. In the Forensic Dilemma described at the start of this chapter, the individual may have had difficulty accessing care due to the barriers of finding treatment for substance-using pregnant individuals, but local laws may not allow her to be turned away. It may be useful to educate patients about these laws where they exist.

Given the high prevalence of individuals with SUDs in the correctional system, it is not surprising that issues for incarcerated pregnant women can be difficult to navigate. Laws and policies related to incarcerated pregnant women and inmate labor and delivery are balanced against policies related to safety and security. SUD treatment for pregnant women in prison settings has a long history and is beyond the scope of this chapter. In short, methadone has traditionally been the mainstay of treatment. In recent years, more carceral settings are also offering buprenorphine to pregnant women. Unfortunately, following delivery, medications for these women (and for other inmates) are often stopped, and they are forced to go through withdrawal with symptom management "comfort" measures only. Clearly, this is another area of needed policy and practice development. In addition to these broad issues, in Chapter 10, we describe how SUDs are managed in correctional settings.

Of women who enter prison and jail, approximately 75% are mothers of minor children, and as many as 10,000 incarcerated women may be pregnant at any given time (Clarke and Adashi 2011). An estimated 2,000 babies are born annually to incarcerated women (Clarke and Simon 2013). Most correctional systems rely on external obstetrical and gynecological services to provide care for inmates, which may require transportation to outside clinics and hospitals for prenatal care and delivery.

Shackling of pregnant women during transport, labor, and delivery and after delivery is another area of legal regulation that has drawn attention (Clarke and Simon 2013). Some states have passed legislation prohibiting the use of restraints for pregnant women and women in labor, and others have passed similar policies. However, not all states enforce their own policies and laws, and 27 states regularly shackle pregnant women and women in labor (Clarke and Simon 2013). Shackles may be placed at the wrists, ankles, and even around the waist. This practice has been viewed as medically risky for both pregnant women and unborn children (American College of Obstetricians and Gynecologists 2011). Despite the ruling in *Estelle v. Gamble* (1976) stating that deliberate indifference of the health care needs of a prisoner constituted a constitutional violation under the Eighth Amendment, this shackling practice has continued in many places. In addition, many carceral settings will separate the newborn from the mother within 24 hours after delivery, which can be psychologically traumatizing and has been associated with heightened recidivism risk (Clarke and Simon 2013; Margolis and Kraft-Stolar 2006). Clarke and Simon (2013) reported that some states have established prison nursery units, and one state (Massachusetts) offers a community-based alternative. Also, prison and jail diversion programs for pregnant or postpartum women may be available.

Because of the high co-occurrence of trauma, SUDs, and criminal involvement and because many women entering into prisons and jails are in their reproductive years, more work is needed to examine the legal and regulatory parameters that can affect their well-being and that of their children. Practitioners, forensic evaluators, and systems consultants should understand the various laws and policies that may be at play and affect outcomes.

# Substance Use Among Children and Adolescents: Delinquency, Juvenile Court, and Legal and Regulatory Modulators and Responses

Substance use among children and adolescents is a major public health concern. The most recent data from the 2021 National Survey on Drug Use and Health (NSDUH) showed that 8.5% of adolescents ages 12–17 reported substance use that may meet criteria for an SUD (Substance Abuse and Mental Health Services Administration 2021). Screening starting at age 9 years is one way to try to prevent SUDs from emerging among youth or to address them early. The CDC reported that before the COVID-19 pandemic, approximately half of students between the ninth and twelfth grades had used marijuana, two-thirds of students had tried alcohol by twelfth grade, and about 20% of twelfth-graders had used prescription medication without a prescription (Jones et al. 2020). Furthermore, the earlier the use, the greater the likelihood of problems from substance use. The intergenerational impact of substance use is also critical: attention to fetal alcohol syndrome for girls and women of reproductive age, and recognizing it in early development, is of growing interest.

A host of downstream negative effects related to youth substance use can occur. For example, poor school performance, missed classes, and school dropout can be the beginning of a downward spiral; accidents, injuries, suicides, and other early deaths are often tragic realities for some. Co-occurring mental health issues also contribute to negative outcomes without treatment. For example, 2021 NSDUH data showed that adolescents ages 12–17 with a major depressive episode in the past year were more than twice as likely to have also used illicit drugs versus those without a major depressive episode (27.7% vs. 10.7%) (Substance Abuse and Mental Health Services Administration 2022). The multiple ways in which this can affect other areas of function is highlighted by one study reporting that young people truant from school engaged in more substance use, and the escalation of truancy affected escalation of substance use and was mediated in part by increased risky unsupervised time with peers (Henry and Thornberry 2010).

For practitioners working with children and adolescents with SUDs, it is important to recognize certain challenges, because these individuals may be at heightened risk of arrest and justice system involvement. One report identified that delinquent behavior and SUDs are tied together but also correlated with school and family problems, involvement with negative peer influences, poor neighborhood social controls, and exposure to physical and sexual abuse (Crowe and Bilchik 1998). A review of 2009–2014 NSDUH data showed that adolescents ages 12–17 with justice involvement had a significantly higher prevalence of SUDs, co-occurring mood disorders, and sexually transmitted infections and other health conditions; African American adolescents in the study were less likely to have substance use or mood disorders than physical health disorders (Winkelman et al. 2017). In a study by Holloway et al. (2022), peer deviancy as reported by caregivers predicted recidivism 2 years later, and alcohol use increased recidivism risk. The intersection of being of younger age, male gender, charged with a delinquent offense, and Black, Latinx, or of multiple races or ethnicities was also associated with recidivism. In a review of data from the National Longitudinal Youth Survey, antisocial behaviors in early adolescence (ages 14–15) were more highly correlated with late adolescent alcohol and drug use 4 years later (ages 18–19), especially for male individuals across several behaviors (but this was also true for female individuals, especially related to property offenses), and early adolescent substance use was a significant predictor of later alcohol and drug use (Windle 1990).

With regard to the intersection of youth substance use and law/regulation, it is important to have some background information. Separate legal interventions for youth with behavioral challenges date back more than 100 years with the emergence of the juvenile justice system, starting with the Cook County courthouse in Chicago (Center on Juvenile and Criminal Justice 2023). The goal of the juvenile system was to help attend to youth needs rather than provide punishment. Language in juvenile justice for actions that break laws that would be considered criminal by adults is distinct from adult language. For example, youth are found "delinquent," not guilty; their cases are given a "disposition," not a sentence. Although processes for youth were more informal originally, cases such as *In re Gault* (1967) and *Kent v. United States* (1966) gave youth more legal protections when involved in juvenile justice as the informal processes became fraught with more punitive approaches.

Separate from delinquency matters, there is a whole class of offenses that do not apply to adults. These are referred to as *status offenses* and include truancy, drinking underage, running away, being "incorrigible," not following parental or caretaker control, and violating curfew. They are not considered crimes or delinquency matters, but they are prohibited by law for minors and thus can lead to involvement of juvenile and family courts. Although desistance from these behaviors is most common (Office of Juvenile Justice and Delinquency Prevention 2015), these behaviors can be early warning signs that a young person may become criminally involved as an adult. Laws have been created to help society address these issues.

Truancy from school, for example, has been a focus of legal intervention ever since states began to establish mandated school attendance. Arrest powers for truancy followed, and by 1918, every state had mandatory school attendance laws (Goldstein 2015). Children in Need of Services (CHINS) (or Persons in Need of Supervision) laws became common and reflected systems in which parents, schools, and police could seek help when a child was engaging in risky behavior (Children's Law Center of Massachusetts 2023). Generally, parents and the child must meet with some state entity, such as a social service agent or probation officer, who works to resolve the issue and keep the child out of court (often called *diversion*). If this effort is unsuccessful, the pathway opens for the filing of a petition to ask for a court order for legal supervision or mandated treatment for the child (American Academy of Pediatrics 2016).

CHINS petitions filed in court would then result in access to services and support. These petitions commonly involve youth with substance use needs, but often they can include involvement of child welfare and, at times, other consequences such as removal from the home or significantly escalating sanctions against the youth and family disruptions. Consequences for repeated school absence include being assigned a probation officer (initially seen as a means to access services and monitor adherence) and even being detained. Although the goal of CHINS petitions is to help children, families, and communities, responses over time range from prosecution to other sanctions. There is a push and pull with regard to best approaches, and one report indicated that sanctions are getting tougher (Goldstein 2015). At the same time, some states have embarked on CHINS reform (Children's Law Center of Massachusetts 2023) to help at-risk families and youth access services more directly. It is important for practitioners in their own jurisdiction to understand the available legal interventions, as well as their risks, benefits, and requirements, for court-involved young patients and the effects on their families.

# SUDs, the Education System, and the Law

Laws protecting the educational needs of children who may have serious emotional disturbances include Section 504 of the Rehabilitation Act (1973), which prohibits discrimination on the basis of disability for federal services. The ADA of 1990 (as amended in 2008) expanded protections for people with disabilities by prohibiting discrimination more uniformly (Americans With Disabilities Act 1990, 2008). Finally, the Individuals With Disabilities Education Act (2004; IDEA) mandated that public schools make available free and appropriate education in the least restrictive manner to all students, including those with disabilities (U.S. Department of Education 2023). IDEA requires public schools to develop and use an individualized education program (IEP) for each child, tailored to their unique needs. It is important to realize that alcohol and drug use are not specifically considered disabilities under the IDEA or Section 504 of the Rehabilitation Act (1973), yet a student's use of substances does not exclude them from the protections these laws provide, and students cannot be excluded from special education based on addiction (Konkler-Goldsmith and Lukach Bradley 2023).

In all of these laws, disabilities are defined, including that there must be a condition that causes impairment in major life activities. Although Section 504 excludes from the definition of disability a student actively engaged in illegal drug use, there may be exceptions for youth who are no longer using drugs but have SUDs and are in a rehabilitation program. Students using alcohol may be able to have Section 504 protections, but the school may also take disciplinary action against them, making the landscape quite complicated (U.S. Department of Education 2023). When IDEA applies to a youth who qualifies, emerging legal cases have pushed schools to maximize the potential success of any youth with a disability. In *Endrew F. v. Douglas County School District* (2017), the U.S. Supreme Court held that under IDEA, a public school must tailor an IEP to do more than the de minimus to enable a child to make progress specific to the child's unique circumstances. Although this case involved a youth with autism spectrum disorder, it marked a line that helped advocates push schools further for supports for similarly situated youth with unique needs to help those with disabilities meet developmental and academic milestones to the extent possible (McKenna 2017). Similarly, it is critical to keep in mind the high co-occurrence of SUDs and mental illness in youth and what these laws might mean for youth with needs that are not being met at school.

For the clinician treating a youth with an SUD, it may be important to con- nect with the child's school to see whether the patient has an IEP and to help inform its contours given the substance use issues that may be involved. Fur- thermore, there may be a benefit to the family securing an education advocate if complicated issues surface about whether the child or adolescent qualifies as having a disability, or if they seem to be excluded from protections due to ad- diction when they have other qualifying conditions. Other options to support youth with SUDs or co-occurring conditions in particular regions can include recovery high schools, which are set up specifically to address the needs of youth with these disorders (Association of Recovery Schools 2023). For foren- sic evaluators looking at whether a youth or family was given the proper sup- ports, understanding of these laws and their limits can be helpful. Working with specializing attorneys can be beneficial in applying clinical data to the le- gal parameters.

## Treatment Issues to Consider for Families and Youth

Weisleder (2004) pointed to inconsistencies in state laws with regard to the age at which minors can consent to substance use treatment and the information used to help write the underlying laws (Weisleder 2007). He noted, for example, that some states allow confidential SUD treatment to be granted to any minor of any age, whereas others have age specifications (such as 12–16) when a minor can consent on their own to confidential substance use care. In another review, Kerwin et al. (2015) examined state laws looking at parental and adolescent de- cision-making for mental health and substance use treatment. They found that parental consent was sufficient in most states for mental health treatment, more so than for substance use treatment, as well as inpatient versus outpatient treat- ment (Kerwin et al. 2015). On the youth side, the same study reported that state laws favored giving minors the right to access drug treatment without parental consent, even at younger ages than they could for mental health treatment. De- spite these differences, the authors noted that few adolescents seek drug treat- ment on their own and that parental pressure is associated with entering into treatment, even though parents are not commonly seeking it (Kerwin et al. 2015).

One challenging situation is when a parent consents, but a minor refuses to go to treatment. Kerwin et al. (2015) noted that even in states where a legally authorized representative can consent to treatment on behalf of a youth, the state may allow for the youth to discharge themselves from treatment, leaving parents to consider involving other peers and family to pressure the youth, call on the legal system (e.g., a CHINS petition) or religious leaders, transport children to other states with different legal allowances, or just accept that they cannot get their child into treatment (Kerwin et al. 2015).

Separate from consent to treatment is the issue of who can gain access to information about a youth's SUD treatment. Some states allow parental notification when a minor consents to treatment independently, although this may make young people less willing to enter treatment. Generally, confidentiality related to SUD treatment is governed by 42 C.F.R. Part 2, which is stricter than the Health Insurance Portability and Accountability Act of 1996. Part 2 requires specific consent, for example, rather than broad consent. Because laws allow minors to seek treatment for an SUD with or without a parent's involvement, the rules of confidentiality may restrict information access for caregivers and legally authorized individuals with parental responsibilities. In custody issues in divorce contexts, one parent may wish to keep information from another. In general, parents have the right to information equally (i.e., when that information is available and not otherwise protected, such as when a youth does not consent to sharing information in an SUD treatment context), but this can become complicated depending on the nature of the relationship of the parental figures.

In the landmark case of *United States v. Windsor* (2013), the U.S. Supreme Court held that federal prohibitions against recognizing same-sex marriage were unconstitutional, which allowed same-sex partners to sign consent on behalf of their incompetent or deceased spouse for disclosure of information under 42 C.F.R. Part 2 (Substance Abuse and Mental Health Services Administration 2022). This ruling is important to consider, as same-sex partners may seek to access information related to youth treatment.

Overall, practitioners should be aware of the legal options related to consenting to treatment for youth or parents with or without the youth's assent. They would do well to also know the state rules about their right to access information (even just the fact of the child being in treatment itself) for children and adolescents with SUDs. There are numerous barriers to helping young people with these conditions, although the laws may facilitate or deter treatment. Knowledge of the legal landscape may help provide clarity around the legal regulation of substance use treatment for youth in what can otherwise be a painful family situation.

# Conclusions

SUDs affect families and tear down family structures. Federal laws, state laws, and legal cases have established certain standards that set the stage for numerous ways in which people with SUDs are affected with regard to custody and child removal. Pregnant women with SUDs may need to be reported; in some states, they may be at risk of criminalization or at heightened risk of child removal, and perhaps ultimately, termination of parental rights. Achieving a balance between child welfare and protection and effecting positive treatment potential for people with SUDs is critical to maximizing safe and healthy environments for children and ensuring appropriate family preservation. Similarly, youth in need of substance use care should be able to access it early. Clinicians working with individuals with SUDs would do well to understand the laws related to SUDs and family systems and to help all patients understand the risks and realities of their ongoing substance use. At the same time, forensic experts should have an understanding of SUDs, the law, and family-related issues. The complex interplay of SUDs and child welfare, education, juvenile justice, and custody issues can lead to critical life-altering decisions for children and their parents and must not be taken lightly.

# Key Points

- Child removals are increasingly related to alcohol and drug use by parents, pointing to the need for improved access to treatment and supports to help promote safe family preservation.
- Termination of parental rights is a permanent decision for which substance use disorders (SUDs) can be a risk.
- Child custody decisions are based on the best interests of the child.
- Child abuse reporting laws vary across states with regard to substance use in pregnancy (separate from other child abuse that may be happening).
- Intentional harm caused to an unborn child (separate from abortion) can be criminalized. Some states have criminalized the use of substances by the pregnant mother.
- *Dobbs v. Jackson Women's Health Organization* (2022), the U.S. Supreme Court decision that reversed *Roe v. Wade* (1973), will have major implications with regard to abortion access, and women with SUDs may be particularly vulnerable to unwanted pregnancy, which will become another layer of challenge. Clinicians should stay abreast of evolving laws related to these issues in their jurisdictions.
- SUDs among youth are a serious concern, and many will have co-occurring mental health conditions.

- Juvenile justice, child welfare, education, and other systems all interplay and have various laws and regulations that can affect outcomes for children and families with SUD issues.

# References

Abel EL, Kruger M: Physician attitudes concerning legal coercion of pregnant alcohol and drug abusers. Am J Obstet Gynecol 186(4):768–772, 2002 11967505

Adoption and Safe Families Act of 1997 (P.L. 105–89)

American Academy of Pediatrics: Out-of-control teens: PINS petitions and the juvenile justice system. HealthyChildren.org, February 26, 2016. Available at: https://www.healthychildren.org/English/health-issues/conditions/emotional-problems/Pages/When-a-Teenager-is-Out-of-Control.aspx. Accessed January 15, 2023.

American College of Obstetricians and Gynecologists: ACOG Committee Opinion No. 511: health care for pregnant and postpartum incarcerated women and adolescent females. Obstet Gynecol 118(5):1198–1202, 2011 22015908

American College of Obstetricians and Gynecologists: ACOG Committee Opinion no. 711: opioid use and opioid use disorder in pregnancy. Obstet Gynecol 130(2):e81–e94, 2017 28742676

Americans With Disabilities Act of 1990 (P.L. 101–336), 104 Stat. 327 (codified as amended at 42 U.S.C. § 12101 note [2008])

Americans With Disabilities Act Amendments Act of 2008, 42 U.S.C. § 12101 note

Association of Recovery Schools: What is a recovery high school? Available at: https://recoveryschools.org/what-is-a-recovery-high-school/. Accessed January 15, 2023.

Azar ST, Lauretti AF, Loding BV: The evaluation of parental fitness in termination of parental rights cases: a functional-contextual perspective. Clin Child Fam Psychol Rev 1(2):77–100, 1998 11324303

Beltran v Strachota et al., Case No. 13-C-1101 (E.D. Wis. Sep. 30, 2014)

Bonbrest v Kotz, 65 F. Supp. 138 (D.D.C. 1946)

Bosk EA, Paris R, Hanson KE, et al: Innovations in child welfare interventions for caregivers with substance use disorders and their children. Child Youth Serv Rev 101:99–112, 2019 32831444

Boudreaux JM, Thompson JW: Maternal-fetal rights and substance abuse: gestation without representation. J Am Acad Psychiatry Law 43(2):137–140, 2015 26071501

Brice M, Generes WM: Dialectical behavior therapy (DBT) for addiction treatment. American Addiction Centers, September 14, 2022. Available at: https://americanaddictioncenters.org/therapy-treatment/dialectical-behavioral-therapy. Accessed on January 15, 2023.

Caffey J: Multiple fractures in the long bones of infants suffering from chronic subdural hematoma. AJR Am J Roentgenol 56(2):163–173, 1946 20995763

Canfield M, Radcliffe P, Marlow S, et al: Maternal substance use and child protection: a rapid evidence assessment of factors associated with loss of child care. Child Abuse Negl 70:11–27, 2017 28551458

Center on Juvenile and Criminal Justice: Juvenile justice history. Available at: https://www.cjcj.org/history-education/juvenile-justice-history. Accessed January 15, 2023.

Child Abuse Prevention and Treatment Act of 1974 (P.L. 93–247)

Child Welfare Information Gateway: Child Welfare Practice to Address Racial Disproportionality and Disparity. U.S. Department of Health and Human Services, 2021.
Available at: https://www.childwelfare.gov/pubs/issue-briefs/racial-
disproportionality/. Accessed January 15, 2023.

Child Welfare Information Gateway: Indian Child Welfare Act (ICWA). U.S. Department of Health and Human Services. Available at: https://www.childwelfare.gov/
topics/systemwide/diverse-populations/americanindian/icwa/. Accessed January
15, 2023.

Children's Law Center of Massachusetts: Children in Need of Services cases. Available at:
http://hbgc.org/phocadownload/Parents_Support/child%20in%20need%20of%20
services%20cases.pdf. Accessed January 16, 2023.

Clarke JG, Adashi EY: Perinatal care for incarcerated patients: a 25-year-old woman
pregnant in jail. JAMA 305(9):923–929, 2011 21304069

Clarke JG, Simon RE: Shackling and separation: motherhood in prison. Virtual Mentor
15(9):779–785, 2013 24021108

Coleman E: Many states prosecute pregnant women for drug use. New research says
that's a bad idea. The Center for Child Health Policy, Vanderbilt University Medical
Center, December 5, 2019. Available at: https://www.vumc.org/childhealthpolicy/
news-events/many-states-prosecute-pregnant-women-drug-use-new-research-
says-thats-bad-idea. Accessed January 16, 2023.

Crowe AH, Bilchik S: Drug identification and testing in the juvenile justice system: consequences of youth substance abuse. Office of Juvenile Justice and Delinquency
Prevention, May 1998. Available at: https://ojjdp.ojp.gov/sites/g/files/xyckuh176/
files/pubs/drugid/ration-03.html. Accessed November 8, 2023.

Davis CS, McNeer E, Patrick SW: Laws forbidding pregnancy discrimination in substance use disorder treatment are not associated with treatment access. J Addict
Med 16(3):364–367, 2022 34282081

Davis J: State laws treat mother's substance use during pregnancy as child abuse, but
should they? Council of State Governments, Midwestern Office, February 13, 2020.
Available at: https://csgmidwest.org/2020/02/13/state-laws-treat-mothers-
substance-use-during-pregnancy-as-child-abuse-but-should-they/. Accessed
November 8, 2023.

Desai RJ, Hernandez-Diaz S, Bateman BT, et al: Increase in prescription opioid use
during pregnancy among Medicaid-enrolled women. Obstet Gynecol 123(5):997–
1002, 2014 24785852

DeShaney v Winnebago Cty. Dept. Soc. Serv., 489 U.S. 189 (1989)

DeVille KA, Kopelman LM: Fetal protection in Wisconsin's revised child abuse law: right
goal, wrong remedy. J Law Med Ethics 27(4):332–342, 1999 11067615

Dietrich v Inhabitants of Northampton, 138 Mass. 14 (1884)

Dobbs v Jackson Women's Health Organization, 142 S. Ct. 2228 (2022)

Endrew F. v Douglas County School District, 580 U.S. 386 (2017)

Epstein J: The pregnant imagination, fetal rights, and women's bodies: a historical in-
quiry. Yale J Law Humanit 7:139–162, 1995

Estelle v Gamble, 429 U.S. 97 (1976)

Faherty LJ, Kranz AM, Russell-Fritch J, et al: Association of punitive and reporting state
policies related to substance use in pregnancy with rates of neonatal abstinence syndrome. JAMA Netw Open 2(11):e1914078, 2019 31722022

Gjelten EA: How alcohol and drug use affects custody decisions. DivorceNet. Available at: https://www.divorcenet.com/resources/how-alcohol-and-drug-use-affects-custody-decisions.html. Accessed January 15, 2023.

Goldstein D: Inexcusable absences. The New Republic, March 6, 2015. Available at: https://newrepublic.com/article/121186/truancy-laws-unfairly attack-poor-children-and-parents#:~:text=By%201918%2C%20every%20state%20had,as%20high%20school%20graduation%20rates. Accessed November 8, 2023.

Guttmacher Institute: State Responses to Substance Abuse Among Pregnant Women. Available at: https://www.guttmacher.org/sites/default/files/pdfs/tables/gr030603t.html. Accessed June 21, 2024.

Henry KL, Thornberry TP: Truancy and escalation of substance use during adolescence. J Stud Alcohol Drugs 71(1):115–124, 2010 20105421

Hirai AH, Ko JY, Owens PL, et al: Neonatal abstinence syndrome and maternal opioid-related diagnoses in the US, 2010–2017. JAMA 325(2):146–155, 2021 33433576

Hoff PM: The Uniform Child-Custody Jurisdiction and Enforcement Act. Juvenile Justice Bulletin, December 2001. Available at: https://www.ojp.gov/pdffiles1/ojjdp/189181.pdf. Accessed November 8, 2023.

Holloway ED, Folk JB, Ordorica C, et al: Peer, substance use, and race-related factors associated with recidivism among first-time justice-involved youth. Law Hum Behav 46(2):140–153, 2022 35073113

Hong JS, Ryan JP, Hernandez PM, et al: Termination of parental rights for parents with substance use disorder: for whom and then what? Soc Work Public Health 29(6):503–517, 2014 25144693

Huebner RA, Willauer T, Hall MT, et al: Comparative outcomes for Black children served by the Sobriety Treatment and Recovery Teams program for families with parental substance abuse and child maltreatment. J Subst Abuse Treat 131:108563, 2021 34256968

In re Gault, 387 U.S. 1 (1967)

Indian Child Welfare Act of 1978, U.S.C. §§ 1901–1963

Individuals With Disabilities Education Act of 1990 (P.L. 100–76), 104 Stat. 1141 (codified as amended at 20 U.S.C. § 1400 [2004])

Jarlenski M, Hogan C, Bogen DL, et al: Characterization of U.S. state laws requiring health care provider reporting of perinatal substance use. Womens Health Issues 27(3):264–270, 2017 28129942

Johnson v State, 602 So.2d 1288 (Fla. 1992)

Jones CM, Clayton HB, Deputy NP, et al: Prescription opioid misuse and use of alcohol and other substances among high school students: Youth Risk Behavior Survey, United States, 2019. MMWR Suppl 69(1):38–46, 2020 32817608

Justia: Grandparent custody and visitation laws. Available at: https://www.justia.com/family/child-custody-and-support/child-custody/grandparent-custody-and-visitation/. Accessed October 1, 2022.

Kempe CH, Silverman FN, Steele BF, et al: The battered-child syndrome. Child Abuse Negl 9(2):143–154, 1985 3891032

Kent v United States, 383 U.S. 541 (1966)

Kerwin ME, Kirby KC, Speziali D, et al: What can parents do? A review of state laws regarding decision making for adolescent drug abuse and mental health treatment. J Child Adolesc Subst Abuse 24(3):166–176, 2015 25870511

Ko JY, D'Angelo DV, Haight SC, et al: Vital signs: prescription opioid pain reliever use during pregnancy: 34 U.S. Jurisdictions, 2019. MMWR Morb Mortal Wkly Rep 69(28):897–903, 2020 32673301

Konkler-Goldsmith H, Lukach Bradley J: Drug and alcohol abuse by students with disabilities. Available at: https://mcandrewslaw.com/publications-and-presentations/articles/drug-and-alcohol-abuse-by-students-with-disabilities/. Accessed January 15, 2023.

Landeros v Flood, 551 P.2d 389 (Cal. 1976)

Legal Action Center: Department of Justice Addresses MAT Discrimination. Washington, DC, U.S. Department of Justice, January 31, 2019. Available at: https://www.lac.org/resource/department-of-justice-addresses-mat-discrimination. Accessed November 8, 2023.

Legal Action Center: Cases Involving Discrimination Based on Treatment With Medication for Opioid Use Disorder (MOUD). Washington, DC, U.S. Department of Justice, January 12, 2022. Available at: https://www.lac.org/assets/files/Cases-involving-denial-of-access-to-MOUD.pdf. Accessed June 6, 2022.

Liu M, Hensley E: Mississippi County is prosecuting some pregnant women and new moms. Mississippi Today, May 11, 2019. Available at: https://mississippitoday.org/2019/05/11/delivering-justice/. Accessed November 8, 2023.

Margolis JK, Kraft-Stolar T: When "Free" Means Losing Your Mother: The Collision of Child Welfare and the Incarceration of Women in New York State. New York, Correctional Association of New York, February 2006. Available at: https://www.ojp.gov/ncjrs/virtual-library/abstracts/when-free-means-losing-your-mother-collision-child-welfare-and. Accessed November 8, 2023.

Marsh JC, Smith BD: Integrated substance abuse and child welfare services for women: a progress review. Child Youth Serv Rev 33(3):466–472, 2011 21499525

McKenna L: How a new Supreme Court ruling could affect special education. The Atlantic, March 23, 2017. Available at: https://www.theatlantic.com/education/archive/2017/03/how-a-new-supreme-court-ruling-could-affect-special-education/520662/. Accessed November 8, 2023.

Myers JEB: A short history of child protection in America. Fam Law Q 42(3):449–463, 2008

National Center on Substance Abuse and Child Welfare: Child Welfare and Substance Use Statistics. Rockville, MD, Substance Abuse and Mental Health Services Administration, 2023. Available at: https://ncsacw.acf.hhs.gov/research/child-welfare-statistics/interactive-statistics-series/1-2-prevalence-aod-removal/. Accessed November 7, 2023.

Office of Juvenile Justice and Delinquency Prevention: Status offenders literature review: a product of the Model Programs Guide. September 2015. Available at: https://ojjdp.ojp.gov/sites/g/files/xyckuh176/files/media/document/status_offenders.pdf. Accessed November 8, 2023.

Painter v Bannister, 140 N.W.2d 152 (Iowa 1966)

Patrick SW, Davis MM, Lehmann CU, et al: Increasing incidence and geographic distribution of neonatal abstinence syndrome: United States 2009 to 2012. J Perinatol 35(8):650–655, 2015 25927272

Public Broadcasting Service: Failure to protect: the Adoption and Safe Families Act of 1997. Frontline, 2003. Available at: https://www.pbs.org/wgbh/pages/frontline/shows/fostercare/inside/asfa.html. Accessed November 8, 2023.

Rehabilitation Act of 1973 (P.L. 93–112), 97 Stat. 355 (codified as amended at 29 U.S.C. § 701)

Roe v Wade, 410 U.S. 113 (1973)

Safe Harbor Act of 2019, S.B. 289 (Mon.)

Santosky v Kramer, 455 U.S. 745 (1982)

Saunders JB, Jarlenski MP, Levy R, et al: Federal and state policy efforts to address maternal opioid misuse: gaps and challenges. Womens Health Issues 28(2):130–136, 2018 29183818

Seay K: How many families in child welfare services are affected by parental substance use disorders? A common question that remains unanswered. Child Welfare 94(4):19–51, 2015 26827475

Stone R: Pregnant women and substance use: fear, stigma, and barriers to care. Health Justice 3:2, 2015

Substance Abuse and Mental Health Services Administration: Highlights for the 2021 National Survey on Drug Use and Health. 2021. Rockville, MD, Substance Abuse and Mental Health Services Administration. Available at: https://www.samhsa.gov/data/sites/default/files/2022-12/2021NSDUHFFRHighlights092722.pdf. Accessed December 2, 2022.

Substance Abuse and Mental Health Services Administration: Substance Abuse Confidentiality Regulations: Frequently Asked Questions (FAQs) and Fact Sheets Regarding the Substance Abuse Confidentiality Regulations. Rockville, MD, Substance Abuse and Mental Health Services Administration. Available at: https://www.samhsa.gov/about-us/who-we-are/laws-regulations/confidentiality-regulations-faqs. Accessed June 17, 2022.

Texas Health and Human Services Commission: Pregnant and parenting intervention. January 15, 2023. Available at: https://www.hhs.texas.gov/services/mental-health-substance-use/adult-substance-use/pregnant-parenting-intervention. Accessed November 8, 2023.

Unborn Victims of Violence Act of 2004 (P.L. 108–212), 118 Stat. 568 (codified at 18 U.S.C. 1841 note)

Uniform Child-Custody Jurisdiction and Enforcement Act of 1997, 9(1A) U.L.A. 657 (1999)

United States v Windsor, 570 U.S. 744 (2013)

U.S. Department of Education: Individuals With Disabilities Education Act: about IDEA. 2023. Available at: https://sites.ed.gov/idea/about-idea/. Accessed January 15, 2023.

Weisleder P: The right of minors to confidentiality and informed consent. J Child Neurol 19(2):145–148, 2004 15072109

Weisleder P: Inconsistency among American states on the age at which minors can consent to substance abuse treatment. J Am Acad Psychiatry Law 35(3):317–322, 2007 17872552

Windle M: A longitudinal study of antisocial behaviors in early adolescence as predictors of late adolescent substance use: gender and ethnic group differences. J Abnorm Psychol 99(1):86–91, 1990 2307771

Winkelman TNA, Frank JW, Binswanger IA, et al: Health conditions and racial differences among justice-involved adolescents, 2009 to 2014. Acad Pediatr 17(7):723–731, 2017 28300655

Wolfe EL, Davis T, Guydish J, et al: Mortality risk associated with perinatal drug and alcohol use in California. J Perinatol 25(2):93–100, 2005 15496968

# CHAPTER 7

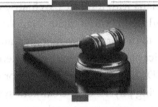

# PRACTICAL ASPECTS OF CIVIL CASE EVALUATIONS INVOLVING SUBSTANCE USE DISORDERS

## Introduction

Numerous issues in civil litigation come before the courts in which substance use and substance use disorders (SUDs) are at issue. For example, one common civil case evaluation for a forensic psychiatrist is a personal injury matter involving the use of particular substances and the aftermath. In this litigation, the courts are looking for whether there was intentional or negligent infliction of emotional distress, which necessitates attaching responsibility for an injury to the responsible agencies, the plaintiff themselves, or some combination thereof. This difficult task often warrants exploration of the nature of volition in addictive disorders, the growing understanding of the biological bases for SUDs, and the requirement for self-mitigation of consequences for the person with an SUD.

Civil cases for driving under the influence (DUI) offenses, usually demanding compensation for an injured party or property damage, can be brought against individuals who may or may not also have been convicted of DUI charges in a criminal court. The rapidly changing legal responses to cannabis in the United States have promoted similarly rapid change in law enforcement's response to drivers who are (or appear to be) intoxicated with cannabis. When there is a question as to whether a decedent took their own life in the context of substance use or direct suicidal thinking and intent, psychological autopsies are best carried out by clinicians with forensic psychiatric expertise who are proficient in the diagnosis and treatment of dually diagnosed individuals and have an understanding of how to perform a psychological autopsy. Malpractice cases examining clinical practices also arise frequently when the treatment revolved around patients with SUDs in which there was a poor outcome that the plaintiffs ascribe to the practicing physician or treatment system. Suicide, substance use, and addictive conditions often run together, sometimes eliciting legal disputes about whether the care delivered to the decedent was at or above the minimum standard of care. Larger tort matters, often involving class action suits against pharmaceutical manufacturers, require an understanding of the science of the matter but also the economics, politics, and public health policy as they relate to SUDs. Numerous civil litigations have arisen in recent years regarding the lack of treatment for SUDs within carceral settings.

All of these are just some examples in which civil law and psychiatry related to SUDs run together. This chapter provides a review of these issues.

## FORENSIC DILEMMA

A 43-year-old male bartender driving home from his 5 P.M. to 2 A.M. shift sustained serious back and neck injuries when he drove through a malfunctioning traffic light and another car struck his car from the side. The bartender sued the local village, claiming that the malfunctioning traffic light caused him to drive into a busy intersection, although others had successfully navigated the same intersection moments earlier. Attorneys for the village point out that the bartender acknowledged having had two or three 12-oz beers over the course of his shift, and his blood alcohol level (BAL) was 0.04 mg/dL in a nonforensic blood test drawn in the emergency department 3 hours after the accident. He has not been charged with DUI or any other criminal charge.

Consider the following:

1. What was the bartender's BAL at the time of the accident?
2. Who would be useful collateral informants in this matter?

In court, defense attorneys for the village present a publicly available chart (Gillette 2023) that reads, "Your body can get rid of one drink per hour." They reason that the bartender's BAL would have been above the legal limit for driving at the time of the accident, and this made him liable for the accident.

3. What would be a more accurate method for estimating the bartender's BAL at the time of the accident?
4. What role might physiological tolerance play in this matter?

Useful collateral informants would be anyone in the bar who witnessed and could testify to how much alcohol the bartender had actually consumed, reliable informants on the bartender's demeanor when he left the bar and got into his car, and the police officers and emergency medical services personnel who saw him after the accident.

> The plaintiff's attorneys counter that an actual retrospective estimation of the bartender's BAL would necessitate using the Widmark equation, including the variables of the bartender's gender and weight, and having certain knowledge of the grams of alcohol he had consumed and precisely when he had consumed them (Maskell et al. 2017). Their expert witness, a toxicologist, estimates that the bartender's ingestion of even three 12-oz beers over the course of the evening would have resulted in a BAL below the legal driving limit at the time of the accident. In addition, the toxicologist points out that the bartender habitually drinks several 12-oz beers during his shift, he has never had any legal or other consequences resulting from his drinking, and no witness can recall him appearing impaired by alcohol, ever. The bartender's tolerance to alcohol, the toxicologist opines, would have rendered him clinically—if not legally—sober at the time of the accident.

# Personal Injury Involving SUDs

As demonstrated in this chapter's Forensic Dilemma, legal responsibility for injuries associated with substance use is often determined in the civil court system. Unquestionably, people who use mind-altering substances have an elevated risk of injury and death in the workplace (Coggon et al. 2010) and elsewhere (Cherpitel et al. 2012). The question of how much of this use is under the user's volitional control is fascinating and elicits academic papers quoting Socrates and Coleridge (Campbell 2003) as well as closely argued treatises defending (Leshner 1997) or attacking (Heyman 2013) the brain disease model of SUDs. However, legal disputes require concrete decisions that assign responsibility for injuries, so the decisions are necessarily much more prosaic, as the following examples show.

Personal injury claims involving alcohol or drug use must make some assessment of how the substance use affected the parties. In a case governed by international law, which was (literally) in the slip-and-fall category, a cruise passenger slipped on some liquids on the dance floor of the *Norwegian Sky* and injured his shoulder (*Salazar v. Norwegian Cruise Lines Holdings, Ltd. et al.* 2016a, 2016b). His lawsuit alleged that in failing to clean up the wet floor, the ship crew's negligence directly caused his shoulder injury. Attorneys for the cruise line claimed that plaintiff Salazar acknowledged having imbibed three to four beers before dinner and two glasses of wine at dinner, rendering him intoxicated and responsible for the fall. Although the cruise line was granted summary judgment because the liquid spill was "open and obvious" and Salazar had not demonstrated that the cruise line knew about the spill, his likely intoxication would have been the cruise line's main argument in avoiding culpability had the case proceeded.

Parties to a personal injury case may argue that alcohol or drug use affected the events, although courts may treat the substance use as so irrelevant and unfairly prejudicial as to require exclusion from the case. Intoxication and impairment are quite distinct from the use of intoxicating substances. For example, in *Bedford v. Moore* (2005b), truck driver Rita Moore was accused of causing a fatal accident after she struck Edwin Bedford's car with the gravel truck she was driving. Although many other issues were involved, Moore's postaccident drug screen was positive for methamphetamine in her system, which an expert witness testified was "at least a minute amount" of drug. The expert witness was not allowed to testify about how that amount of drug would affect most individuals and did not opine that the methamphetamine had actually affected Moore's ability to drive. In excluding the expert's testimony, the trial judge wrote the following:

> [The expert] could not tie the presence of methamphetamines in Moore's body to impairment at the time of the accident, and therefore could not connect the presence of the drug to causation. Further, because [the expert] could not identify any particular level of the drug in Moore's system at the time of the accident or state that the amount of the drug in her system was at a level at which any impairment could be adduced, there was no evidence that the presence of the drug was a causative factor in the accident. (*Bedford v. Moore* 2005a)

Evidence of use of a potentially addictive drug, which could certainly cause impairment at some dosages, was determined to be inappropriate for presentation to the jury.

Although the court excluded a positive drug test result and presumptive use as irrelevant in *Bedford*, other cases have been resolved differently. In *Harris v. Kubota Tractor Corp.* (2006), the plaintiff injured himself while removing a rotary tiller from his tractor, to the point of needing a leg amputation. Although Harris initially denied using any drugs during the previous week, a urine drug screen revealed the presence of cocaine metabolites and cannabinoids. Harris argued that these urine drug screen results should be withheld from the jury because they were unfairly prejudicial, as they related to his past (preaccident) drug use and did not show that he was impaired at the time of the accident. Because Harris's method of removing the rotary tiller was "contrary to common sense" (the tiller was in operation and elevated), his state of mind at the time of the accident was an important issue for the jury to consider. Therefore, the previous positive drug screen and Harris's apparent prevarication about his own drug use were relevant. In short, according to the presiding judge, "the probative value of the evidence is not substantially outweighed by the prejudice it may cause. Hence, the test results are relevant, probative, and admissible in this case" (*Harris v. Kubota Tractor Corp.* 2006).

In addition to arguments about the causation of an injury, evidence of an SUD can be used to mitigate the cost of damages. In *Zwinge v. Neylan* (2017) in Canada, plaintiff Zwinge, a 46-year-old man who earned a living installing drywall, was injured in a head-on collision with defendant Neylan. No alcohol was involved in the crash, but the plaintiff had multiple physical injuries from the crash as well as depression, PTSD, and anxiety. However, given the plaintiff's long history of alcohol problems, the defendant argued that the plaintiff's ongoing use of alcohol reduced his earning potential and slowed his recovery from his injuries to the point that the plaintiff was not taking reasonable measures to cure the various injuries for which he was seeking compensation. Therefore, the defense argued that plaintiff showed a "failure to mitigate damages," which then should pave the way for a decrease in monetary damages awarded. Although the judge agreed that the ongoing alcohol use should be considered, he observed that the plaintiff's work had been only marginally affected by his alcohol problems, he had received treatment in 2013, and his drinking had been "somewhat moderated" in the months before the accident. As such, evidence of the plaintiff's alcohol use was excluded.

# Driving Under the Influence: Alcohol and Cannabis

The majority of U.S. arrests for DUI are related to alcohol, although the rolling legalization and decriminalization of cannabis may change that proportion. In any case, injuries and deaths associated with alcohol-related DUIs can result in legal action in criminal and civil courts, and clinical experts, including addiction specialists, are often called on to review records, render opinions, and sometimes testify. In 2019, 10,142 Americans died in drunk-driving accidents; although the number of fatalities has been decreasing over the past 10 years, the death and devastation remains staggering (National Highway Traffic Safety Administration 2022). *Intoxication* itself is a broad term, but legally 49 U.S. states define a blood alcohol concentration (BAC) of 0.8 mg/dL as intoxication for the purpose of DUI criminal charges; Utah has set a limit at 0.5 mg/dL. Notwithstanding these legal limits, 1,775 people died in 2019 in accidents in which the driver had a BAC of 0.1–0.7 mg/dL, below the generally accepted level for legal intoxication with alcohol.

Although law enforcement officers may use blood, saliva, and urine tests in traffic stops, interpretation of the results can be quite complex. For example, forced drawing of a blood sample is generally not done because it contradicts the Fourth Amendment right for freedom from unwarranted search and seizure and would require a warrant; an individual could theoretically volunteer to give their blood sample at the time of a police stop. Standardized field sobriety tests (SFSTs) are allowable. When a person agrees to such a test, they are implying consent; without agreement, license violations can be issued. SFSTs are described in manuals produced by the National Highway Traffic Safety Administration (NHTSA) and the International Association of Chiefs of Police (National Highway Traffic Safety Administration 2018). In addition to tests of the driver (described later in this chapter), stops for DUI themselves can be challenged related to road conditions, officer actions, and other factors. Nevertheless, experts examining civil litigation for either the prosecution or defense should understand some of the tests used and clinical aspects of these matters.

The use of breath alcohol levels is very common in police traffic stops. Since modern breathalyzer technology was first developed in 1954, it has faced multiple legal challenges, some fanciful and some quite effective. Unlike the inexpensive breathalyzers available on the retail market, those that function at the level necessary for law enforcement purposes are termed *evidential breath test* (EBT) devices (Swotinsky 2015). EBTs use fuel cell technology to produce an electric current to break down alcohol molecules, infrared spectrometry, or gas chromatography and cost $1,500 to $7,000. Production of stored results and a printed readout are mandatory, although a U.S. Supreme Court ruling determined that there is no need to retain the breath sample itself (*California v. Trombetta* 1984).

Legal challenges to EBT results typically focus on operator training, anomalies in device maintenance or calibration, testee use of mouthwash or candies just before the test, or arguments about the legal justification for the "search" implied by the EBT itself. In one New Jersey Supreme Court case (*State v. Cassidy* 2008) that essentially negated the results of more than 20,000 EBT tests, a state police sergeant was found to have falsified calibration records for the EBTs used in 5 of New Jersey's 21 counties. The presiding judge ruled that the responsible sergeant's failure to actually perform one of the steps in the calibration procedure contaminated the entire calibration, rendering invalid any tests done on those machines. The judge reasoned as follows:

> [P]roof of the good working order of the (EBT) device has been required as mandatory foundational evidence to allow a breath test reading in evidence

[and] that proof is established by the production of the coordinators' certification, attesting to the fact that he or she performed the calibration in accordance with all required procedures. (*State v. Cassidy* 2018)

The SFSTs developed by the NHTSA and administered by police officers usually consist of the horizontal gaze nystagmus test and the walk-and-turn and one-leg stand tests. Despite their ubiquity at late-night roadside traffic stops and their general acceptance in courtrooms, these tests have ambiguous scientific validation, at best. In a review of the tests' scientific and legal underpinnings, Rubenzer (200820082008, p. 293) concluded that "the research that supports their use is limited, important confounding variables have not been thoroughly studied, reliability is mediocre, and their developers and prosecution-oriented publications have oversold the tests." Although SFSTs have likely ensured the convictions of many intoxicated drivers, defense attorneys have made the obvious argument that medical, orthopedic, or obesity issues may interfere with the SFST results (Levow DWI Law 2022).

In addition to testimony about the accuracy and meaning of breathalyzers and SFST results, clinicians serving as experts can provide meaningful information about the estimated levels of risk for reoffending with subsequent DUI arrests. This type of sentence mitigation sometimes relies on advising the fact finder of the defendant's remorse, the addiction treatment they are receiving, and the reasons for the addictive condition in the first place. One published rubric for determining the likelihood of reoffending with an alcohol- or drug-related offense is promulgated by the Central States Institute on Addiction and categorizes levels of risk as follows (Cavaiola and Wuth 2022).

- *Minimal*: no prior convictions or court-ordered supervision for DUI; no prior statutory summary suspension; no prior reckless driving invocations reduced from DUI; a BAC of less than 0.15 g/dL at the time of the arrest for DUI; and not meeting diagnostic criteria for an SUD
- *Moderate*: no prior conviction or court orders or supervision for DUI; no prior statutory summary suspension; no prior reckless driving conviction reduced from DUI; a BAC of 0.15–0.19 g/dL or refusal of chemical testing at the time of the index DUI arrest; and not meeting diagnostic criteria for an SUD
- *Significant*: one prior conviction or court-ordered supervision for DUI, one prior statutory summary suspension, or one prior reckless driving conviction reducing DUI; and/or 0.20 g/dL or higher at the time of the index DUI and/or meeting diagnostic criteria for an SUD
- *High*: meeting diagnostic criteria for an SUD, no prior arrest
- *High+*: two prior convictions or court-ordered supervision for DUI, two prior statutory summary suspensions, or two prior reckless driving convic-

tions reduced from DUI within a 10-year period from the date of the most
current (third) arrest

- *High++*: meeting diagnostic criteria for an SUD and two prior convictions,
  or two prior statutory summary suspensions, or two prior reckless driving
  convictions reduced from DUI within a 10-year period from the date of the
  most current (third) arrest

DUI matters involving alcohol have produced a relatively well-documented
body of laws, regulations, and case law. For DUI offenses involving cannabis,
the rapidly changing legal structure in the United States around the drug has resulted in a confusing patchwork of driving laws and regulations, with few legal
precedents. The presence of an agreed-on national standard for driving while
under the influence of alcohol (usually 0.8 mg/dL) will likely not be matched
with legislation addressing driving while under the influence of cannabis. Because cannabis can remain detectable in human tissue long after intoxication
has passed, law enforcement faces a conundrum in trying to keep roads safe
while respecting the right of adults to engage in any legal behaviors they wish.

It is clear from laboratory simulation studies (Hartman and Huestis 2013)
and studies of actual driving performance (Bondallaz et al. 2016) that cannabis
use impairs skills necessary for good driving, including psychomotor skills,
quick reflexes, ability to divide attention, lane tracking, and various cognitive
functions, at least among nonhabitual cannabis users (Brooks-Russell et al.
2021). A summary of the relevant data follows:

> [D]riving simulator tests have shown that drivers who are high on marijuana re-
> act more slowly, find it harder to pay attention, have more difficulty maintaining
> their car's position in the lane, and make more errors when something goes
> wrong than they do when they're sober. But such tests have also shown mari-
> juana-impaired drivers are likely to drive at lower speeds, make fewer attempts
> to overtake, and keep more distance between their vehicle and the one ahead of
> them. (Insurance Institute for Highway Safety 2021)

The actual effect of cannabis decriminalization and legalization on highway
safety and the subsequent change in population-wide cannabis use defy easy
quantification. One insurance industry study (Highway Loss Data Institute
2020) reviewed data through 2019 and examined the effect of cannabis legalization in four western states. The authors found that cannabis legalization was
associated with a statistically significant 3.8% increase in collision claim frequency, a measurement of the cost of crash damage to vehicles and property,
and injuries to people. Colorado, Washington, and Nevada had increases in collision claims, whereas Oregon showed a decrease.

In an analysis of drug tests performed on drivers involved in fatal car
crashes in Washington State during 2008–2019 (Tefft and Arnold 2021), the
proportion of drivers with a positive Δ-9-tetrahydrocannabinol (THC) screen

approximately doubled after the legalization of recreational cannabis in December 2012. The authors acknowledged that the base rate of cannabis use had, of course, also increased, and that the heavier cannabis use was statistically associated with fatal car crashes rather than necessarily causative of those crashes. Several reviews of large data sets appear to show that the combination of alcohol and cannabis intoxication confers greater risk than DUI of either substance alone (Lira et al. 2021; Sewell et al. 2009).

The toxicological determination of THC levels by law enforcement has been stymied by the absence of a well-tested, if challengeable, technology available for roadside alcohol testing. Although 24 states have statutes that authorize the use of oral fluid specimens for roadside drug testing, only a few have actual programs in place to do so. Alabama and Indiana regularly conduct these tests, Michigan has a program in five counties, and Colorado ran an oral testing program from 2015 to 2018 (National Conference of State Legislatures 2021).

Although the techniques available for law enforcement officers to recognize and document drug intoxication are nowhere near as codified as those for identifying alcohol intoxication, a substantial body of knowledge exists. For instance, certification of drug recognition experts (DREs) is under the aegis of the International Association of Chiefs of Police, with support from the NHTSA and the U.S. Department of Transportation (National District Attorneys Association 2020). Certification is earned in three phases, including DRE preschool, which takes 16 hours; DRE school, which takes 56 hours; and a required field certification, which takes 40 hours. This substantial educational process allows the expert (usually a police officer) to deliver an expert opinion as to 1) whether a particular examinee was so impaired that they should not operate a motor vehicle, 2) whether the impairment was due to drug use or an injury or medical problem, and 3) which drug or category of drugs would be most likely to cause the impairment.

The DRE arrives at those opinions by performing a breath alcohol test, an interview, and a directed observational examination of the individual involved, and they sometimes request further toxicological testing. Although the signs and symptoms of stimulant or opioid use are arguably more distinct than those for cannabinoids, the DRE is instructed to look for a lack of eye convergence and an inability to shift attention, suggestive of intoxication with cannabinoids.

An up-to-date listing of state marijuana laws is maintained by the Insurance Institute for Highway Safety (2024). A similar compilation focused on marijuana-impaired driving laws was created by the National Alliance to Stop Impaired Driving (2024). The state responses to cannabis on the roads vary widely (National Conference of State Legislatures 2021). Some states (Arizona, Delaware, Georgia, Indiana, Iowa, Michigan, Oklahoma, Pennsylvania, Rhode Island, South Dakota, Utah, and Wisconsin) have zero-tolerance laws, which consider any positive drug test result, including for THC, to be evidence of intoxication. Five states (Illinois, Montana, Nevada, Ohio, and Washington) have per se laws, which establish a legal THC limit of 2–5 ng/mL and automatically define any person with a drug test result above that level as intoxicated. Colorado has a "reasonable inference" law, which allows drivers with a level above the limit of 5 ng/mL to present an affirmative defense that despite the THC level in their body, they were not in fact intoxicated. The Massachusetts legislature considered a bill (the Trooper Thomas Clardy Law, named for a Massachusetts state trooper killed by an allegedly marijuana-intoxicated driver) that would have equalized alcohol and marijuana impairment cases, make "open containers" of marijuana illegal, suspend the license of any driver who declines a requested chemical test for impairment, and explicitly allow the testimony of DREs (Commonwealth of Massachusetts 2021). However, the bill remains stalled after opposing lawmakers complained that there is no reliable device to assess cannabis intoxication and that the 6-month suspension is unfair (Young 2022).

In addition to the difficulties just described with assessing the results of THC testing and roadside drug-related sobriety testing, toxicologists testifying regarding accusations of cannabis-impaired driving can expect questions on the practical meaning of any particular level of THC. One Colorado judge (Celeste 2017) suggested that these questions should include

1. Is there a set THC blood concentration that equates to marijuana driving impairment?
2. Do SFSTs apply to marijuana driving impairment?
3. What was the potency of the marijuana used?
4. How do age, gender, weight, dosage, use, tolerance, metabolism, ingested food, absorption, distribution, and excretion rate of THC affect impairment?

Although this case does not set precedent for all future cases, experts working on these types of litigation matters may benefit from preparation that includes answers to these and related questions.

# Psychological Autopsies When an SUD Is Involved

Sera: Are you saying that your drinking is a way to kill yourself?
Ben: Or, killing myself is a way to drink?
Sera: Very clever.

—*Leaving Las Vegas* (Figgis 1995)

This dialogue from *Leaving Las Vegas*, in which the protagonist, Ben, drinks himself to death, demonstrates the ambiguous intent to harm oneself often seen in the person dependent on or using a particular substance at a particular time. Deaths that appear to be completed suicides sometimes necessitate a psychological autopsy, in which the decedent's intent to take their own life is assessed. An assessment as to whether suicide was the cause of death can be important in criminal matters, life insurance policy claims, emotional closure for survivors, and clarification of population-wide risk factors in the hope of preventing future suicides and substance-related deaths.

When a mind-altering substance is present in the body and the decedent used the substance around the time of death, the situation becomes complicated in terms of intent, correlation, and causation. There is an undeniable association between suicidal behavior and use of addictive substances. Previous meta-analyses reported that suicide risk is 5–10 times higher in individuals with SUDs than in the general population (Harris and Barraclough 1997; Voss et al. 2013). Alcohol use disorder and opioid use disorder (OUD) are associated with suicidality as demonstrated by elevated standardized mortality rates (SMRs) for suicide, but intravenous use of any drug, mixed drug use, and even heavy drinking show similarly elevated SMRs (Wilcox et al. 2004). Approximately 22% of U.S. suicide deaths involve alcohol intoxication (Substance Abuse and Mental Health Services Administration 2016). A meta-analysis of 11 studies evaluating 23,317 individuals reported that young adult cannabis users were 3.46 times more likely to attempt suicide than nonusers (Gobbi et al. 2019).

The COVID-19 pandemic is widely considered to have fueled an increase in suicide rates as a result of increased isolation and "deaths of despair." There is some doubt as to whether suicide rates have actually risen, although it is quite clear that drug overdose rates have increased sharply (Friedman and Hansen 2022; Rahimi-Ardabili et al. 2022). Distinguishing between intentional suicide and substance use that is so careless as to closely simulate suicide is difficult but important—an essential element of the psychological autopsy must be a clear determination of the decedent's intent. This intent may be difficult to ascertain and ambiguous, even to the decedent, who can no longer speak for themselves. Although every user of illicit substances may evidence some disregard for their own well-being, the relevant question is whether the decedent specifically intended to take their own life with the action that completed the suicidal act. Family members who say, for instance, that an individual "was slowly killing himself with alcohol" may be speaking metaphorically, and the decedent's demise may have been entirely unintentional. In more acute instances, such as motor vehicle accidents involving a car being driven into a tree or someone falling asleep on train tracks, there can be further questions of intent. Where there is litigation, the intent may become highly relevant.

The risk factors for suicidal behavior promoted by alcohol—both alcohol use disorder and intoxication—have been well delineated (Hufford 2001). Alcohol use 1) worsens psychological distress, 2) increases aggressiveness, 3) promotes the transformation of suicidal ideation to suicidal action because of suicide-specific alcohol expectations, and 4) impairs the cognition necessary for forming alternative coping strategies. Alcohol often lowers inhibitions at the exact moment that the drinker feels at their worst and can grievously harm themselves, such as while driving.

Given the high prevalence of fentanyl contamination of illicit opioids and the concomitant high rate of fatal overdose, use of any illicitly obtained opioid certainly appears to be a near-suicidal act. However, many individuals with OUD do not, in fact, intend to kill themselves. In an emergency department review of adult patients, Bohnert et al. (2018) found that 12% reported a prior serious overdose in the previous years. Of those individuals, 61% denied any intent for self-harm. However, those who used one drug in the previous years were 1.8 times more likely to actually experience a medically serious overdose, those who used two drugs from separate categories were 5.8 times more likely, and those who used four drugs were 25.1 times more likely. An interesting Swedish study (Brådvik et al. 2019) reviewed the deaths of 365 subjects who had received treatment for prescription opioid use. The researchers found that those who qualified for a "misuse" diagnosis were more likely to die by suicide than those who had met full criteria for an OUD.

Although the correlation between illicit dangerous substances and suicide may seem obvious, behavioral addictions (especially gambling) are also associated with suicidal ideation and behavior. In addition to its correlation with lower quality of life, financial problems, and psychiatric comorbidity, a diagnosis of gambling disorder confers an increased risk of completed suicide (Andreeva et al. 2022). A cohort of French treatment-seeking "problem gamblers" (Guillou-Landreat et al. 2016) were 3.4 times more likely than the general population to attempt suicide, and major depressive disorder and anxiety disorder predicted suicidal risk, along with the perception that stopping gambling was impossible. In a case series of suicides associated with pathological gambling, Wong et al. (2010) found that unmanageable debt and major depressive disorder strongly correlated with completed suicide. None of the 17 decedents had sought or received treatment for their symptoms, and the authors pointed out that pathological gambling is a modifiable risk factor for suicide.

The usual practice of psychological autopsy (Isometsä 2001; Snider et al. 2006) includes structured interviews of survivors, especially family members, relatives, and friends of the decedent. Health care workers who attended to the decedent, both before and after the fatal event, may also have important information. All medical and psychiatric records, including those from the physical autopsy, are relevant to the psychological autopsy. Of course, particular dilemmas often exist when conducting a psychological autopsy of a person with an SUD. Close friends and relatives may have used substances with the decedent and may consciously or unconsciously minimize the effect of substances on the decedent. Witnesses are understandably reluctant to disclose illegal or dangerous behavior to investigators after a death. In some circumstances, the medicalized view of suicide and addictive disorders itself may prevent a full understanding of the decedent's death, and narratives curated by lay interviewers may be more effective (Gavin and Rogers 2006).

Specific SUD-related legal cases, such as life insurance matters, malpractice claims, personal injury claims, and criminal prosecutions, may require a psychological autopsy, but raw data culled from psychological autopsies may also have broader, population-wide implications. For instance, one study pooled results from deaths in which the postmortem toxicology results showed opiate use and evaluated three groups: those who died by suicide, those who died by accident, and those who died from natural causes (Athey et al. 2020). Those who died by suicide had more serious depressive disorders and were more likely to have previously attempted suicide than the other groups. Both of these markers, if replicated, could become part of a clinical algorithm for defining suicide risk in individuals with OUD.

# Malpractice Claims Involving Questions of Substance Use and Treatment

Clinical work in addiction psychiatry presents multiple opportunities for committing, or being accused of committing, medical malpractice. Patients with SUDs are among the most volatile within psychiatry and are prone to endanger themselves, harm others, and generally break societally accepted norms. Thus clinicians who treat individuals with SUDs must ensure that they practice psychiatry within clinical standards that are appropriate and informed by evidence. It is also important that they appropriately document that care and prepare themselves for litigious patients, family members, and government agencies.

Addiction treatment providers and addiction treatment facilities can present as easy targets for malpractice cases, at least in part because of the remaining miasma of stigma that hovers around SUDs themselves. The addicted person's high risk of suicide, overdose, and catastrophic relapse makes their treatment a high-stakes activity for all involved. Other potential causes for malpractice include failure to recognize the need for inpatient treatment, careless (or even criminal) prescribing of controlled substances such as buprenorphine, and breach of the numerous and sometimes arcane laws, regulations, and rules that govern the treatment of people with SUDs (reviewed also in Chapter 8).

As with other types of malpractice, an addiction psychiatry malpractice case has four elements: 1) the physician had a duty to the patient, 2) there was some dereliction or negligence related to that duty, 3) actual damages resulted, and 4) there was a direct connection from the dereliction or negligence to the damage experienced by the patient (Preskorn 2014). As Justice Oliver Wendell Holmes Jr. famously reminded a junior lawyer arguing a case in front of the U.S. Supreme Court, "This is a court of law, young man, not a court of justice." This quote underlines the fact that practicing addiction psychiatry necessitates more than just delivering evidence-based or evidence-informed and competent care: one must consider the clinical implications of case law, the administrative policies of medical boards, and where exactly the boundary of cutting-edge treatment lies. The external appearance of the treatment delivered may carry the day in a courtroom or an administrative hearing.

Boundaries are important, given the potential for complications in treating individuals who use substances, who may or may not receive an SUD diagnosis, and who may have a penchant for getting caught up with the law. Clinicians treating these patients must pull on the mantle of authority and reassure and guide them, perhaps more than in other specialties. However, conflicting obligations complicate adherence to laws and regulations. When should confidentiality be breached for the person with an SUD who is harming themselves with drugs or alcohol? Different clinicians, quite naturally, have different thresholds for what constitutes enough of an emergency to warrant a no-permission call to the patient's family or 911. Although medication dosages should usually adhere to published guidelines, most clinicians occasionally prescribe dosages outside those guidelines or use medications off-label in hopes of better helping their patients. These efforts can then be questioned with regard to acceptable practices. The best path usually lies somewhere in between the poles of the simplistic (and simplifying) dichotomies that clinicians fashion for themselves.

In addition to obtaining the right education and experience for treating people with addictive disorders, clinicians must remain cognizant of the rules and regulations that form the boundaries for clinical interactions. Patients with addictive disorders, more than most patients, can present challenges—they may break rules and test boundaries, whether because of the nature of their substance use or underlying personality characteristics, and this requires the clinician to be vigilant. For example, prescription drug monitoring programs (PDMPs) were developed as a way to help prescribers know when a patient has sought addictive substances from other prescribers. This technological support mechanism can promote a healthy respect for boundaries and potentially lead to interventions that may be more helpful to the patient.

In addiction malpractice cases, the relevant matter sometimes becomes whether there was an actual doctor-patient relationship. An investigation is sometimes confused by loose boundaries within the addiction treatment world, which includes peer-support groups like Alcoholics Anonymous, informal treatments where medical records are less than ideal or even nonexistent, and a plethora of unlicensed and sometimes uncredentialed addiction treatment providers. The knotty issue of volition can often come to the fore, as blaming a clinician for a fatal relapse can be a convenient way to discharge the anger and rage the patient's family may feel.

Specific malpractice risks for addiction professionals include patient relapse and overdose (including overdose on prescribed medications for OUD [MOUD]), vicarious liability for staff members who participate in treatment, and breaches of confidentiality for protected health information. Telepsychiatry, ubiquitous since the COVID-19 pandemic, presents special challenges for the addiction professional. Patient suicide in the context of addictive disorders can elicit complaints of malpractice against the clinician.

Although overdoses and relapses to drug or alcohol use are unfortunately common among individuals with SUDs, the treating clinician's care may be challenged and civil liability may be attached if the care does not appear to meet the minimum standard. Of course, lawsuits occur even if the care was superb, and those types of lawsuits cannot be prevented. However, the clinician must provide proper approaches to care and good documentation that can best explain the treatment decisions made. In addition to practicing good medicine, clinicians should 1) ensure that patients, and their families, have a reasonable way to contact them when difficulties arise and 2) develop a standard action plan for foreseeable emergencies. In the multidisciplinary world of addiction treatment, clinicians should maintain clear communications with others on the treatment team, and they should ensure that all clinicians function well within the bounds of their own discipline and licensure. The extra confidentiality ascribed to SUD records under 42 C.F.R. compared to the Health Insurance Portability and Accountability Act of 1996 is now gaining increased attention and may evolve. Yet given the profound stigma still attached to SUDs and their treatment, clinicians should clarify all medical information requests and ask for legal advice if there is any uncertainty as to the legality of the request to share SUD diagnoses and other protected health information.

Prominent malpractice risks can be associated with prescribing MOUD, particularly methadone and buprenorphine. These include challenges to proper care delivery when the patient may be engaging in medication diversion (e.g., a patient legitimately prescribed buprenorphine sells or gives their medication to another). The clinician can minimize, although not eliminate, this risk by checking the state's PDMP, seeing the patient at least once per month, conducting urine toxicology tests, and adhering to treatment guidelines. PDMPs that obligate authorized prescribers to check whether patients have received other prescriptions of controlled substances before prescribing a controlled substance can help mitigate some risks. A few exceptions to that obligation include provision of a 5-day supply from an emergency department, from hospice care, or as a result of a power outage. Obligated or not, it is certainly a good idea to check the PDMP before prescribing, as doing so provides clear evidence of good clinical care on the part of the prescribing physician and would certainly be useful in the defense of a malpractice matter. Clinicians may check the PDMP only for clinical reasons and only for current patients. Clinicians are typically not allowed to look at the PDMP for forensic matters, personal matters (e.g., to see what their spouse is taking), or any other nonclinical reasons. The PDMP systems record the IP (internet protocol) addresses from which information requests are made, if the ethical and legal rationales are not convincing enough and a related matter is being scrutinized.

Adhering to treatment guidelines for buprenorphine is important, especially because the U.S. Drug Enforcement Administration (DEA), not the FDA, oversees this medication. Buprenorphine prescribers are well aware that they are subject to random DEA checks of their offices, procedures, and patient lists. Popular reports that accuse buprenorphine prescribers of "replacing one addiction with another" may foretell suits against prescribers. Still, clinically prescribing MOUD is considered a standard of care even with its own risks. And failure to treat OUD patients with MOUD might itself be a reason for a malpractice lawsuit if there is a poor outcome. Clearly, the complexities of opioid treatment, especially when there are tragic outcomes, can provoke highly charged emotional responses that can make litigation a path of recourse for those affected.

Telehealth in SUD treatment is another area that can be brought to bear in malpractice litigation. Long before the COVID-19 pandemic, telehealth had been in use to provide care in distant state hospitals since the 1950s, and telemedicine has been used for space shuttle missions, battlefield triage, and treatment of researchers on the South Pole. However, caution is indicated, especially in the case of addictive disorders. Two important questions are, 1) Does the clinician need any additional license to prescribe via telepsychiatry? 2) Can the clinician actually meet the patient's needs?

Although rules were relaxed during the height of the COVID-19 pandemic, it is generally expected that a physician maintain a license in the state in which the patient is sitting, to comply with the laws of licensure and medical board requirements related to patient care. When they are unable to be physically present with the patient, clinicians are unable to see many useful markers of addictive disorders (e.g., lethargy, constricted or dilated pupils, and sweating) during telehealth sessions. In email or text exchanges, it is not possible to tell whether the person writing the email or text is who they claim to be. Although this may not be a likely problem in other subspecialties, requesting a prescription can be a very real issue for the patient with an addictive disorder. Even via videoconferencing services, the clinician cannot smell the patient or check their blood pressure. For any clinician who has asked a supposedly sober teenager why their office smells like marijuana as soon as the patient walks in, this can be a relevant deficit.

Although these challenges must be acknowledged when telehealth is inevitable, they should be considered as the clinician decides whether telehealth treatment is viable for a particular patient or context. Some settings have hybrid approaches, such as requirements for first appointments to be in person. Again, many of these requirements were waived during the pandemic because of greater concerns that patients would lose access to life-saving medications. Thus, there can be a critical balancing act, and the prescriber should be cognizant of that balance and document their rationale when choosing or refusing to offer a telepractice option. Similarly, a forensic expert must review the facts and circumstances to determine whether the care fell below the standard by virtue of the telepsychiatry intervention itself or other factors that caused the poor outcome, such as the treatment provider's inherent clinical practices themselves.

A patient's death by suicide can also be a substantial malpractice risk for the treating physician. The National Institute of Mental Health (2020) defines *suicide* as "death caused by self-directed injurious behavior with intent to die as a result of the behavior," a *suicide attempt* as "non-fatal, self-directed, potentially injurious behavior with intent to die as a result of the behavior," and *suicidal ideation* as "thinking about, considering, or planning suicide." These definitions, while useful pedagogically, fall short in the context of addictive disorders. For the person with an SUD, the extent to which the compulsive substance use is volitionally self-directed is murky, as is the individual's ability to form any coherent intent other than to continue using the addictive substance. This complexity is a bit difficult to explain to a judge or jury and, indeed, to any person without substantial experience with SUDs.

Clinicians are vulnerable to malpractice actions for not preventing (or at least anticipating, through a careful risk assessment) the suicidal behavior or act. However, suicide itself remains a relatively rare act, making it difficult to predict. Substance use is only one of many risk factors that should lead the clinician to consider suicide risk. The CDC listed SUDs among 10 risk factors for suicide that clinicians should consider; others included previous suicide attempt, mental illness, social isolation, and serious illness (Centers for Disease Control and Prevention 2022).

The clinician treating a patient who misuses substances or has symptoms that meet the full criteria for an SUD should always screen and assess the patient's suicide risk and then consider whether any risk mitigation strategies are indicated (Pinals 2019). In addition to considering the full panoply of these types of strategies (e.g., hospitalization, admission to an intensive outpatient program, or involuntary detention via civil commitment), the clinician treating a patient with substance use issues should ensure that the patient has access to peer supports such as Alcoholics Anonymous, knowledge of hotline numbers such as 988 (which is intended for all types of crises, including suicide and substance use crises), and a full understanding of what to do should suicidal thoughts emerge. Understanding of whether the patient engages in regular, chronic substance use or a more episodic binge pattern might inform planning for the possibility of thoughts of self-harm or suicide and ways to mitigate risk, such as helping the patient understand that substance use itself or using while alone heightens risk.

There is potential for physician malpractice liability after opioids have been tapered for some patients. Because there has been a decrease in physician willingness to prescribe opioids for pain (as well as literature about changes in practice standards) in the context of the prescription opioid epidemic, opioids may be tapered to a lower dosage or tapered off entirely for some patients who are not ready for tapers, or tapers may be done too quickly. According to some, the subsequent emotional turmoil has "caused needless suffering and, increasingly, suicide" (Rothstein and Irzyk 2022). Prescribing physicians should therefore carefully consider the clinical utility and potential emotional consequences of this type of "nonconsensual taper" (Rieder 2020), and they should stay abreast of the latest practice guidelines regarding how best to clinically manage these situations. Experts reviewing these matters will look at a variety of contextual variables and the prescribing decisions codified in patient records and recorded in depositions to render opinions about whether the standard of care was met and whether any deviation resulted in the poor outcomes.

# Examples of Malpractice Cases and Court Decisions

In an instructive case, *Price v. Divita* (2006a, 2006b), patient Price was referred to psychiatrist Divita by a psychologist who said that the patient had a "high ADD test" and needed medication. After evaluating the patient, Divita prescribed Adderall, gradually titrating it up to 45 mg/day. Price, an attorney, subsequently began a gambling spree in which he spent $2 million, much of it from client funds. He claimed that the Adderall prescribed by Divita made him impulsive and manic, feel invincible, abuse alcohol, gamble compulsively, take illegal drugs (including other amphetamines), consort with prostitutes, divorce his wife, and estrange himself from his family. Price received a 6-year prison term for the theft of client funds.

Divita was granted summary judgment in the malpractice case, despite the testimony of two expert witnesses who suggested that the Adderall prescription was below the minimum standard of care. The court found that Price's failure to report past addictive problems gave Divita no way to know about a possible propensity for future addictive problems. The legal testimony seems to show that Divita did a careful assessment, in addition to what a clinic psychologist had told him, and prescribed well within the usual clinical boundaries. The case against Divita did not go forward.

In an expensive and tragic case about methadone prescription (*David Lingren et al. v. John Stroemer et al.* 2016), an addiction treatment clinic and its prescribing physician settled a case for $8.5 million with the families of two road workers who were killed by a patient leaving a methadone clinic in Minnesota. According to news reports, the patient acknowledged injecting her methadone dose in the Brainerd clinic just before getting into her car and beginning the 100-mile drive back home to Cloquet. She crossed the center line of the highway and caused the accident, killing the road workers. The prescribing physician was accused of failing to examine the patient or even look at her records before allowing a take-home dose of methadone. As a side note, records show that he was prescribing Suboxone to 300 patients despite being authorized to prescribe it to only 30 patients. This case demonstrates that the horrific nature of the damages, and at least the appearance of carelessness, led to an indefensible position for the clinic and the prescriber.

# Industry Lawsuits About Substance Use

Class action and other industry lawsuits regarding addiction often require expert testimony about the scientific basis for claims, the intricacies of addiction treatment, and the suffering caused by the addictive disorders, as well as determination of whether other actors (e.g., state policymakers or system consultants) contributed to systemic poor outcomes. These types of matters often feature a team of content experts on each side, with the case decided by deposition and trial testimony over many months.

The case against Purdue Pharma and the Sackler family for their part in promoting the prescription opioid epidemic ended (at least in its first iteration) with dissolution of the company and a $4.5 billion payment by the Sacklers. The payment was intended to be used to mitigate the effects of the opioid epidemic. The (widely challenged) rationale for the relatively low amount and the decision to eschew further criminal prosecution of the Sackler family was to make certain that the funds would arrive to communities and individuals for treatment before further damage ensued (Hoffman 2021).

Numerous addiction experts participated in the various legal proceedings. Joshua Sharfstein, M.D., who served as an unpaid expert witness in the City of Baltimore's suit against Purdue Pharma, advocated for learning from the mistakes made with the $200 billion settlement received in settlement funds from tobacco companies as part of the 1998 Master Settlement Agreement. Rather than again allowing 90% of the funds to be used by states to pay debts, reduce taxes, and pay for tobacco-related projects, Sharfstein argued, the opioid settlement monies should actually go toward mitigating the opioid crisis and compensating the victims (Sharfstein and Olsen 2020). Such settlement dollars are starting to be distributed in this way toward communities.

A project chaired by Sharfstein at the Johns Hopkins Bloomberg School of Public Health and funded by Bloomberg Philanthropies promulgated some thoughtful principles about how exactly the funds from opioid litigation settlements should be disbursed. In coming up with these five principles, Sharfstein and colleagues tried to avoid what they describe as the "missed opportunity" that occurred with the tobacco settlement funds:

- Principle 1: Spend the money to save lives.
- Principle 2: Use evidence to guide spending.
- Principle 3: Invest in youth prevention.
- Principle 4: Focus on racial equity.
- Principle 5: Develop a fair and transparent process for deciding where to spend the funding.

These principles are expanded on the project's website (Johns Hopkins Bloomberg School of Public Health 2023).

Addiction experts have testified both in support of and against the tobacco industry in industry lawsuits, usually on the nature of nicotine itself and how much responsibility the smoker bears for their use of nicotine. Especially in the early days of tobacco litigation, the industry defendants hired experts who would testify to the nonaddictive nature of smoking cigarettes in support of the defendant tobacco companies. For instance, in 1988, Theodore Blau, a psychologist and former president of the American Psychological Association, testified as follows on deposition:

> Q: You believe that, uh, it is easy to stop smoking?
> A: Do I believe it is?
> Q: Hum-hum.
> A: Yes, sir, for most people.
> Q: For some people it's not?
> A: Only those who don't want to stop.
> Q: But there's nothing in cigarette smoke itself that has an effect on a person's ability to discontinue the use of cigarettes; is that correct?
> A: I've never seen any definitive data to suggest that. (Henningfield et al. 2006)

In later cases, a witness for the plaintiffs, Judith Prochaska, an addiction psychologist and professor at the Stanford University Prevention Research Center, testified in 17 separate cases against tobacco companies R.J. Reynolds and Philip Morris. Videos of her testimony are archived on the LexisNexis legal website (LexisNexis 2022). In *Neff v. Philip Morris* (2021), Prochaska testified about the link between smoking tobacco and SUDs and cancer-related death. She was able to identify nicotine as the addiction-causing agent and the fundamental reason that the decedent, Neff, continued smoking for nearly 60 years. Prochaska testified to the efficacy of the tobacco company's advertising and the typical signs of addictive disorders manifested by the decedent over her lifetime. The jury, evidently convinced by Prochaska's testimony, awarded $10 million to the decedent's family.

Unsurprisingly, both sides in the tobacco industry litigation developed sophisticated courtroom strategies and hired expert witnesses to use those strategies in espousing views most helpful to their cause. In a computational linguistics assessment of the tactics used in closing arguments by defense and plaintiffs' lawyers in the Big Tobacco cases, Risi and Proctor (2020, p. e41) found that attorneys defending the tobacco industry "seek to place the smoker on trial, using their friends and family members to demonstrate that he or she must have been fully aware of the harms caused by smoking." The testimony of experts and the attorneys' documents often used terms (or ideas) like *free choice*, *common knowledge*, and *personal responsibility*. By contrast, plaintiff's attorneys attempted to refocus agency and responsibility onto the tobacco industry itself. Lessons from these cases include the important role of expert witnesses and the guiding ethical principles of honesty and striving for objectivity, as enumerated in the ethics guidelines of the American Academy of Psychiatry and the Law (2005) that are applicable to any psychiatrist practicing in a forensic role.

# Class Action and Individual Civil Litigation in Correctional Settings

Aspects of SUD treatment in correctional settings are described more fully in Chapter 10 and are thus covered only briefly here. In general, recent litigation has ensued against many correctional facilities for failure to provide MOUD as per community standards (American Civil Liberties Union 2021). This litigation can require experts to testify about community and correctional standards. Guidelines for treatment of SUDs in criminal legal and carceral settings are increasingly available from the American Society of Addiction Medicine (2022), the National Commission on Correctional Health Care (2021), and the Substance Abuse and Mental Health Services Administration (2019). How these guidelines will play out in litigation remains to be seen, but they will undoubtedly help support expected standards both from a systems perspective and from an individualized treatment perspective. Thus, practitioners working in correctional settings should be familiar with emerging data and expected care practices. Although systemic issues may create barriers for individual practitioners, civil liability can attach to an individual even in complex systems of care. Expert witnesses (especially in federal civil claims) may also be asked to review not only the practices of practitioners but also policies, staff qualifications, and roles of other actors (e.g., correctional staff and others) in delivering acceptable care to inmates.

# Conclusions

Civil liability matters involving SUDs often require a comprehensive examination of the person engaged in the substance use, the treatment that was or was not offered or received, and an understanding of the relevant law in a particular matter. The particular legal case may hinge on the specific responsibility of the person using the substance for a particular act or may seek to shift responsibility and liability to other actors, which may be murky. Treatment providers will be scrutinized for whether they followed the standard of care or deviated from it. In forensic contexts, evaluators may need to insist on access to the most comprehensive possible examination of the subject, relevant documents, interviews of collateral informants during the evaluation process, and depositions and other data as available in discovery. This will allow the forensic psychiatrist to produce a report or testimony that comes as close to the truth as possible.

# Key Points

- Personal injury matters involving substance use and substance use disorders (SUDs) often interrogate the substance user's level of responsibility for the harm.

- State laws for driving under the influence regarding cannabis vary widely: some states presume that any level of cannabis denotes impairment, whereas others require testimony that the driver was actually impaired.

- Psychological autopsies for decedents whose death involves substances often produce ambiguous results.

- Increases in opioid overdose rates necessitate attention to the medicolegal aspects of treatment for SUDs.

- Class action lawsuits regarding SUDs often require expert consultation on the present understanding of the addictive process.

# References

American Academy of Psychiatry and the Law: Ethics guidelines for the practice of forensic psychiatry. May 2005. Available at: https://www.aapl.org/ethics.htm. Accessed December 22, 2022.

American Civil Liberties Union: ACLU releases report on treatment for incarcerated people with opioid use disorder. Press Release, June 30, 2021. Available at: https://www.aclu.org/press-releases/aclu-releases-report-treatment-incarcerated-people-opioid-use-disorder. Accessed December 23, 2022.

American Society of Addiction Medicine: Treatment in Correctional Systems Toolkit. Available at: https://www.asam.org/advocacy/advocacy-in-action/toolkits/treatment-in-correctional-settings. Accessed December 23, 2022.

Andreeva M, Audette-Chapdelaine S, Brodeur M: Gambling-related completed suicides: a scoping review. Addict Res Theory 30(6):391–402, 2022

Athey AJ, Beale EE, Overholser JC, et al: Acute stressors and clinical characteristics differentiate death by suicide, accident, or natural causes among illicit and prescription opiate users. Drug Alcohol Depend 208:107847, 2020 31951908

Bedford v Moore, 166 S.W.3d 454, 461 (Tex. App.-Fort Worth 2005a, no pet.)

Bedford v Moore, Appellees No. 2-03-377-CV (2005b)

Bohnert ASB, Walton MA, Cunningham RM, et al: Overdose and adverse drug event experiences among adult patients in the emergency department. Addict Behav 86:66–72, 2018 29198490

Bondallaz P, Frat B, Chtioui H, et al: Cannabis and its effects on driving skills. Forensic Sci Int 268:92–102, 2016 27701009

Brådvik L, Löwenhielm P, Frank A, et al: From substance use disorders in life to autopsy findings: a combined case-record and medical-legal study. Int J Environ Res Public Health 16(5):801, 2019 30841557

Brooks-Russell A, Brown T, Friedman K, et al: Simulated driving performance among daily and occasional cannabis users. Accid Anal Prev 160:106326, 2021 34403895

California v Trombetta, 467 U.S. 479 (1984)

Campbell WG: Addiction: a disease of volition caused by a cognitive impairment. Can J Psychiatry 48(10):669–674, 2003

Cavaiola A, Wuth C: Assessment and Treatment of the DWI Offender. Binghamton, NY, Haworth Press, 2022, pp 164–165

Celeste MA: A judicial perspective on expert testimony in marijuana driving cases. J Med Toxicol 13(1):117–123, 2017 27541956

Centers for Disease Control and Prevention: Risk and protective factors: many factors contribute to suicide risk. 2022. Available at: https://www.cdc.gov/suicide/factors/index.html. Accessed August 4, 2022.

Cherpitel CJ, Ye Y, Watters K, et al: Risk of injury from alcohol and drug use in the emergency department: a case-crossover study. Drug Alcohol Rev 31(4):431–438, 2012 21824208

Coggon D, Harris EC, Brown T, et al: Occupation and mortality related to alcohol, drugs and sexual habits. Occup Med (Lond) 60(5):348–353, 2010 20407041

Commonwealth of Massachusetts, House Docket No. 45866, No. 4255 (2021)

David Lingren, Angela Lingren, and James Gamache, trustees, v John Stroemer, et al., Case No.: 09-CV-13-215 (D. Mo. 2016)

Figgis M: Leaving Las Vegas. MGM/UA Distribution Company, 1995

Friedman JR, Hansen H: Evaluation of increases in drug overdose mortality rates in the US by race and ethnicity before and during the COVID-19 pandemic. JAMA Psychiatry 79(4):379–381, 2022 35234815

Gavin M, Rogers A: Narratives of suicide in psychological autopsy: bringing lay knowledge back in. J Ment Health 15(2):135–144, 2006

Gillette H: BAC facts: impairment starts at the first drink. Healthline, 2023. Available at: https://www.healthline.com/health/alcohol/blood-alcohol-level-chart. Accessed May 5, 2024.

Gobbi G, Atkin T, Zytynski T, et al: Association of cannabis use in adolescence and risk of depression, anxiety, and suicidality in young adulthood. JAMA Psychiatry 76(4):426–434, 2019 30758486

Guillou-Landreat M, Guilleux A, Sauvaget A, et al: Factors associated with suicidal risk among a French cohort of problem gamblers seeking treatment. Psychiatry Res 240:11–18, 2016 27078754

Harris EC, Barraclough B: Suicide as an outcome for mental disorders: a meta-analysis. Br J Psychiatry 170:205–228, 1997 9229027

Harris v Kubota Tractor Corp., WL 2734460 (W.D. La. 2006)

Hartman RL, Huestis MA: Cannabis effects on driving skills. Clin Chem 59(3):478–492, 2013 23220273

Henningfield JE, Rose CA, Zeller M: Tobacco industry litigation position on addiction: continued dependence on past views. Tob Control 15(Suppl 4):iv27–iv36, 2006 17130621

Heyman GM: Addiction and choice: theory and new data. Front Psychiatry 4:31, 2013

Highway Loss Data Institute: Recreational marijuana and collision claim frequencies. HLDI Bulletin, December 2020. Available at: https://www.iihs.org/media/f5fb46ff-d4b7-47b5-9c2c-951f2a30e0a6/8W5rpg/HLDI%20Research/Bulletins/hldi_bulletin_37-20.pdf. Accessed May 14, 2022.

Hoffman J: Purdue Pharma is dissolved and Sacklers pay $4.5 billion to settle opioid claims. The New York Times, September 17, 2021. Available at: https://www.nytimes.com/2021/09/01/health/purdue-sacklers-opioids-settlement.html. Accessed November 9, 2023.

Hufford MR: Alcohol and suicidal behavior. Clin Psychol Rev 21(5):797–811, 2001

Insurance Institute for Highway Safety: Crash rates jump in wake of marijuana legalization new studies show. June 17, 2021. Available at: https://www.iihs.org/news/detail/crash-rates-jump-in-wake-of-marijuana-legalization-new-studies-show. Accessed May 14, 2022.

Insurance Institute for Highway Safety: Marijuana laws. January 2024. Available at: https://www.iihs.org/topics/alcohol-and-drugs/marijuana-laws-table. Accessed April 22, 2024.

Isometsä ET: Psychological autopsy studies: a review. Eur Psychiatry 16(7):379–385, 2001 11728849

Johns Hopkins Bloomberg School of Public Health: Principles for the use of funds from the opioid litigation. 2023. Available at: https://opioidprinciples.jhsph.edu. Accessed April 22, 2024.

Leshner AI: Addiction is a brain disease, and it matters. Science 278(5335):45–47, 1997 9311924

Levow DWI Law: 20 ways to challenge a DWI. Available at: https://www.newjerseydwilawyer.com/20-ways-to-challenge-a-dwi.html. Accessed May 15, 2022.

LexisNexis: LexisNexis® Courtroom Cast. Available at: https://courtroomcast.lexis nexis.com/witnesses/prochaska-dr-judith. Accessed May 7, 2022.

Lira MC, Heeren TC, Buczek M, et al: Trends in cannabis involvement and risk of alcohol involvement in motor vehicle crash fatalities in the United States, 2000-2018. Am J Public Health 111(11):1976–1985, 2021 34709858

Maskell PD, Alex Speers R, Maskell DL: Improving uncertainty in Widmark equation calculations: alcohol volume, strength and density. Sci Justice 57(5):321–330, 2017 28889860

National Alliance to Stop Impaired Driving: State laws. 2024. Available at: https://nasid.org/state-laws. Accessed April 22, 2024.

National Commission on Correctional Healthcare: Opioid use treatment in correctional settings. 2021. Available at: https://www.ncchc.org/opioid-use-disorder-treatment-in-correctional-settings-2021/. Accessed on December 23, 2022.

National Conference of State Legislatures: Drugged driving/marijuana-impaired driving. 2021. Available at: https://www.ncsl.org/research/transportation/drugged-driving-overview.aspx. Accessed May 14, 2022.

National District Attorneys Association: Investigation and prosecution of cannabis-impaired driving cases. National Traffic Law Center, July 2020. Available at: https://ndaa.org/wp-content/uploads/Investigation-and-Prosecution-of-Cannabis-Impaired-Driving-Cases-Final.pdf. Accessed May 14, 2022.

National Highway Traffic Safety Administration: DWI Detection and Standardized Field Sobriety Testing: Instructor Guide. February 2018. Available at: https://www.nhtsa.gov/sites/nhtsa.gov/files/documents/sfst_full_instructor_manual_2018.pdf. Accessed December 12, 2022.

National Highway Traffic Safety Administration: Drunk driving: how alcohol affects driving ability. Traffic Safety Facts and Data Publications, 2022. Available at: https://www.nhtsa.gov/risky-driving/drunk-driving. Accessed May 15, 2022.

National Institute of Mental Health: Suicide. 2020. Available at: https://www.nimh.nih.gov/health/statistics/suicide#:~:text=Suicide%20is%20defined%20as%20death,might%20not%20result%20in%20injury. Accessed August 4, 2022.

Pinals DA: Liability and patient suicide. Focus Am Psychiatr Publ 17(4):349–354, 2019 32047380

Preskorn SH: Clinical psychopharmacology and medical malpractice: the four Ds. J Psychiatr Pract 20(5):363–368, 2014 25226197

Price v Divita, 224 S.W.3d 331 (2006a)

Price v Divita, 224 S.W.3d 331, 336 (Tex. App. – Houston [1st Dist.] 2006b, pet. denied)

Rahimi-Ardabili H, Feng X, Nguyen P-Y, et al: Have deaths of despair risen during the COVID-19 pandemic? A systematic review. Int J Environ Res Public Health 19(19):12385, 2022 36232135

Rieder TN: Is nonconsensual tapering of high-dose opioid therapy justifiable? AMA J Ethics 22(1):E651–E657, 2020 32880351

Risi S, Proctor RN: Big tobacco focuses on the facts to hide the truth: an algorithmic exploration of courtroom tropes and taboos. Tob Control 29(e1):e41–e49, 2020 31519796

R.J. Reynolds Tobacco Co. v Neff, 325 So. 3d 872 (Fla. Dist. Ct. App. 2012)

Rothstein MA, Irzyk J: Physician liability for suicide after negligent tapering of opioids. J Law Med Ethics 50(1):184–189, 2022 35243987

Rubenzer SJ: The standardized field sobriety tests: a review of scientific and legal issues. Law Hum Behav 32(4):293–313, 2008

Salazar v Norwegian Cruise Line Holdings, Ltd. et al., 188 F. Supp. 3d 1312 (S.D. Fla. 2016a)

Salazar v Norwegian Cruise Line Holdings, Ltd. et al., U.S. District Court, S.D. Florida (2016b)

Sewell RA, Poling J, Sofuoglu M: The effect of cannabis compared with alcohol on driving. Am J Addict 18(3):185–193, 2009 19340636

Sharfstein J, Olsen Y: How not to spend an opioid settlement. JAMA Health, January 24, 2020. Available at: https://jamanetwork.com/journals/jama/fullarticle/2762895. Accessed May 17, 2022.

Snider JE, Hane S, Berman AL: Standardizing the psychological autopsy: addressing the Daubert standard. Suicide Life Threat Behav 36(5):511–518, 2006 17087630

State v Cassidy, 235 N.J. 482, 197 A 3d 86 (2018)

Swotinsky RB: The Medical Review Officer's Manual, 5th Edition. Beverly Farms, MA, OEM Press, 2015

Substance Abuse and Mental Health Services Administration: Substance Use and Suicide: A Nexus Requiring a Public Health Approach. Rockville, MD, Substance Abuse and Mental Health Services Administration, 2016. Available at: https://store.samhsa.gov/sites/default/files/d7/priv/sma16-4935.pdf. Accessed July 31, 2022.

Substance Abuse and Mental Health Services Administration: Use of Medication-Assisted Treatment for Opioid Use Disorders in Criminal Justice Settings. Rockville, MD, Substance Abuse and Mental Health Services Administration, 2019. Available at: https://store.samhsa.gov/product/Use-of-Medication-Assisted-Treatment-for-Opioid-Use-Disorder-in-Criminal-Justice-Settings/PEP19-MATUSECJS. Accessed December 23, 2022.

Tefft BC, Arnold LS: Estimating cannabis involvement in fatal crashes in Washington State before and after the legalization of recreational cannabis consumption using multiple imputation of missing values. Am J Epidemiol 190(12):2582–2591, 2021 34157068

Voss WD, Kaufman E, O'Conner SS, et al: Preventing addiction related suicide: a pilot study. J Subt Abuse Treat 44(5):565–569, 2013 23375569

Wilcox HC, Conner KR, Caine ED: Association of alcohol and drug use disorders and completed suicide: an empirical review of cohort studies. Drug Alcohol Depend 76(Suppl):S11–S19, 2004 15555812

Wong PW, Chan WS, Conwell Y, et al: A psychological autopsy study of pathological gamblers who died by suicide. J Affect Disord 120(1–3):213–216, 2010 19395046

Young C: Family of fallen Massachusetts state police trooper pushes for passage of law in his name. WCVB-5, February 8, 2022. Available at: https://www.wcvb.com/article/push-for-trooper-thomas-clardy-law-february-8-2022/39018130. Accessed December 23, 2022.

Zwinge v Neylan, 2017 BCSC 1861, Branch, J. [British Columbia, Canada], 2017

# PART 3

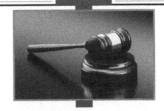

# CRIMINAL ISSUES

# CHAPTER 8

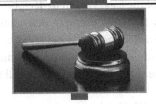

# CRIMINAL CASE EVALUATIONS IN SUBSTANCE USE DISORDERS

## Introduction

Although the effects of drug and alcohol use on the mind and body are clear, the associations among substance use disorders (SUDs), violence, and criminal offending are multifaceted and multidirectional. Individuals with SUDs are more likely to perpetrate general crime (often interrelated with drug possession, drug dealing, and other crimes associated with acquiring drugs), as well as crimes of violence, which, in part, leads to the overrepresentation of individuals with SUDs in the criminal justice system (Cloud et al. 2014). Socioeconomic status is another contributing factor to the associations among SUDs, violence, and criminal offending. Consequently, SUDs have societal and financial burdens at the local, state, and federal levels and should be thoroughly evaluated to minimize such effects.

One important element in the quest to decrease SUD-related crimes is a better understanding of their genesis. Such crimes may best be understood through Paul Goldstein's structure of criminal behavior, which highlights three main types of substance-related criminal activity: economic-related crime, use-related crime, and system-related crime (Goldstein 1985). In understanding the basis of substance-related crime, legal, mental health, and medical professionals can begin to shield perpetrators and the population at large from the effects of substance-related criminal activity. The model of SUDs as a brain disease further complicates the question of responsibility in legal matters, as it suggests essentially the rewiring of some decision-making pathways of the brain. Thus it must be the foundation of the legal system to decipher the role of SUDs in substance-related criminal activity. For example, defendants may consider criminal defenses such as diminished capacity, dissociative amnesia, or even temporary insanity as grounds for innocence. SUDs are introduced in various places in criminal case processes and must be considered in all their complexity.

## FORENSIC DILEMMA

A 34-year-old man experiencing homelessness was arrested for the attempted murder of a stranger he allegedly tried to push onto a subway track. The man acknowledges that he was intoxicated with phencyclidine (PCP) at the time of the event, and he notes that his memory of what happened is "fuzzy." He has a long criminal record of petty crimes, including trespassing and minor theft, and has been detained in city jails more than 10 times since moving to the state 6 years ago. He reports a long history of excessive alcohol use and use of cocaine, PCP, and marijuana; he also recently started injecting heroin. During processing procedures, the man receives a diagnosis of being positive for HIV and hepatitis C virus, both of which were negative a year ago.

Consider the following:

1. What risk factors increase this man's likelihood of engaging in criminal acts?
2. What type of crime is this man most likely to be involved in?
3. What considerations should be accounted for related to this man's social context?

The man's primary risk factor for violence is his substance use, especially intoxication with PCP. Although he is charged with attempted murder, people with SUDs are more often involved with crimes related to obtaining money for their substance use or dealing drugs to others. Important psychosocial factors include his homelessness and serious, untreated medical illness.

In court, the man's attorney presents an affirmative defense. The attorney argues that as a result of intoxication with PCP, the defendant did not know what he was doing and did not know it was wrong in the commission of the instant offense. The attorney also argues that the man's use of PCP was not voluntary because it was driven by his SUD diagnoses.

4. Can the man's use of substances and SUDs negate that his use was voluntary? If not, can the effects of his voluntary intoxication serve as an exculpatory affirmative defense?
5. What role does the defendant's inability to recall what happened during the instant offense play in his defense?

Case law makes it clear that voluntary intoxication cannot be used as the sole reason that a defendant could not form the intent to commit a particular crime. However, if the defense can show that the defendant, in fact, did not form the intent to commit a crime when it was a specific intent crime, voluntary intoxication can mitigate punishment or even exculpate the defendant. The "I don't remember" defense is notoriously weak, as external evidence may be sufficiently strong to yield a conviction. SUDs are generally not, in and of themselves, sufficient to establish that taking the substances is "involuntary" unless someone is given a substance and ingested it unknowingly, which is not the case in this scenario. Individual jurisdictions will have their own definitions for what might constitute an insanity defense, but intoxication as the sole reason is generally excluded.

# Alcohol, Drugs, Violence, and Crimes

Drug and alcohol intoxication (and to a lesser extent, withdrawal) typically causes a combination of diminished behavioral and cognitive control, poor insight, impaired judgment, and interpersonal and intrapersonal disinhibition in addition to anxiety, grandiosity, paranoia, and irritability. However, different substances may affect these phenomena differently. As one might expect, any permutation of such effects may lead to aggressive behaviors, commission of illegal acts, or both. Indeed, the relationship between drug or alcohol use (and consequently, an SUD) and violent behaviors is well documented, as evidenced by the exponential increase in academic publications investigating this connection beginning in the 1990s (Duke et al. 2018). In a meta-analysis of 32 meta-analyses examining the effects of drug or alcohol use on violence, Duke et al. (2018) found a consistent significant positive effect of substance intoxication on violence perpetration across different models of violence, including intimate partner violence, community violence, violent crimes, and laboratory-based measures of aggression. The authors noted that this connection was even stronger in those who were male and those with psychotic diagnoses. Interestingly, they also identified an association between increased risk of violence victimization and alcohol use, but not drug use. These findings are in line with the outcomes of the National Institute of Mental Health Epidemiologic Catchment Area surveys (Swanson et al. 1990) and the MacArthur Violence Risk Assessment Study (Steadman et al. 1998). Indeed, Steadman et al. (1998) concluded that the interaction between untreated SUDs with other serious mental illnesses was a predictor of violence more so than each condition alone. Similarly, Steadman et al. found that although persons with non-SUD psychiatric disorders were more likely to be victims of, rather than perpetrators of, violence (in fact, their risk of engaging in violent behaviors was lower than that of the general population), those with comorbid SUDs had a dramatically higher risk of violence perpetration. This risk further increases with treatment noncompliance. For example, previous studies reported that persons with untreated SUDs who continue to use drugs or alcohol are more likely to not be compliant with their general psychiatric treatment, which in turn could increase their risk of violence (Swartz et al. 1998; Torrey 1994).

As one might expect, findings for criminal behaviors show a significant positive relationship between drug or alcohol use (and SUD diagnosis) and criminal offending. This association is reflected in the overrepresentation of those with SUDs in the criminal legal system at every level—jails, prisons, parole, probation, whether state or federal—and for both male and female adults as well as young people (Bronson and Stroop 2017). The same study further demonstrated that justice-involved women and non-Hispanic White individuals were more likely to meet diagnostic criteria for SUDs than any other group. According to the survey data, nearly 4 in 10 persons arrested were intoxicated with drugs or alcohol at the time of commission of the offense, and 6 in 10 had positive drug or alcohol findings on urine drug screens. Moreover, nearly one-third of all arrests involved people committing an offense with the purpose of obtaining the financial means to purchase drugs or alcohol. These findings are further supported by data from the 2007 National Crime Victimization Survey, demonstrating that upward of 750,000 violent crimes were committed under the influence of drugs or alcohol (Bureau of Justice Statistics 2008). Such findings are not unique to the United States. In fact, one international meta-analysis using homicide data from nine countries identified that roughly half of murder perpetrators were intoxicated with alcohol at the time of the offense (Kuhns et al. 2014).

Drug and alcohol use is more likely to be associated with nonviolent property crimes or substance-related crimes than with violent crimes. Interestingly, it appears that alcohol use is more closely connected to violent crime perpetration than illicit drug use. Similarly, it appears that alcohol use, more so than illegal drugs, is strongly associated with drug-related crimes, robberies, and property crimes (Pierce et al. 2015). It may be that the disinhibition associated with alcohol use correlates with criminal behavior, as opposed to the lethargy and stimulation often associated with drug use.

Finally, driving under the influence (DUI) of drugs or alcohol is a crime. Data from the Federal Bureau of Investigation show that approximately 1.4 million individuals annually are charged with a DUI offense. Unfortunately, this number appears to be a significant underestimate of the actual DUI incidence, given that survey data indicate that upward of 100 million Americans per year admit to DUI (Zador et al. 2000).

The impact of substance use on crime and societal costs is tremendous. One analysis estimated that in the United States, the annual price tag associated with drug- and alcohol-related crimes is upward of $205 billion (Miller et al. 2006). This estimate includes mental health costs, property loss, loss of future earnings, public services resulting from the crimes such as adjudication, and sanctioning costs. Interestingly, the cost of alcohol-related crimes was nearly double that of drug-related crimes. Similarly, although the majority of drug- or alcohol-related crimes were nonviolent, the cost of violent crimes represented nearly 85% of the total price tag (here again, the authors noted that the price tag of alcohol-related violent crimes was four times that of drug-related crimes). These findings should guide public policy and legislative priorities, whereby policies aiming at reducing national spending related to criminal behaviors should heavily target prevention of alcohol use disorder and other SUDs.

Given the intimate relationship among substance use, SUD, violence, and criminal offending, public policy measures aimed at reducing crime should be based on a meaningful understanding of its etiology. Longitudinal studies investigating the direction of this causality examine rates of criminal offending before and after initial substance use. The findings demonstrate that the initiation of drug or alcohol use leads to a significant increase in subsequent criminal offending (Hayhurst et al. 2017). Interestingly, individuals who develop an SUD are more likely to have engaged in criminal activities before they first initiated substance use, compared with those who never develop an SUD (Pierce et al. 2017). As such, drug or alcohol use initiation contributes to the initiation of one's risk for criminal offending but also exacerbates preexisting levels of one's criminal proclivity. This relationship is true among both men and women but is more pronounced among women (Pierce et al. 2017). Together, these findings suggest that individuals with particular vulnerabilities have a shared etiological pathway for criminal offending and development of SUDs.

# The Intimate Connection Between Crimes and SUDs

Functionally, the causal relationship between criminal behaviors and substance use is memorialized through the taxonomy framework first introduced by Paul Goldstein in 1985. The framework recognizes common driving factors for the co-occurrence of substance use and criminal acts as follows (Goldstein 1985):

1.  *Economic-compulsive crimes* (or *economic-related crime*): This classification re-
    lates to criminal acts whose purpose is to generate money to fund the use of
    drugs or alcohol. In these contexts, violent or criminal acts allow one to gain ac-
    cess to the intoxicating substance *(e.g., stealing money to pay for drugs)*.
2.  *Psychopharmacological crimes* (or *use-related crimes*): This classification re-
    lates to the effects of these substances on one's thoughts and behavior:
    a.  Using drugs or alcohol results in physical, cognitive, or intellectual im-
        pairments that in turn lead to the commission of illegal acts or other
        criminally sanctioned behaviors *(e.g., physically assaulting another per-
        son after using stimulant drugs)*; or
    b.  Using drugs or alcohol to become more disinhibited or have the courage
        to commit the crime *(e.g., drinking alcohol before breaking into an apart-
        ment)*.
3.  *Systemic crime* (or *system-related crime*): This classification relates to crim-
    inal acts that are intrinsic to the drug trade, including the production, man-
    ufacture, transportation, and sale of substances. In these contexts, violent or
    criminal acts allow one to gain access to the intoxicating substance or to re-
    solve disputes over them *(e.g., gang members selling drugs)*.

The temporal relationship between using substances and the commission of
the criminal act can be further used to classify it to better understand the causal
relationship (Bennett and Holloway 2009). For example, situations in all three
categories just described can fall into three subcategories:

1.  *Forward causation*: Substance use leads to criminal activity.
2.  *Reverse causation*: Involvement with criminal behaviors leads to substance use.
3.  *Confounding*: Crime and substance use share a common set of causes and
    influence each other.

In this context, understanding of the intimate relationship among substance
use, SUD, violence, and criminal offending can be used to assess and rehabilitate
criminal offenders. This is well exemplified in the *risk-need-responsivity model*
developed by Donald Andrews and James Bonta. The risk-need-responsivity
model is premised on the principle that the levels and intensity of mitigating
measures aimed at minimizing the criminogenic needs of criminal offenders
should be modeled based on their risk factors and needs as follows (Bonta and
Andrews 2007):

1.  *Risk principle*: Static (e.g., age at first arrest, history of arrest, or gender) and
    dynamic (e.g., SUDs or other psychiatric diagnoses) reoffending risk factors
    should be used to match the level of service required.

2. *Need principle*: The assessment of criminogenic needs allows for their targeting in treatment interventions.
3. *Responsivity principle*: The offender's ability to learn from a rehabilitative intervention is maximized by providing cognitive-behavioral treatment and tailoring the intervention to their learning style, motivation, abilities, and strengths.

# Social Determinants of Health in the Context of Crimes and SUDs

Factors such as poverty, homelessness, residential segregation, racism, and incarceration or other criminal involvement history are more than mere consequences of substance use. They represent social factors that affect the sociolegal outcomes of using intoxicating substances. Such factors shape the divergent consequences of substance use, affect the likelihood of risky substance use behaviors, and increase the health consequences of substance use. When viewed through this lens, it becomes apparent that an individual's health (including whether they use drugs or alcohol and develop SUDs) is determined partially by their access to social, cultural, and economic opportunities. Indeed, such access plays a primary deterministic role in shaping the health and lives of substance users. This concept of understanding how one's lived social environment affects one's health, functioning, and quality of life outcomes is referred to as *social determinants of health*.

Although it seems easy to conceptualize how drug or alcohol use causes poverty, homelessness, or criminal behavior, the relationship is not that straightforward. In fact, such factors also represent social circumstances that are responsible for shaping health differentials among substance users. Studies report that the cycle of incarceration followed by release or reentry, particularly among people from lower-income backgrounds, increases morbidity and mortality for incarcerated substance users (Binswanger et al. 2012; Galea and Vlahov 2002). As a result of their history of legal involvement and limited financial resources, these individuals have less access to SUD treatment resources and are more likely to lack financial and emotional resources. As a result, they become more likely to be noncompliant with treatment, engage in behaviors that worsen their prognosis (e.g., trading sex for drugs and money or engaging in high-risk sex acts), and contract infectious diseases (Galea and Vlahov 2002). These consequences are compounded by the increased rates of contracting HIV and hepatitis C virus, developing AIDS, and experiencing drug-related morbidity and mortality (including fatal overdoses and drug-related homicides) among underrepresented racial and ethnic minority groups and those who have not completed high school. In turn, for people with SUDs, experiencing homelessness increases the risks of being involved in criminal activities, of being inappropriately criminalized, and of being held longer in incarceration. Furthermore, in a previous study, investigators found that incarceration increases the risk of initiating high-risk substance use behaviors. Specifically, for every year spent incarcerated, the risk of injecting drugs increased by 17% (McNiel et al. 2005). Similarly, having a history of early trauma or exposure to violence, as is common in racially segregated communities, was associated with a significant increase in the likelihood of using drugs as an adult (Carliner et al. 2016).

Finally, it is worth noting that incarceration has significant effects on recovery. Indeed, individuals with SUDs who were abstinent while in the controlled environment of detention carry an elevated risk of postrelease relapse. The stressors associated with being an ex-convict create a set of social circumstances that make it difficult not to experience relapse (Chandler et al. 2009). These stressors include the following:

- Stigma associated with being labeled an ex-offender
- Difficulties in finding housing and legitimate employment
- The stress of reunifying with one's family
- The stress caused by the strict supervision requirements (with conditional release)
- Returning to the same neighborhoods associated with preincarceration drug use (i.e., environments rich in drug-related cues)
- Molecular and neurobiological adaptations resulting from chronic drug use that can persist for many months after drug discontinuation

# Criminal Forensic Evaluations Involving SUDs

## CRIMINAL RESPONSIBILITY

The U.S. justice system is founded on the principle that criminal responsibility requires two elements, the *actus reus* and the *mens rea*. The former refers to the "evil" act itself, or the behavior one engages in that violates the laws; the latter refers to having a guilty state of mind with intent to commit the criminal act. Every state and jurisdiction can decide for themselves how they define criminal responsibility. In fact, in *Kahler v. Kansas* (2020), the U.S. Supreme Court reaffirmed the rights of states to have their own statutory schemes that can accept, redefine, or even reject an insanity defense. Nevertheless, it is useful to understand how laws have been crafted to examine criminal responsibility related to substances.

One classic example of this can be seen through the Model Penal Code. This code was published in 1962 by the American Law Institute and was designed as a not-legally-binding law; rather, it is a guiding framework to standardize the penal code in the United States. Since publication of the Model Penal Code, more than half of states have enacted criminal codes that borrow heavily from it (American Law Institute 1985). The Model Penal Code introduced a formal classification of the different levels of mental state required to ascertain culpability for each specific crime based on the *mens rea:* 1) purposely, 2) knowingly, 3) recklessly, and 4) negligently. Each is defined as follows:

- *Purposely*: Criminal elements requiring this level of mental state are defined by having a conscious awareness of the illegality of one's conduct or of its consequences and the pursuit of such outcomes.
- *Knowingly*: Criminal elements requiring this level of mental state are defined by having a conscious awareness of the illegality of one's conduct or of its consequences and by acting in spite of and in disregard of such outcomes (not in pursuit, as in *purposely*).
- *Recklessly*: Criminal elements requiring this level of mental state are defined by consciously disregarding substantial or unjustifiable risk in deviation from the conduct that an average law-abiding citizen would follow.
- *Negligently*: Criminal elements requiring this level of mental state are defined by any level of awareness of substantial risk associated with one's conduct in deviation from the conduct that an average law-abiding citizen would follow.

Securing a criminal conviction and subsequent sentencing for any given crime would be contingent on proving beyond a reasonable doubt that the defendant engaged in willful misconduct when engaging in behaviors that violate the law and met the required mental state level for the offense or *mens rea*. Failing to prove beyond a reasonable doubt that the individual intended to commit a crime would result in an acquittal unless they were then charged with lesser offenses. Intent to commit a crime can be specific (knowingly or willingly engaging in criminal conduct) or general (recklessly engaging in conduct whose primary purpose is not to violate the law despite knowledge that the consequences of such conduct may be illegal). In contrast, negligently engaging in conduct whose consequences might be illegal generally does not constitute criminal intent. Hence, intending to commit a crime would require one's capacity to form the requisite criminal intent to be intact.

Viewed in this context, the insanity defense in criminal matters would provide a complete acquittal from criminal responsibility for individuals who committed a criminal act, while laboring under mental disease or defect lacking substantial capacity to know or appreciate the nature and consequences of such conduct or that such conduct was wrong (the specific standard varies among states). The Model Penal Code proposes the following elements for an insanity defense in section 4.01 (Mental Disease or Defect Excluding Responsibility):

1. A person is not responsible for criminal conduct if at the time of such conduct as a result of mental disease or defect he lacks substantial capacity either to appreciate the criminality [wrongfulness] of his conduct or to conform his conduct to the requirements of law.
2. As used in this Article, the terms "mental disease or defect" do not include an abnormality manifested only by repeated criminal or otherwise anti-social conduct. (American Law Institute 1985)

# CRIMINAL RESPONSIBILITY AND DIMINISHED CAPACITY IN MATTERS INVOLVING INTOXICATION OR SUDS

The presence of intoxication or SUDs is frequently cited in various criminal matters in courts. The Model Penal Code provides the following framework for delineating the role of drug or alcohol intoxication in adjudicating criminal matters in section 2.08 (Intoxication):

1. Except as provided in Subsection (4) of this Section, intoxication of the actor is not a defense unless it negates an element of the offense.
2. When recklessness establishes an element of the offense, if the actor, due to self-induced intoxication, is unaware of a risk of which he would have been aware had he been sober, such unawareness is immaterial.
3. Intoxication does not, in itself, constitute mental disease within the meaning of section 4.01.
4. Intoxication which (a) is not self-induced or (b) is pathological is an affirmative defense if by reason of such intoxication the actor at the time of his conduct lacks substantial capacity either to appreciate its criminality [wrongfulness] or to conform his conduct to the requirements of law. (American Law Institute 1985)

This framework carries implications for insanity defense forensic evaluations in which voluntary intoxication with drugs or alcohol would not qualify for the affirmative defense of insanity. Indeed, despite the direct behavioral and cognitive effects of such substances rendering a person unable to understand or appreciate the nature and quality of their acts or to conform to the requirements of the law, a person's ability to refrain from intoxication invalidates such a defense. Successful insanity defenses are rare, and cases involving drugs or alcohol render such a defense even less likely to succeed, so it is not uncommon for lawyers to pursue a diminished capacity partial defense instead, at least in those jurisdictions that allow for them.

Diminished capacity to form criminal intent is distinct from a total affirmative defense (such as a defense of not guilty by reason of insanity). Not all states consider diminished capacity defenses, but in general this defense is considered as a result of partial impairment or a global inability. Forensic psychiatrists may be called on to perform evaluations and provide testimony for diminished capacity to form a criminal intent in specific cases. This is particularly relevant to the practice of forensic addiction psychiatrists, because the effects of intoxicating drugs and alcohol include impairments in insight, judgment, and cognitive abilities, including memory formation (Bergman 1997). Many states restrict or completely bar this defense and thus would also bar related forensic psychiatric testimony (Miller 2010). It is worth noting that any forensic evaluation of intent would be incomplete without assessing the relationship between intent formation and individual responsibility, discussed further later in this chapter.

# INTOXICATION AS A DEFENSE

The question of whether intoxication with drugs or alcohol may prevent one from forming a specific intent to engage in a criminal act is complex and further complicated when the individual has an SUD. Those with SUDs may have an impaired ability to exercise restraint in using or experiencing relapse of drug or alcohol use and subsequently prevent the occurrence of potentially illegal adverse consequences of their substance use. Although one may easily comply with societal norms if sober (or conversely, form specific intent to commit an illegal act), an SUD resulting in the compulsive use of alcohol or drugs is likely to prevent that sort of compliance. Indeed, the direct cognitive and behavioral effects of these substances increase the likelihood that these individuals will engage in illegal activities they may not have if they had been sober; those with SUDs are likely to compromise their ability to form the specific intent required to secure a guilty conviction. SUDs are brain disorders that involve a cognitive preoccupation with seeking and consuming intoxicating substances despite any negative consequences of such consumption, whether related to health status or social or legal functioning. In that context, relapsing to using intoxicating substances as a drive among those with SUDs is evidence of the impaired sense-of-control component of the disorder. It is worth reiterating that control is not wholly lost but rather partially compromised, rendering the individual less capable of resisting the urge to use. This is the basis for the U.S. Supreme Court decisions in *Robinson v. California* (1962a, 1962b), which codified that having an SUD as a status may not be criminalized, and in *Powell v. Texas* (1968), which found that substance-related behaviors may be criminalized (these decisions are discussed in more detail in Chapters 1 and 2).

Indeed, in *Robinson*, the majority opinion famously noted the following:

> Even one day in prison would be a cruel and unusual punishment for the "crime" of having a common cold....But I do not see how under our system being an addict can be punished as a crime. If addicts can be punished for their addiction, then the insane can also be punished for their insanity. Each has a disease, and each must be treated as a sick person. (*Robinson v. California* 1962a, 1962b)

Contrast this with the majority opinion in *Powell*, which noted the following:

> Traditional common-law concepts of personal accountability lead us to disagree with appellant. We are unable to conclude, on the state of this record or on the current state of medical knowledge, that chronic alcoholics...suffer from such an irresistible compulsion to drink and to get drunk in public that they are utterly unable to control their performance of either or both of these acts and thus cannot be deterred at all from public intoxication. (*Powell v. Texas* 1968)

In another oft-discussed case, *People v. Saille* (1991), Saille threatened to get a gun and kill a security guard who told him he could no longer drink at a bar because of his visible intoxication. Saille went home and got his firearm, brought it to the bar, shot at the guard, and killed a patron. His blood alcohol content was 0.19 mg/mL at the time of the crime. California law did not permit the use of voluntary intoxication or mental disorder as a defense to reduce murder charges to involuntary manslaughter. Saille disagreed, arguing that "voluntary intoxication, like the heat of passion upon adequate provocation, could negate express malice," which was required in determining whether he had premeditated and deliberated the act for a murder conviction.

The California Supreme Court disagreed and held that the California statutes abolishing the defense of diminished capacity in cases of voluntary intoxication were reasonable but recognized that defendants in such matters were still free to demonstrate that as a result of mental illness or voluntary intoxication, they did not form malice aforethought. In other words, the California Supreme Court ruled that Saille's deliberate intention to kill met the required standard for a murder conviction for this specific intent crime, without the need for additional mental state findings to establish malice aforethought. As such, in California, voluntary intoxication may not be proffered as a global defense but rather to rebut a specific element of a crime.

The *Saille* ruling, although limited to California, exemplifies the jurisprudential concept that voluntary intoxication with drugs or alcohol does not, on its face, qualify for a diminished capacity defense. Note that this contrasts with the involuntary intoxication defense, a temporary insanity defense defined by a state of intoxication from the actions of others or similar clandestine means (when individuals engage in acts that result from unknowingly reaching a state of intoxication without intending to do so). Similarly, idiosyncratic intoxication (having an unanticipated intoxicating reaction from consumption of a substance) or medical syndromes caused by chronic and excessive substance use (e.g., Wernicke-Korsakoff encephalopathy or delirium tremens) may serve as the basis for a diminished capacity defense (Watterson 1991). Beyond asserting diminished capacity at trial, many individuals with SUDs are ultimately convicted or plead guilty to their criminal charges, but they may look toward forensic experts to help establish SUDs as mitigating circumstances at the time of the crime. Chapter 9 reviews situations in which criminal sentencing may be mitigated in view of an addictive disorder diagnosis.

# Blackout as a Criminal Defense

Consuming large amounts of alcohol may lead to states of dissociation marked by impairments in the integration of the different elements of consciousness including identity, memory, and motor function. *Alcohol-induced dissociative amnesia* or *blackout* is a phenomenon that refers to the loss of memory of important events that occurred while drinking alcohol. Although the signs and symptoms associated with alcohol intoxication are well known and easily recognizable, blackout episodes may present as markedly different. Indeed, excessive alcohol users experiencing a blackout episode may behave in manners inconsistent with intoxication. In fact, it is not uncommon during a blackout episode for an individual to engage in activities requiring high levels of executive function or in meaningful conversations while appearing perfectly sober to an outside observer; blackout impairs memory registration, but the alcohol use at the time does not necessarily cloud one's consciousness (van Oorsouw et al. 2004). Thus, an individual can engage in well-coordinated legal and illegal activities, deviantly or nondeviantly, and then later describe a blackout where they do not recall what they did or what occurred (White et al. 2002).

Depending on its severity, a blackout can be further categorized as fragmentary or complete (en bloc), with the former indicating partial loss of memories and the latter a global memory loss. Moreover, a blackout can also be categorized depending on whether the individual appears intoxicated externally. Blackouts are generally marked by a profound impairment of state-dependent retrieval when sober of memories acquired while intoxicated (Fillmore et al. 1999). Memory loss resulting from a blackout is typically irreversible but may be partially recovered when the individual is exposed to cues of the lost memories (Pressman and Caudill 2013). Reports of recovered memories are subject to attribution and confirmation biases, whereby inappropriate or upsetting acts can be attributed to the effect of alcohol. Similarly, expectancy effects related to one's expectation of their conduct under the influence of alcohol can either shape the content of such reconstituted memory or shape one's behaviors in a blackout as a self-fulfilling prophecy.

In the context of alleged criminal behaviors, it is not uncommon for defendants to assert an inability to recall the events of the instant offense. In fact, it is estimated that one in four defendants makes such claims, often citing drug or alcohol use as the cause for the amnesia (Cima et al. 2004). The appeal of such claims is obvious, as a convenient strategy to assert a lack of criminal responsibility for illegal conduct. This is complicated, however, by the fact discussed earlier, that voluntary intoxication is not an acceptable defense for substance-related conduct. Recall that in contrast, involuntary intoxication could serve as an effective defense. This therefore raises important questions: Is a blackout episode evidence of the absence of mens rea? Could a blackout, as an involuntary unexpected state, be akin to a state of involuntary intoxication, or is it no more than the product of a voluntary intoxication? The former may excuse the conduct, whereas the latter would not (Merikangas 2004).

To analyze these questions, one should review the neurobiological effects of alcohol on intellectual and cognitive functions. Indeed, alcohol-mediated effects on the frontal lobe result in impairments in executive functioning, impulse control, decision-making, and complex task planning. Similarly, through its functional effect on the hippocampus, alcohol negatively affects short-term memory formation and interferes with information storing without affecting old memories. As such, it may be argued that during a blackout, one's ability to comport oneself in line with a previously instilled understanding of rules of acceptable conduct should remain unaffected. This is consistent with court decisions related to excluding amnesia as a global criminal defense, because amnesia does not imply impaired levels of consciousness, awareness, or attention during the commission of the offense (van Oorsouw et al. 2004). For these reasons, Pressman and Caudill (2013) concluded that despite the fact that blackouts interfere with one's memory, they should not be construed as a negation of mens rea during the episode. In contrast, Merikangas (2004) classified acts carried out during an alcoholic blackout as "automatisms" and concluded that "alcoholic blackouts are states of absence of mind that should be recognized by the law as exculpatory in cases in which they are the unanticipated result of social drinking, when intoxication was neither desired nor expected" (p. 377). This argument would require proof once again of what comprised voluntary ingestion and the anticipated outcomes of such ingestion.

## The Tarasoff Principle and SUDs

The *Tarasoff principle* derives from *Tarasoff v. Regents of University of California* (1976a, 1976b), in which the California Supreme Court ruled in 1976 that mental health providers had a responsibility to take affirmative action to protect ascertainable third parties from foreseeable dangers by patients they evaluated. In their opinion, the justices wrote the following:

> When a therapist determines, or pursuant to the standards of his profession should determine, that his patient presents a serious danger of violence to another, he incurs an obligation to use reasonable care to protect the intended victim against such danger. The discharge of this duty may require the therapist to take one or more of various steps, depending upon the nature of the case. Thus, it may call for him to warn the intended victim or others likely to apprise the vic-

tim of the danger, to notify the police, or to take whatever other steps are reasonably necessary under the circumstances. (*Tarasoff v Regents of University of California* 1976a)

As such, the elements of the Tarasoff duty involve foreseeability of danger and an ascertainable victim. The Tarasoff principle has since been adapted and incorporated into statute by some, but not all, state legislatures.

Given the relationship between SUDs and violent behaviors discussed earlier, it is evident that application of the Tarasoff duty may be complicated in patients with SUDs. There is a lack of clear and unequivocal legal guidance from the courts or from state or federal legislatures as to whether SUDs should be treated any differently from other psychiatric disorders in terms of applying the Tarasoff duty. The Washington State Supreme Court weighed on this issue in *Petersen v. State* (1983), ruling that a hospital was liable for damages caused by a recently discharged patient who struck a car while in a state of drug-induced psychosis. Indeed, in that matter, the court found that the dangers the defendant posed were predictable, given that when he was allowed to go home for Mother's Day (the day before his ultimate discharge), he was apprehended by hospital security personnel while spinning his car in circles and driving on the hospital grounds in a reckless fashion. Thus, the court ruled that the hospital had failed to discharge their duty when they released the patient.

Although the *Tarasoff* and *Petersen* cases are decades old and unique to their particular jurisdictions, they continue to teach important lessons. To that end, there remain many situations in which a clinician or a practitioner may develop concerns that a person with an SUD will cause harm to others. In these situations, it may be helpful to consult a colleague with forensic expertise or to review the facts and circumstances with a risk management attorney. The option to have the individual evaluated if there is a mental illness of concern is available, either voluntarily or involuntarily, in all states, which can further the ability to ascertain the proper facts to analyze any needed action steps to mitigate the risk of harm to others.

# Conclusions

The intimate relationship between violence perpetration and criminal behaviors on the one hand and drug or alcohol use and SUDs on the other is well documented and multifactorial. Understanding the causal and co-occurring dynamics behind this connection allows for the development and utilization of appropriate services to mitigate an offender's recidivism risk. In evaluating criminal behavior through a forensic lens, it is important to understand how drug or alcohol intoxication may affect criminal responsibility.

# Key Points

- There is a significant intensifying effect of drug or alcohol intoxication on violence perpetration.

- Drug and alcohol use is more likely to be associated with nonviolent property crimes or substance-related crimes than with violent crimes (but alcohol is more commonly associated with violent crimes than drugs).

- Social determinants of health, such as poverty, homelessness, residential segregation, racism, incarceration, or other criminal involvement history, play a significant role in substance use and associated outcomes.

- Despite the direct behavioral and cognitive effects of drugs and alcohol that render one unable to understand or appreciate the nature and quality of their acts or conform to the requirements of the law, one's ability to refrain from intoxication invalidates the insanity defense in such contexts.

# References

American Law Institute: Model Penal Code: Official Draft and Explanatory Notes: Complete Text of Model Penal Code as Adopted at the 1962 Annual Meeting of the American Law Institute, Washington, DC, May 24, 1962. 1985. Available at: https://www.legal-tools.org/doc/08d77d/pdf. Accessed November 10, 2023.

Bennett T, Holloway K: The causal connection between drug misuse and crime. Br J Criminol 49:513–531, 2009

Bergman B: Responsibility for crime and injury when drunk. Addiction 92(9):1183–1188, 1997 9374018

Binswanger IA, Nowels C, Corsi KF, et al: Return to drug use and overdose after release from prison: a qualitative study of risk and protective factors. Addict Sci Clin Pract 7(1):3, 2012 22966409

Bonta J, Andrews DA: Risk-need-responsivity model for offender assessment and rehabilitation. 2007. Available at: https://www.publicsafety.gc.ca/cnt/rsrcs/pblctns/rsk-nd-rspnsvty/rsk-nd-rspnsvty-eng.pdf. Accessed November 10, 2023.

Bronson J, Stroop J: Drug Use, Dependence, and Abuse Among State Prisoners and Jail Inmates, 2007–2009. Washington, DC, Bureau of Justice Statistics, June 2017

Bureau of Justice Statistics: Criminal Victimization in the United States, 2007. Washington, DC, Bureau of Justice Statistics, 2008

Carliner H, Nijman H, Merckelbach H, et al: Childhood trauma and illicit drug use in adolescence: a population-based National Comorbidity Survey Replication–Adolescent Supplement study. J Am Acad Child Adolesc Psychiatry 55(8):701–718, 2016 27453084

Chandler RK, Fletcher BW, Volkow ND: Treating drug abuse and addiction in the criminal justice system: improving public health and safety. JAMA 301(2):183–190, 2009 19141766

Cima M, Nijman H, Merckelbach H, et al: Claims of crime-related amnesia in forensic patients. Int J Law Psychiatry 27(3):215–221, 2004 15177990

Cloud DH, Parsons J, Delany-Brumsey A: Addressing mass incarceration: a clarion call for public health. Am J Public Health 104(3):389–391, 2014 24432940

Duke AA, Smith KM, Oberleitner L, et al: Alcohol, drugs, and violence: a meta-meta-analysis. Psychol Violence 8(2):238–249, 2018

Fillmore MT, Vogel-Sprott M, Gavrilescu D: Alcohol effects on intentional behavior: dissociating controlled and automatic influences. Exp Clin Psychopharmacol 7(4):372–378, 1999 10609972

Galea S, Vlahov D: Social determinants and the health of drug users: socioeconomic status, homelessness, and incarceration. Public Health Rep 117(Suppl 1):S135–S145, 2002 12435837

Goldstein P: The drugs/violence nexus: a tripartite conceptual framework. J Drug Issues 15:493–506, 1985

Hayhurst KP, Pierce M, Hickman M, et al: Pathways through opiate use and offending: a systematic review. Int J Drug Policy 39:1–13, 2017 27770693

Kahler v Kansas, 589 U.S. __ (2020)

Kuhns JB, Exum ML, Clodfelter TA, et al: The prevalence of alcohol-involved homicide offending: a meta-analytic review. Homicide Stud 18:251–270, 2014

McNiel DE, Binder RL, Robinson JC: Incarceration associated with homelessness, mental disorder, and co-occurring substance abuse. Psychiatr Serv 56(7):840–846, 2005 16020817

Merikangas J: Commentary: alcoholic blackout—does it remove mens rea? J Am Acad Psychiatry Law 32(4):375–377, 2004 15704621

Miller NS: Principles of Addictions and the Law. New York, Academic Press, 2010

Miller TR, Levy DT, Cohen MA, et al: Costs of alcohol and drug-involved crime. Prev Sci 7(4):333–342, 2006 16845591

People v Saille, 54 Cal.3d 1103 (Cal. 1991)

Petersen v State, 100 Wn.2d 421 (Wash. 1983)

Pierce M, Hayhurst K, Bird SM, et al: Quantifying crime associated with drug use among a large cohort of sanctioned offenders in England and Wales. Drug Alcohol Depend 155:52–59, 2015 26361712

Pierce M, Hayhurst K, Bird SM, et al: Insights into the link between drug use and criminality: lifetime offending of criminally active opiate users. Drug Alcohol Depend 179:309–316, 2017 28837946

Powell v Texas, 392 U.S. 514 (1968)

Pressman MR, Caudill DS: Alcohol-induced blackout as a criminal defense or mitigating factor: an evidence-based review and admissibility as scientific evidence. J Forensic Sci 58(4):932–940, 2013 23692320

Robinson v California, 370 U.S. 660 (1962a)

Robinson v California, 370 U.S. 660, 82 S. Ct. 1417 (1962b)

Steadman HJ, Mulvey EP, Monahan J, et al: Violence by people discharged from acute psychiatric inpatient facilities and by others in the same neighborhoods. Arch Gen Psychiatry 55(5):393–401, 1998 9596041

Swanson JW, Holzer CE 3rd, Ganju VK, et al: Violence and psychiatric disorder in the community: evidence from the Epidemiologic Catchment Area surveys. Hosp Community Psychiatry 41(7):761–770, 1990 2142118

Swartz MS, Swanson JW, Hiday VA, et al: Violence and severe mental illness: the effects of substance abuse and nonadherence to medication. Am J Psychiatry 155(2):226–231, 1998 9464202

Tarasoff v Regents of University of California, 17 Cal.3d 425 (1976a)

Tarasoff v Regents of University of California, 17 Cal.3d 425, 131 Cal. Rptr. 14, 551 P.2d 334 (Cal. 1976b)

Torrey EF: Violent behavior by individuals with serious mental illness. Hosp Community Psychiatry 45(7):653–662, 1994 7927289

van Oorsouw K, Merckelbach H, Ravelli D, et al: Alcoholic blackout for criminally relevant behavior. J Am Acad Psychiatry Law 32(4):364–370, 2004 15704619

Watterson RT: Just say no to the charges against you: alcohol intoxication, mental capacity, and criminal responsibility. Bull Am Acad Psychiatry Law 19(3):277–290, 1991 1777689

White AM, Jamieson-Drake DW, Swartzwelder HS: Prevalence and correlates of alcohol-induced blackouts among college students: results of an e-mail survey. J Am Coll Health 51(3):117–119, 122–131, 2002 12638993

Zador PL, Krawchuk SA, Voas RB: Alcohol-related relative risk of driver fatalities and driver involvement in fatal crashes in relation to driver age and gender: an update using 1996 data. J Stud Alcohol 61(3):387–395, 2000 10807209

# CHAPTER 9

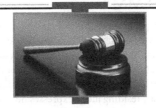

# SUBSTANCE USE DISORDERS AND SPECIALTY COURTS, JAIL DIVERSION, AND ALTERNATIVES TO INCARCERATION PROGRAMS

## Introduction

The relationship between substance use disorders (SUDs) and criminal behavior is complicated, and academic interest in this nexus has increased exponentially over the past two decades. Individuals with SUDs are overrepresented in the criminal justice system. Bureau of Justice Statistics survey data from a 2017 study suggested that almost two-thirds of convicted inmates in jails and prisons met diagnostic criteria for SUDs (Bronson et al. 2017). Those on parole or probation were three times more likely than the general population to have an SUD, according to the same data. Bronson et al. (2017) also reported that 40% of inmates were in a state of intoxication at the time of their offense, and one-third committed the offense to obtain money to purchase drugs. Interestingly,

SUDs were more prevalent among inmates convicted of property offenses or drug-related offenses than violent or other public-order offenses (Bronson et al. 2017). These data are consistent with findings from the National Crime Victimization Survey, which identified upward of 750,000 violent crimes in the United States in 2007 in which the offender was believed to be intoxicated with drugs or alcohol (Maston and Bureau of Justice Statistics 2010). Thus, the need for sophisticated SUD treatment within the legal system is obvious.

## FORENSIC DILEMMA

A 32-year-old woman experiencing homelessness in a small Indiana town has been charged 13 times with offenses such as heroin dealing, prostitution, and trespassing over the course of a calendar year. Each time she has gone before the court, she is sentenced to fines and brief jail sentences, both of which she accepts without comment. In her latest appearance before the court after being again arrested for trespassing, the presiding judge expresses her frustration with the frequent arrests, and the defendant blurts out, "I got to get the smack, Judge." This outburst prompts the judge to refer the defendant to the drug court session, which is held every 2 weeks on Friday afternoon and is presided over by a different judge.

Consider the following:

1. What obligation does the court have to look into the presence of SUDs or other mental health issues in making determinations regarding criminal acts?
2. Is an SUD automatically exculpatory for criminal acts?

Directing individuals with mental illness, including those with SUDs, toward treatment when appropriate to the legal situation can be a function of the courts. Some might argue that it should always be a priority for the courts, if examined from the perspective of a public health response.

In this case, the defendant readily agrees to attend the drug court, in hopes that she will receive a lighter sentence. However, when she arrives at the drug court, she is obligated to undergo a 90-minute assessment with the resident substance abuse professional and then wait for three other defendants to be heard in court. The presiding judge imposes a suspended sentence of 7 days for the trespassing but requires the defendant to attend an intensive outpatient treatment program and to return to the courtroom in 2 weeks with a urine drug screen result in hand. During the court proceeding, the judge comes off the bench and talks with the defendant, the district attorney, and the substance abuse professional in an in camera discussion at a conference table at the back of the courtroom.

3. Can courts mandate SUD treatment?
4. Should defendants be sanctioned for failure to maintain sobriety?

Courts can mandate attendance at treatment, although engaging with the defendant and supporting them is much more effective than simply ruling as the main approach to care.

> The defendant in this case expressed surprise and some gratitude that the judge had taken the time to listen to her particular issues and appeared to be concerned for her well-being. Although sanctioning a defendant for positive drug screens is best avoided, keeping sanctions—including jail time—in abeyance for continued inability to remain sober is an effective strategy.

# The Need for Legally Mandated Treatment of SUDs in Criminal Contexts

Substance-related and substance-attributable crimes have a significant economic burden, which is estimated at upward of $200 billion annually in the United States alone (Miller et al. 2006). In a meta-analysis of 32 meta-analyses examining the link between violent behaviors and SUDs, Duke et al. (2018) identified a significant association between alcohol or illicit drug use on violence perpetration in intimate partner violence, community violence, violent crimes, and laboratory-based measures of aggression. The researchers noted that this relationship was even stronger for male individuals and those with co-occurring psychotic illnesses. Similarly, the results suggested a significant association between alcohol use and experiencing violent victimization.

Government agencies are interested in identifying effective interventions that target criminal recidivism and violent behaviors among the substance-using population. Social circumstances and social determinants also contribute to the relationship among SUDs, violence, and criminal justice system involvement. Individuals with SUDs are often faced with the effects of racial and ethnic disparities, precarious living circumstances, poverty, trauma, and social association with people with criminal records. These factors may catalyze circumstances that culminate in criminal behavior and introduce a person to the justice system, potentially leading to a cycle of incarceration, probation, or parole and further compromised socioeconomic situations, in turn subjecting them to experiences that further increase their risk of violence.

# Therapeutic Jurisprudence

Therapeutic jurisprudence reflects a notion that at times and in certain ways, the courts can play a role in furthering therapeutic goals (Hora et al. 1999). It has evolved to be used more widely as a legal principle that melds the coercive aspect of the courts with clinical treatment needs of individual defendants to assert an obligation to participate in treatment beyond what would traditionally be permitted by the law, as a vehicle to singly arbitrate disputes and hold people accountable for violating social rules (Hora et al. 1999). The theory of therapeutic jurisprudence was introduced by David Wexler in 1987, who asserted that the law may and should be operating as a therapeutic agent, defined as follows:

> The study of the extent to which substantive rules, legal procedures, and the roles of lawyers and judges produce therapeutic or antitherapeutic consequences for individuals involved in the legal process…by taking a non-adversarial approach to the administration of justice. (Wexler and Winick 1991, p. 981)

In essence, therapeutic jurisprudence is an understanding of laws applied to mental health treatment as a force harnessed to promote therapeutic consequences and prevent antitherapeutic outcomes. To achieve the most effective disposition to criminal acts committed by people with therapeutic needs, therapeutic jurisprudence calls for the identification of areas in which effective therapeutic options are available as an alternative to traditional judicial case processing. Avoiding antitherapeutic consequences of a legal decision in favor of a more constructive referral to treatment when indicated is believed to further the prosocial goals of increased personal and societal well-being, all while reducing criminal behavior.

With that in mind, there has been growing interest in therapeutic jurisprudence as a vehicle that is legally permissible for mandated treatment for individuals in various settings. For example, individuals with SUDs who were criminally charged may be offered treatment in lieu of a traditional punishment sentence; this process is known as diversion and is discussed in the next section. This chapter reviews the interface among the law, SUD treatment, and alternatives to traditional punishments that use a combination of strategies.

# Diversion and the Sequential Intercept Model

Justice-involved people and those with SUDs are two groups that traditionally receive limited clinical services. Indeed, the majority of those with SUDs who would benefit from treatment do not receive it, owing to lack of access or an erroneous belief that they do not need treatment (Lipari et al. 2016) or to other factors that make it difficult to sustain treatment for the individual. Similarly, justice-involved individuals are less likely than the general population to receive medical treatments and supportive social services because of substantial barriers. Trends toward criminalizing SUDs in policies and laws have led to increases in populations that are unable to access sustained care. Many current policies are aiming to shift tides from criminalization to decriminalization of SUDs (see Chapter 2). For individuals involved in the criminal system, there are efforts to identify and intercept these otherwise "inaccessible" people, combined with a system of legal incentives for treatment. Individuals with SUDs are overrepresented at every level of the criminal justice system, providing an opportunity for interception to channel them toward treatment as an alternative to incarceration or other punishments. *Diversion* is a general term to describe these procedures aiming at redirecting persons in need of treatment into treatment as an alternative strategy to incarceration.

It is important to note other technical uses of the term *diversion*. Here, *jail diversion* might be considered the redirecting of an individual at the level of filing charges or at the level of a prosecutor determining a case is appropriate for rerouting. *Drug diversion*, in contrast, is the redistribution of prescribed substances usually for illicit purposes. With regard to criminal case processes, some would argue that once an individual is arraigned and has a criminal charge, *alternatives to incarceration* would then be more proper terminology. In this book, *jail diversion* in this context is used more generically as the *redirection to treatment* at any stage of criminal case processing.

The *sequential intercept model* (SIM) was first introduced in 2006 in a seminal article by Munetz and Griffin (2006). Although the model's name is agnostic as to the nature of the interventions it may include or some of the desired goals, the authors noted that SIM seeks to "prevent individuals with mental illness from entering or penetrating deeper into the criminal justice system" (Munetz and Griffin 2006, p. 544). The authors suggested that diversion from the justice system and linkage to clinical services allows for the decriminalization of mental illness. With that goal in mind, they described a conceptual framework for intercepting justice-involved individuals with mental illness mapped along the justice continuum.

Every step of the arrest-incarceration-release process is a point of interception, according to this framework, where unique diversion strategies may be used. In 2017, Abreu and colleagues added intercept 0, in recognition of the role that crisis services can play when initial contacts with individuals with behavioral health crises can lead to arrest or be deflected toward treatment (Abreu et al. 2017). The six intercept points along the justice continuum include

0. community-level interventions
1. law enforcement and emergency services
2. initial detention and initial hearings
3. jail, courts, forensic evaluations, and forensic commitments
4. reentry from jails, state prisons, and forensic hospitalization
5. community corrections and community support

Advocates of the model have promoted its use across the United States, and its general principles have been applied in many localities. The model has been expanded and used for individuals with mental illnesses and SUDs, co-occurring or alone, since it was first described (Bonfine et al. 2018; Pinals and Carey 2019); these conditions are now more commonly referred to as *behavioral health conditions* to be more inclusive. This is premised on the assumption that untreated mental disorders (including SUDs) lead to criminal behaviors and more frequent encounters with the justice system. Some studies have suggested that treatment might not be enough, failing to identify any reductions in criminal or violent outcomes between offenders with mental illness who receive treatment and those who do not (Hagan et al. 1997), including offenders who receive specialized treatment for SUDs (Rothbard et al. 1999). Such findings suggest that a one-size-fits-all approach to providing treatment to offenders with psychiatric disorders including SUDs might be insufficient. They may further signify that medical treatment interventions may need to be paired with nonclinical interventions addressing social determinants to prevent recidivism to criminal behaviors.

SIM seeks to reduce criminal justice system involvement among people with behavioral health challenges more broadly. This chapter identifies three dimensions whereby SIM is also being expanded and considered for individuals with SUDs specifically, and it further examines other potential avenues of prevention of negative outcomes for individuals who are criminally involved, as follows:

1. Include non-diversion-type (but early intercept 0–type) prevention interventions that may further serve the same goal of reducing criminal involvement.
2. Examine the outcomes sought by the model beyond reducing criminal justice involvement. Additional valid goals may include improving health outcomes, engaging in harm reduction, and improving quality of life and social productivity.
3. Continue adapting the model to subpopulations, specifically, for people with SUDs.

This chapter aims to add contours to an expanded model based on SIM, specifically designed to address the needs of the substance-using population across intercepts, looking at clinical and nonclinical interventions along the justice continuum for individuals with SUDs. The extended SIM described in this chapter focuses in more detail on clinical outcomes for people with SUDs. This is an important focus, given that such outcomes can further drive individuals toward criminal charges and worse health outcomes overall. For example, relapse in drug or alcohol use (a clinical outcome) may lead to criminal activity or violation of the terms of probation or parole (with legal consequences). As such, the expanded model will examine the clinical outcomes (e.g., substance use, overdoses, or medical complications) and the nonclinical outcomes (e.g., criminal recidivism, or the economic burden on society) of the different interventions.

Studies of services that offer jail diversion or alternatives to incarceration as part of the original SIM examine primarily criminal justice outcomes (e.g., decreased arrest and decreased days in jail) of the specific interventions. As such, clinical interventions designed to address the treatment needs of those with SUDs are often assessed on whether they affect criminal recidivism, with the clinical outcomes considered as secondary outcomes if at all. For example, diversion strategies seek to connect justice-involved persons with SUDs to treatment; by definition, this would alleviate the symptoms of the SUDs. A medically driven conceptualization of interventions for SUDs would ask whether they improve substance use and associated SUD outcomes. Any reductions in criminal behavior achieved as a result of such interventions would be considered an added benefit. However, the success of diversion interventions appears to be linked to whether individuals offered diversion are less likely to engage in criminal behavior, rather than whether they become less likely to use substances. These outcomes will ultimately determine which interventions will be implemented and utilized in their communities.

This approach of linking interventions with criminal recidivism outcomes differs significantly from the way clinical interventions for other disorders are delivered. For example, providing treatment for diabetes or depression is unlikely to be made contingent on whether it reduces criminal behavior. This highlights a lack of parity between SUDs and other psychiatric and nonpsychiatric disorders, whereby clinical interventions are held hostage to whether they reduce criminal behavior. An alternative model would conceptualize SUDs as a public health problem. This conceptualization would allow for a greater focus on outcomes beyond criminal recidivism through greater resource allocation and more meaningful collaborations between governmental agencies and health care providers.

By focusing on SUDs as a primary target for interventions in SIM and conceptualizing approaches across intercept points, new and unique opportunities for interventions that engage individuals who might not otherwise have been accessible for engagement can be offered. This can lead to reduced justice involvement but also improved health outcomes and social productivity. For example, Brinkley-Rubinstein et al. (2018b) used the SIM framework to present a model of clinical interventions aimed at reducing opioid overdoses among justice-involved people with opioid use disorders (OUDs). That model maps interventions, such as novel approaches to screening for OUD and training in the use of naloxone, along the justice continuum.

The conceptualization of the justice continuum involves multiple points of interception at each level of the person's involvement with the justice system.

Every interception point should be seen as an opportunity to intervene and prevent further justice involvement.

The initial contact with law enforcement officers or emergency personnel is the first opportunity to intercept justice-involved individuals with SUDs. At that level, officers may initiate prearrest interventions, arrest the individual, or both. Arrested individuals are typically detained pending arraignment. Interventions at that stage may offer alleged offenders diversion opportunities as alternatives to adjudication. Individuals moving forward for the process face initial hearings and may be arraigned. Those who do not qualify for interventions at that level may continue to court proceedings. If found guilty (or pleading guilty), some qualified offenders may be offered opportunities for posttrial diversion. Alternatively, offenders may be sentenced to prison or probation time, both of which afford the individual further opportunities to access interventions. Individuals who are incarcerated may benefit from reentry programming before their release. Upon completion of their prison sentence, individuals may be released on parole or unconditionally, which includes further opportunities to intervene (see Figure 9–1).

Diversion strategies are implemented by law enforcement officers at the prebooking level and by the courts before or after adjudication, including in criminal courts and drug courts. Post-adjudication-level diversion in criminal courts is typically enforced through probation as a condition of release. The limited data available appear to demonstrate that diversion strategies are effective at reducing future justice involvement and increasing engagement in treatment (Brinkley-Rubinstein et al. 2018b). The correctional system offers a constrained setting in which people with SUDs may be offered treatment. Therapeutic communities in detention facilities lead to reduced rates of criminal recidivism and improved substance use outcomes (Welsh 2007). Further, studies investigating the use of medications for OUD (MOUD) in correctional settings show that substance use outcomes are positive, whereas criminal outcomes after release are mixed (Gordon et al. 2017; Kinlock et al. 2009). Reentry programming for people released from detention aims to streamline access to clinical services. Data on specific reentry interventions are sparse, and few conclusions as to their effectiveness can be drawn (Hamilton 2010).

Although specific interventions at discrete decision points along the justice continuum can provide adequate tools to address justice involvement and substance use, it is the layering of services at consecutive points that can help stakeholders focus on continuity of treatment to help the individual make more meaningful progress in recovery (Peters et al. 2017). Thus, the model should be viewed as a longitudinal set of interventions that can be mapped along different intercept points, rather than distinct opportunities. However, few data exist on the comparative effectiveness of interventions at different time points or on the cumulative effectiveness of a sequence of interventions. In addition, because

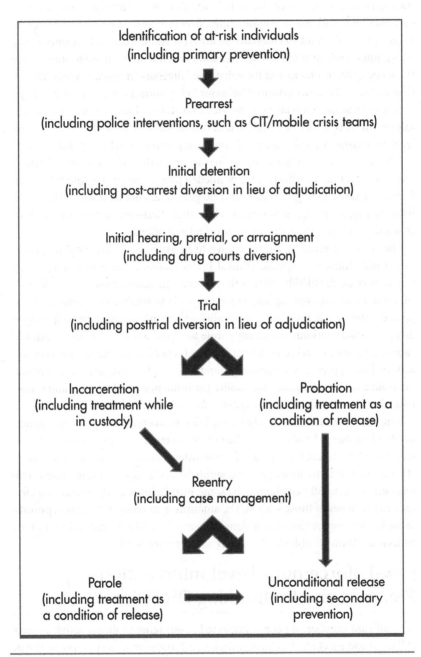

**Figure 9–1.** Framework for the justice continuum as it applies to the sequential intercept model (SIM).

CIT = crisis intervention team.

the interventions may allow some individuals to be redirected out of criminal case processes and others will be routed deeper into the criminal system, outcomes can be difficult to compare. Research is still needed to best understand which interventions might be beneficial for specific offender subgroups. Given the scope of the problem and the substantial diversity in specific SUDs, the nature and severity of the criminal behavior being addressed in the criminal system, and local factors relating to service availability, there is a need to identify interventions that can be effective and can be tailored to a variety of clinical-legal circumstances. For example, people using alcohol might respond to different interventions than those using heroin or methamphetamines. Similarly, interventions that are effective for domiciled people may be less likely to be effective for those facing homelessness. Repeat offenders or those with serious felonies might require different services than first-time offenders or those charged with less serious crimes or drug-related offenses.

Because untreated SUDs are known to be associated with criminal behaviors, withholding appropriate clinical interventions from people with SUDs might increase the likelihood that they reenter the justice system. One obvious situation in which ongoing substance use leads to further involvement in the justice system is the revocation of conditional release for those participating in diversion interventions, including parole and probation. Similarly, continued substance use can lead to recidivism in the form of engaging in new criminal acts, including property crimes to generate income for drug use, crimes resulting from a person's actions while under the influence of substances, and crimes related to the drug distribution system (Bennett and Holloway 2009). This revolving-door situation is clearly exemplified in correctional settings—people need to be sober to be able to exit the justice system. Having access to evidence-based SUD treatment is necessary for individuals to achieve the required sobriety; however, such treatment is often withheld while they are incarcerated. This has been successfully challenged in some jurisdictions as deliberate indifference to the needs of those with SUDs, amounting to cruel and unusual punishment in violation of the Eighth Amendment of the U.S. Constitution and the Americans With Disabilities Act (*Pesce v. Coppinger* 2018).

# Law-Enforcement-Level Interventions: Prearrest and Prebooking Diversion

A significant number of people suspected of engaging in illegal activities have SUDs (Morabito et al. 2017). As such, law enforcement officers serve as the de facto first line of interaction between them and the justice system, and at times, they are the first entry point for clinical interventions. Clinical diversion at this early stage represents a unique opportunity to intervene to improve both substance use outcomes and criminal outcomes (Kopak and Gleicher 2020).

During the initial police encounter, officers may use their discretionary authority to offer some qualified individuals the opportunity to enter treatment in lieu of being charged with a crime. Individuals found to be appropriate for diversion can be identified, taken to a health care facility or an emergency department for clinical assessment, and linked with case management and treatment programs (Lattimore et al. 2003). On the basis of the person's participation in the program, charges may not be filed, charges may be reduced, or proceedings may be continued. Although prebooking diversion is available through a large number of law enforcement agencies, little has been published on the outcomes.

Steadman and Naples (2005) used a quasi-experimental design to examine the outcomes of diversion programs for individuals with co-occurring severe mental illness and SUDs in Tennessee, Pennsylvania, and Oregon. Participants who were not diverted were almost twice as likely to be rearrested within a year and, on average, spent 2 fewer months in the community (i.e., hospitalized or incarcerated) than those who were diverted. Similarly, subjects in the diversion group were more likely to take prescribed medications and attend counseling sessions. Interestingly, those in the nondiverted group were more likely to use residential treatment services for SUDs. Unfortunately, substance use outcomes were not reported.

A crisis intervention team (CIT), as adapted from the original program in Memphis, Tennessee, is a specialized law enforcement response program that includes a collaborative training program for law enforcement officers to acquire mental health knowledge and intervention skills to improve interactions between police and people with mental illness. The training component of a CIT, which is only one element of the program, consists of 40 hours of lectures, role-playing activities, and exposure to clinical situations dealing with various psychiatric disorders. The concept promotes the use of de-escalation strategies and is meant to minimize the use of force in police encounters, promoting the safety of both officers and subjects and facilitating treatment referrals when appropriate (Compton et al. 2014). The CIT model has been adopted widely; however, there are no uniform requirements for the content taught to officers, particularly as it relates to SUDs.

Steadman et al. (2000) compared the CIT model to alternative prebooking interventions, including the community service officer model, mobile crisis teams, and emergency response teams. Their findings suggest that CIT may be more effective than other models in reducing the rates of arrest and in diverting individuals to mental health treatment.

Individuals with SUDs are more likely to be perceived as resisting and disrespectful in police encounters (Novak and Engel 2005). As such, it would be beneficial to examine whether CIT training affects such perceptions and, ultimately, outcomes. Unfortunately, much of the CIT literature examines mental illness without differentiating between SUDs and other disorders or comorbidities. Consequently, little is known about the outcomes of the CIT model for the substance-using population specifically. Broussard et al. (2010) found that CIT-trained officers in Georgia were significantly more likely to refer individuals with SUDs to psychiatric emergency services or family members than non-CIT-trained officers. They did not identify any significant differences among other psychiatric conditions examined. Compton et al. (2014) performed a retrospective analysis of 1,063 police records examining the outcomes of CIT training on encounter disposition and use of force. They found that in police encounters involving individuals with SUDs, CIT-trained officers were more likely to refer to treatment and less likely to arrest or resolve the situation at the scene than non-CIT-trained officers. Interestingly, the effect size for referring individuals to treatment was greater for individuals with SUDs alone than for individuals with a comorbid psychiatric disorder or with mental illness alone. Data from the Portland Police Bureau in Oregon, where all patrol officers had received CIT training, showed that police encounters were more likely to involve the use of force when the individual was perceived as having an SUD (Morabito et al. 2017). Similarly, such individuals were more likely to be perceived as resisting. Unfortunately, those outcomes were not compared with outcomes from officers who had not received CIT training to evaluate the effect of such training on police use of force and police perceptions of individuals with SUDs.

In contrast to CIT, interventions such as mobile crisis teams involve mental health professionals aiding and providing support to law enforcement officers. Collaboration among police officers and clinicians occurs either directly (e.g., co-response ride-along, whereby mental health professionals accompany officers responding to situations potentially involving persons with mental illness) or indirectly (e.g., remote or telephone consultation). Such interventions aim to improve the police/community relationship, improve officers' ability to manage people with mental illness, reduce the use of force, and refer eligible individuals to treatment (Hartford et al. 2006; Scott 2000). Watson et al. (2019) provided a detailed review of the research evidence on the different types of response models. Currently, there are no studies reporting the effects of using mobile crisis teams with the substance-using population.

In Seattle, the Law Enforcement Assisted Diversion (LEAD) program was established to divert those suspected of low-level drug and prostitution offenses to clinical, social, and legal services instead of prosecution. This model is unique in that it uses a harm reduction approach whereby qualified individuals are offered legal support and case management tailored to their needs, including housing, vocational training, and education, as well as SUD treatment. Collins et al. (2017) reported that LEAD intervention was associated with reductions of 60% in subsequent arrests and 39% in felony charges.

In Portland, Oregon, a program similar to LEAD was established to identify individuals with co-occurring addictive and nonaddictive psychiatric disorders who come in contact with law enforcement and to divert them to treatment (Gratton et al. 2001). Compared with nondiverted individuals, program participants had better health outcomes for SUDs and other psychiatric disorders (although the improvements in substance use waned after a year). The diverted group did not have reductions in the rates of criminal recidivism (Gratton et al. 2001).

The landscape of crisis response is evolving rapidly. With the murder of George Floyd in 2020 and increased scrutiny of law enforcement responses to individuals with behavioral health conditions, policymakers are focusing on expanding partnerships and attending to disparate treatment of individuals of underrepresented racial and ethnic minority groups and those with mental illness who encounter law enforcement. Additionally, the development and implementation of the 988 suicide and crisis line, which is not just for people with mental illness and specifically includes individuals with SUDs, will likely lead to further developments at the intercept-0 level of intervention.

# Diversion Preadjudication or at Initial Court Hearings

Individuals who are not eligible for prebooking diversion or who live in communities lacking the resources to develop prebooking diversion programs often move forward along the justice continuum. Initial hearings, including arraignment proceedings, offer another opportunity to intercept justice-involved individuals with SUDs, although eligibility for such programs varies across jurisdictions. At this level, diversion to treatment may be offered as an alternative to or prior to prosecution, but not all prosecutors will look at opportunities similarly. In some jurisdictions, presentencing evaluations will be developed by nonclinicians. In other places, clinicians affiliated with the courts may evaluate arrested individuals for the presence of conditions amenable to treatment for whom diversion may be appropriate. They identify and advise the court on those who may qualify for the program (Munetz and Griffin 2006). It is important to note that the ethics guidelines of the American Academy of Psychiatry and the Law (2005) advise against performing assessments on behalf of the government in criminal contexts where an individual has not had access to a defense attorney. As such, any evaluations for prosecution prior to arraignment or access to counsel would be prohibited.

From the perspective of outcomes by the courts, there are different ways that early diversion can work (Shafer et al. 2004). These include the following:

- *Release on conditions*: Bail statutes generally assess an individual's risk of failure to appear in court and may also assess for risk of violence to the community. If an individual is determined to be of low risk in these areas, they may be released preplea on the conditions that they appear in court and do not engage in further prohibited behavior. Also, individuals with a good track record may be released from jail while awaiting trial postplea, allowing the person to engage in SUD treatment in the community. They are typically required to comply with treatment, have no further arrests, and appear in court for the normal course of proceedings. Violating these conditions may lead to revocation of bail or pretrial release.

- *Deferred prosecution*: In situations in which sufficient facts are available to warrant a finding of guilt, the court may defer further legal proceedings for a period of time (e.g., a year). During this time, individuals are offered probation (albeit prior to adjudication) and are monitored by probation officers who work for and report to the court. The individuals so released are required to comply with treatment as dictated by the court, abstain from substance use, have no further arrests, and appear in court for the normal course of proceedings. Violating these conditions may lead to extensions of the time of oversight, modification of conditions, or resumption of prosecution. Upon successful completion of the program, the charges may be lowered or dismissed. As noted earlier in Chapter 2, this practice was recently challenged in a case heard by the Massachusetts Supreme Judicial Court. In *Commonwealth v. Eldred* (2018), a defendant arraigned on felony charges for larceny was offered probation that required her to submit to outpatient SUD treatment and abstain from drug use. When the defendant was found to have used opioids, the judge ruled that she had violated the conditions of her probation and required her to submit to inpatient SUD treatment instead. The court affirmed the power of the judge to revoke or modify the conditions of probation, noting that this was not a punishment for the violation but had therapeutic intent.

Steadman and Naples (2005) also reported data from three postbooking diversion programs for individuals with co-occurring severe mental illness and SUDs in Arizona, Connecticut, and Oregon. With postbooking diversion, they found that participants who were not diverted were more likely to be rearrested at 1 year and, on average, spent one less month in the community than those who were diverted, similar to their findings with prebooking diversion. Diverted subjects were more likely to be taking prescribed medications and attend counseling sessions and were less likely to use residential treatment services for SUDs. As with many of the studies focused more on mental illness, substance use outcomes were not reported. Still, in this study, prebooking diversion was associated with better outcomes than postbooking diversion.

Conversely, another study from Arizona included individuals with co-occurring SUDs and other mental illnesses and compared outcomes between postbooking diverted subjects and nondiverted subjects (Shafer et al. 2004). The authors identified no differences in criminal or substance use outcomes. The diverted group was noted to be more likely to use emergency room services for mental health needs, including SUDs, compared with the nondiverted group. Overall, as programs emerge across the country, more studies are needed to develop pathways for individuals with SUDs and determine outcomes over time.

# Probation: Postadjudication Diversion

Programs that move individuals with SUDs toward treatment as an alternative to incarceration postadjudication are also critical in the sequential intercept continuum. If they are determined to be eligible, individuals with SUDs who have been convicted of a criminal act may be offered participation in programs in the community in lieu of incarceration. Under these circumstances, probation officers monitor adherence with the terms set forth by the adjudicating court. Such probationers are required to meet regularly with supervising probation officers, attend treatment, abstain from substance use, and have no further arrests. More recently, participation in substance use treatment that may involve use of prescribed medications (e.g., buprenorphine and methadone) is becoming increasingly acceptable. Still, violating any of the conditions may lead to extensions of the mandated supervision time, may result in modification of the probation requirements, or may involve incarceration itself—either for a brief stay or for the duration of the sentence previously avoided.

# Drug Courts

People with SUDs charged with a crime may be deemed appropriate for drug court. The drug court literature describes two major goals: 1) reduction in substance use and 2) reduction in criminal behavior. Drug courts are special-jurisdiction courts modeled to offer participants the opportunity to seek SUD treatment and ongoing monitoring as an alternative to, or as a means of reducing, punishment via incarceration (Huddleston and Marlowe 2011). Since the initial inception of the model, specialized drug courts such as juvenile drug courts, driving while intoxicated courts, or courts for individuals with co-occurring SUDs and nonaddictive psychiatric disorders have emerged. The National Treatment Court Resource Center (2023) estimates that upward of 4,000 drug courts are in operation across the United States. The majority of drug courts receive federal funding; eligibility requires that courts exclude violent offenders (U.S. General Accounting Office 1997). As such, historically, most drug courts restricted program eligibility to those with SUDs who were charged with nonviolent, non-drug-trafficking offenses, without prior serious violent offenses, and with fewer than three prior felony charges (Belenko 1998; Rossman et al. 2011). Although many of these restrictions still apply, studies of the model for individuals also at high risk of recidivism have also shown promise compared with sending these same high-risk offenders through routine probation (Koetzle et al. 2015).

Drug courts allow for the diversion of eligible individuals following one of two tracks: preceding or following adjudication. (Some courts offer both tracks based on the nature of the offense or characteristics of the defendant.) In the first track, defendants are admitted to the court shortly after arrest and waive their right to a speedy trial, with the agreement that their charges will be dropped if they successfully complete the program. In the second track, eligible individuals who have already been adjudicated as guilty through a plea bargain but have not been sentenced may receive a sentence of time served or probation if they comply with the court's requirements and graduate from the program (National Association of Drug Court Professionals 1997; Peters et al. 2017. It is worth noting that drug courts follow a nonadversarial approach and that participating in these programs is voluntary, even if there is the reality of incarceration as the alternative option. This issue of voluntariness is also recognized as important as more drug courts and other criminal justice settings begin to accept the use of MOUD (Hyatt and Lobmaier 2020).

Drug court participants are required to submit to frequent urine testing, attend a treatment program, and appear in court regularly for status hearings, typically for 6–18 months. According to National Association of Drug Court Professionals (NADCP) best practice standards, participant responses are given incentives, and noncompliance with terms may be subject to sanctions. Incentives include verbal praise and phase advancement, graduation, and even rewards; sanctions refer to verbal admonishments, tightened program requirements, stern warnings, community service, short jail stays, or even termination from the program (National Association of Drug Court Professionals 2018). Along the way, the judge and the drug court team may make adjustments to program requirements. The 2018 NADCP standards also put forth a number of different considerations from a racial and ethnic equity perspective to attempt to remove structural biases in how programs operate.

A prospective study examined outcomes of 2,095 patients at 15 U.S. Veterans Affairs intensive 21- or 28-day SUD residential treatment programs across three groups (Kelly et al. 2005). The groups comprised patients who were involved in the justice system and mandated to treatment, were nonmandated and involved in the justice system, and were not involved in the justice system. Mandated patients had a less severe clinical picture at program outset, but even with that distinction, they showed similar or better outcomes. Treatment perceptions were similar across groups. Overall, the authors concluded that mandates may offer offenders with SUDs an opportunity for benefits and access to treatments that may lead to improved outcomes (Kelly et al. 2005). Of course, whether this study's findings would be equivalent in non-veteran-involved contexts is unknown.

As an extension of examining mandated treatments in criminal justice contexts, drug court outcomes have been studied extensively. Methodological limitations and significant variability across these specialized treatment courts limit the generalizability of the findings. Yet a multisite evaluation of 23 adult drug courts spanning 8 states identified significant reductions in drug and alcohol use for drug court participants during program participation versus a comparison group, and the reductions extended for several months after completion (Rossman et al. 2011). Interestingly, reductions were significant for alcohol use, marijuana use, and illegal use of prescription drugs, including methadone, but reductions in cocaine, heroin, and amphetamine use were not significant. Further, participating in these programs led to significant reductions (23%) in criminal reoffending relative to the comparison group. The impact of drug courts was most significant for drug-related crimes, including both possession and trafficking, and continued to be significant for up to 3 months after graduation. Further analysis of these findings suggests that the reduction in criminal behavior was mediated by the reduction in substance use, confirming the nexus between substance use and crime (Rossman et al. 2011).

Mitchell et al. (2012a) published a meta-analysis of 92 studies evaluating drug court outcomes. Their findings were mostly consistent with those noted earlier in this section, showing a 13% reduction in criminal recidivism during drug court participation and for up to 36 months after entering the program. They also noted that courts that had more rigorous requirements (with more frequent status hearings) and that dismissed or expunged charges were likely to see more pronounced reductions in criminal behavior, suggesting that the courts' leverage can effectively motivate behavior change. Interestingly, Mitchell et al. (2012a) found that courts that admit violent offenders may be less effective than those that do not. Finally, unlike the previous study by Rossman et al. (2011), Michell et al. did not identify statistically significant differences in substance use associated with drug courts. This was thought to be due to the scant number of studies that adequately reported the effect of drug court participation on measures of actual substance use (Mitchell et al. 2012a). Nonetheless, this study estimated that just under half of drug court participants graduate successfully from the programs (Mitchell et al. 2012a). Overall, the drug court literature has shown promising outcomes, furthering the efforts to continue to establish these programs, broaden them to additional populations (e.g., as seen with the expansion to veterans' treatment courts), and study how to refine them. The NADCP and its local chapters remain a critical force behind furthering the work for drug courts across the United States as a major alternative to traditional incarceration for particular offenders.

Even with the availability of expanding treatment court programs, including mental health courts and co-occurring courts, data have shown that there are disparities in referrals to treatment courts (higher for White individuals and female individuals compared with their arrests) and graduation rates (higher for White individuals than Black individuals) (Ho et al. 2018). However, policies may be put in place to minimize these disparities. It is important to continuously consider these issues of structural inequities as treatment options are expanded.

# Correctional-Level Interventions

The majority of incarcerated individuals with SUDs do not receive evidence-based SUD treatment (Bronson et al. 2017). Incarceration may constitute an important, if not ideal, setting for the identification and treatment of individuals with SUDs by virtue of accessible medical care and reduced access to drugs and alcohol. However, access to such interventions is often limited because of correctional policies, stigma, and the erroneous belief that being sober while incarcerated is therapeutic in itself, negating the need for further treatment (Wakeman 2017). A multitude of interventions are used to address the clinical needs of people with SUDs in the correctional system, including individual or group counseling, boot camps, prison-based therapeutic communities, and prison-based medication-assisted treatment (MAT) for SUDs. A review of the published literature suggests that the latter two interventions are the most promising emerging correctional approaches (Mitchell et al. 2012b). A detailed review of SUDs in correctional settings is presented in Chapter 10, but the next section provides an overview of the effects of therapeutic interventions in correctional settings on clinical and criminal outcomes for those with SUDs, consistent with the tenets of offering opportunities to intercept and treat individuals presenting at various points along the criminal continuum.

# Therapeutic Communities in Prisons

Therapeutic communities are hierarchical 12- to 18-month residential treatment programs in which the community is used as the agent of behavioral change to promote long-term abstinence (Welsh 2007). The community provides a highly structured prosocial environment, seeking to modify negative thinking and behaviors through reinforcement by positive and negative contingencies. The therapeutic community comprises clinical staff and recovering individuals, using confrontation and behavior modification strategies to foster interaction, assimilation of social norms focused on sobriety, learning of effective coping strategies, and development of self-control and responsibility. Peer influence is shaped through group process, individual therapy, and participation in a therapeutic milieu. Therapeutic communities have been adapted to prison settings and appear to lead to improved substance use and criminal recidivism outcomes.

Assessing the effectiveness of therapeutic community interventions is complicated, because published data frequently present sequential models of individuals assigned to a prison-based therapeutic community followed by a community-based one. This makes appraising the prison-based component as a stand-alone intervention less reliable. For example, older studies from Delaware (Inciardi et al. 2004; Martin et al. 1999), California (Wexler et al. 1999), and Texas (Knight et al. 1999) reported on inmates with SUDs who were nearing release from incarceration and were assigned to a prison-based therapeutic community, followed by a community-based one and subsequent outpatient SUD treatment. Compared with inmates with SUDs who were not assigned to these interventions, the study group was more likely to remain arrest free and less likely to experience drug or alcohol relapse for up to 5 years. Of note, assignment of subjects to the study or comparison groups was not random. Subgroup analysis showed that differences were less marked for participants who completed the prison-based therapeutic community but dropped out of postrelease treatment.

Welsh (2007) studied the outcomes of prison-based therapeutic communities as stand-alone interventions in five Pennsylvania prisons. Inmates with SUDs were assigned to therapeutic communities with a mean duration of 48 weeks prior to release, with or without postrelease interventions. Two years after release, the control group without the therapeutic community intervention was more likely to have been rearrested and reincarcerated. However, there were no significant differences in the rates of relapse between the two groups. Younger age, greater addiction severity, and less employment were associated with more postrelease criminal behaviors in both groups.

A Campbell systematic review and meta-analysis of 35 prison-based therapeutic community studies published between 1980 and 2011 demonstrated that the intervention was associated with relatively consistent but modest improvements in criminal and SUD outcomes (Mitchell et al. 2012a). A reduction in criminal recidivism was associated with participating in a therapeutic community program, with a significant odds ratio of 1.40, among both male and female inmates.

Overall, the collective weight of the literature on prison-based therapeutic communities suggests that they lead to reduced rates of criminal recidivism and improved substance use outcomes, but their effect is not as strong as that of other interventions. Furthermore, because many of the studies predate the height of the opioid epidemic and the methamphetamine surge seen in the

United States, it will be important to continue to pursue research of these programs and examine outcomes across settings.

# Medication Use for the Treatment of SUDs in Correctional Settings

The World Health Organization recommends that medications for the treatment of SUDs be made available to incarcerated individuals, as is frequently the case in Canada, several European countries, Australia, and China, among others (Sharma et al. 2016; World Health Organization 2009). Over the past two decades, there has been great interest in implementing maintenance treatment programs for SUDs using approved pharmacotherapy in correctional settings in the United States. Such programs are meant to go beyond simply providing medically supervised withdrawal management (which was in the past more commonly referred to as *detoxification*). Published research to date focuses primarily on treating OUDs with FDA-approved medications (i.e., methadone, buprenorphine, and extended-release naltrexone). However, very little has been published on the use of medications for the treatment of other SUDs for incarcerated populations, including SUDs for which FDA-approved medications are available, such as alcohol use disorder or nicotine use disorder. Further, studies on the use of MOUDs in correctional settings vary widely based on whether the following are present:

- The target population was being prescribed such medications prior to arrest
- Medications were started early, as soon as the disorder was identified, or not until the prerelease period
- Study outcomes were measured during incarceration or after release
- The study was performed in a jail or prison
- The study examined a particular medication or medications

In Rhode Island (Brinkley-Rubinstein et al. 2018a; Rich et al. 2015), inmates who were already enrolled in a methadone maintenance program at the time of arrest were randomly assigned to continued methadone treatment while incarcerated compared with inmates who received methadone taper. Participants were followed for 12 months after release. Those who continued on maintenance treatment were more likely to return to methadone treatment upon release and less likely to report using opioids outside of prescribed treatment. No differences in reincarceration rates were identified. A retrospective analysis of 960 inmates in New Mexico reported that individuals who continued methadone while incarcerated were less likely to recidivate, took longer to be rebooked (i.e., rearrested), and were more likely to return to their prearrest methadone clinic compared with inmates who were forced to be withdrawn from methadone during incarceration (Westerberg et al. 2016). Finally, in one controlled trial, jail inmates who were not receiving MOUD at the time of arrest were randomly assigned to receive either methadone or buprenorphine (Magura et al. 2009). They maintained the medication for the duration of jail time and at the time of release and were referred to outpatient clinics where they could continue treatment after release. The buprenorphine group was more likely to continue treatment 3 months after release; however, no group differences between self-reported heroin use or reincarceration rates were identified. This study did not include a control group that did not receive medications; as such, the researchers were unable to draw conclusions as to whether being prescribed methadone or buprenorphine while incarcerated increases the likelihood of engaging in OUD treatment after release compared with not prescribing treatment at all. That said, medications are considered life-saving and needed care for OUD, and this study highlights the importance of access to these treatments even for incarcerated populations.

Overall, it appears that the use of prison-based medications for SUD treatments is effective at reducing substance use after release, especially when individuals are connected to care providers for continuity of treatment. However, their role in reducing future criminal behavior is not uniformly covered by the literature and requires further study.

# Reentry-Level Interventions

*Reentry services* refers to programs designed to promote continuity of treatment services for individuals who are released back into the community (sometimes referred to as *returning citizens*). Court rulings in state courts and several federal circuits have mandated some level of discharge service planning (e.g., *Brad H. v. City of New York* 2000; *Wakefield v. Thompson* 1999). Such rulings, along with other factors, have contributed to significant variability in the levels of services available. This section examines more comprehensive models of reentry services that have been postulated to affect criminal recidivism or SUD outcomes. These include programs that use psychosocial interventions such as reentry courts, integrated case management services, and programs that use medications to treat SUDs as part of reentry services.

Factors hindering the delivery of clinical services for SUDs in correctional settings relate to some misconceptions. Indeed, abstinence in confinement is inappropriately equated with cure for SUDs. This uses a conceptual model of SUDs that is similar to infectious diseases in the sense that when symptoms improve, the illness is cured (for example, when influenza symptoms have improved, the infectious process is typically resolved). The same cannot be said for

SUDs. Being in detention—where opportunities for substance use, in principle, are limited—can create some confusion, because being "sober" for the duration of one's sentence does not imply that a person's underlying SUD is cured. Without evidence-based SUD treatment during incarceration or detention and continuity of this treatment upon release, the risks associated with return to illicit substance use are grave. This underscores the importance of providing SUD treatment in prisons. As noted earlier in this chapter, there is a dire need for research on treating other SUDs, such as alcohol use disorder or stimulant use disorders, in correctional settings because of their significant effects on public health and criminal behaviors.

# Reentry Programming Using Psychosocial Interventions

Different models of psychosocial programming exist for individuals with SUDs. They all aim to link the released offender with agencies in the community that can provide mental health and SUD treatment services, assistance with housing and vocational training, and other services. The success of such interventions is increased by fostering effective transfer of information between the detention facility and community agencies, assisting with transportation to initial appointments, and facilitating the enrollment of the subject for benefits such as Medicaid or Supplemental Security Income (Peters et al. 2017). These programs are marked by significant diversity, differing in counseling components and interventions targeting specific subpopulations or family cohesion needs.

The literature examining such interventions specific to persons with SUDs is sparse and, for the most part, examines specific programs instituted in local institutions, which limits the extent to which the effectiveness of each intervention is understood. This is further complicated by the fact that despite including large numbers of subjects with SUDs, studies have not been generally designed to examine the specific outcomes in this population across particular SUDs or needs of subpopulations. As such, some of the models found to be most generalizable are described in this chapter. Of specific interest are integrated case management services and reentry courts.

## INTEGRATED TRANSITIONAL CASE MANAGEMENT

Integrated transitional case management programs for offenders with SUDs have been investigated as part of several local initiatives. These programs typically include a combination of counseling services and case management services to coordinate the complex treatment needs of participating individuals, help transition them to integrated community treatment programs, and reduce factors that may contribute to criminal behavior (Prendergast 2009). They often aid with housing, education, vocational training, transportation documentation, or family support.

The REAL MEN (Returning Educated African American and Latino Men to Enriched Neighborhoods) program from the New York City jails offered a prerelease 30-hour counseling intervention, along with community partnerships, to provide general educational development (GED)-level education, job training, and referrals for health care services for qualifying individuals (Freudenberg et al. 2010). Compared with a control group, people receiving the intervention had an increased likelihood of following up with community-based health organizations, improved substance use outcomes, and less subsequent time spent in incarceration (Freudenberg et al. 2010).

Community Reinforcement and Family Training (CRAFT), a program based on operant conditioning, follows a similar model that incorporates a community reinforcement approach to substance abuse treatment. Eligible individuals are coached to identify new, enjoyable substance-free activities (Miller et al. 2016). A comparison of subjects participating in the CRAFT program and control participants noted that the study group was less likely to recidivate. No substance use outcomes were reported, however (Miller et al. 2016).

Such programs may be integrated with parole, as was done in the Treatment Accountability for Safer Communities (TASC) model. However, specific outcomes for the SUD population were not published (Prendergast 2009).

## REENTRY COURTS

Reentry courts are based on some of the successful components of the drug court model, using judicial oversight and collaborative case management to support individuals released on parole (Hamilton 2010) or probation. In this model, the role of probation or parole officers is expanded to assist the judge in the design of a reentry plan involving a psychosocial assessment and service need identification for SUDs and other mental health treatments, along with vocational and educational training. The court provides an extra layer of oversight, using incentives and sanctions to promote compliance. The program typically lasts 6–12 months, and successful completers are transferred to traditional parole supervision, where they may continue to receive case management services. The Center for Court Innovation published outcomes from one such court in Harlem, New York (Hamilton 2010). Although the author did not specifically examine the impact of this intervention in the SUD population, Hamilton (2010) noted that a large fraction of the program's participants met criteria for SUDs. The author found that the intervention had a positive impact with regard to preventing future criminal behavior, particularly drug-related arrests or convictions.

# Medications for SUD Treatment as a Component of Reentry Services

As discussèd earlier in this chapter, medications for the treatment of SUDs are being used as a component of reentry services. As such, inmates with SUDs nearing the end of their incarceration may be evaluated for the appropriateness of MAT. As in the literature on correctional-based MAT, there are few published data on using medications for nonopioid SUDs. This limitation is more of a concern in reentry settings, because of the risk of relapse to alcohol or tobacco for individuals with alcohol use disorder or tobacco use disorder by virtue of increased access to these substances in the community compared with jails and prisons.

Multiple studies have examined outcomes of using MAT in reentry programming for individuals with OUD. In this context, maintenance treatment using both opioid agonist medications (e.g., buprenorphine or methadone) and opioid antagonist alternatives (e.g., naltrexone) were evaluated. Further, studies varied in whether the medication was started while the individual was still incarcerated or whether reentry staff arranged postrelease referrals for the medications to be started in the community.

Kinlock et al. (2007, 2009) investigated the effects of initiating methadone treatment prerelease among inmates with OUD from a Maryland prison compared with counseling while incarcerated with a referral to methadone treatment in the community postrelease. They found that the study group had an increased likelihood of continuing methadone treatment after release, a longer duration of treatment, and less opioid use, as evidenced by negative urine drug screens for up to 12 months. There were no differences in the rates of reincarceration between the two groups.

In another trial, researchers investigated the effects 12 months after release of initiating treatment with buprenorphine prior to release from incarceration for inmates with OUD (Gordon et al. 2014, 2017). They found that compared with inmates offered counseling only while incarcerated with referral to buprenorphine treatment in the community after release, the study group had a higher number of days in treatment. There were no significant differences between the two groups in opioid- or cocaine-positive urine drug screens or criminal behavior.

Since the introduction of extended-release injectable naltrexone (XR-NTX), there has been interest in using this medication in correctional settings. This interest is likely driven by the fact that XR-NTX is an opioid antagonist without agonist effects at the μ opioid receptor. Lee et al. (2015) conducted a randomized controlled trial that assigned inmates in a New York City jail to XR-

NTX immediately prior to release or to a treatment-as-usual control group without medication. The authors found that 75% of inmates who received XR-NTX prior to release returned for a second injection 1 month after release. Study participants who received the medication were less likely to experience opioid relapse, as demonstrated by urine drug test results. No significant differences were noted between the two groups in terms of participation in community SUD treatment programs or rates of reincarceration. A similar study was conducted in a Massachusetts jail, where inmates with OUD were assigned to XR-NTX initiation immediately prerelease or referral to community treatment for XR-NTX initiation (Lincoln et al. 2018). The former group was more likely to be retained in treatment for up to 6 months. Of the 47 study participants assigned to initiating XR-NTX prerelease, 3 died from an opioid overdose after stopping XR-NTX versus 0 in the comparison group. This finding is consistent with reports of fatal opioid overdoses seen with XR-NTX in community settings, thought to be related to a reduced tolerance to opioids following a period of abstinence (Saucier et al. 2018).

Instead of initiating OUD medications prerelease, some reentry models have relied on providing referrals for eligible individuals to community-based opioid treatment programs. One retrospective study examining the outcomes of this model reported that fewer than 1 in 20 of those referred by a justice agency to community treatment centers for OUD were treated using maintenance medications (Krawczyk et al. 2017). The authors noted that individuals referred from other sources to those same treatment centers were 10 times more likely to receive MAT.

With some of these findings and anecdotal reports, more recent questions have emerged about naltrexone outcomes compared with the use of agonists to treat OUD and the newly available long-acting injectable forms of buprenorphine. To that end, EXIT-CJS is a multisite open-label randomized controlled trial that will compare retention and effectiveness of extended-release buprenorphine and extended-release naltrexone to treat OUD in people who are involved in the criminal justice system (Waddell et al. 2021). It will be important for practitioners of all types to stay abreast of emerging data to ensure proper access to care in carceral settings and beyond. This research will also be important for forensic practitioners who may be examining case outcomes, policies, and practices in contexts involving forensic opinion formation.

# Interventions at the Level of Community Supervision: Probation and Parole

*Parole* is the supervised release of a prisoner. *Probation* is a supervised release, either as a suspended incarceration for a person convicted of a crime or as a portion of a sentence. Probation can also be offered pretrial (as described earlier

in this chapter). Incarcerated offenders may be eligible for early release on parole. Parole is considered a privilege and not a right granted to eligible offenders, who are subject to parole conditions with a set duration. To avoid returning
to correctional custody, parolees are typically required to report regularly to
their parole officers, avoid rearrests, and, for offenders with SUDs, abstain from
alcohol and drug use and engage in SUD treatment. Those who successfully
complete the terms of their parole are eligible for unconditional release.

Parole and probation are similar in many regards: both represent pathways for
offenders to reside in the community instead of prison or jail, both are subject to revocation or modification in the event of noncompliance with the conditions of release, and in both, the individual is required to report regularly to a supervising
officer. However, probation is generally handled through the courts, and parole is
handled via a parole board of sorts through a particular state agency. Some individuals can be released on combined probation and parole, as they are managed dis-
tinctly and may stem from different underlying offenses. Outcomes research
literature frequently combines outcomes from both parole and probation. In this
section, the evidence for both parole and probation interventions will be presented
combined. Note, however, that parolees will have served time in prison prior to being released, which may represent a confounder in the appraisal of interventions
used at this level. Studying the effect of this confounder on substance use and criminal recidivism outcomes in interventions targeting the SUD population would provide valuable information; however, published studies are limited in addressing this
issue. Specific and targeted interventions may be examined within community supervision (Perry et al. 2009). Specialized probation and parole programs in which
the supervising officer serves as a case manager of sorts have been developed with
a focus on treatment and various other interventions of interest, such as using the
TASC model described earlier in this chapter or pairing community supervision
with assertive community treatment team models. Such interventions are generally
published as a proof of concept and are often not replicated.

Kubiak et al. (2006) used data from the National Survey on Drug Use and
Health to study the association between justice involvement and admission into
specialty treatment programs for individuals with SUDs. They found that people with SUDs under conditional release and in community supervision were
most likely to seek treatment. Further, they noted that within that group, those
with a recent arrest were even more likely to engage in treatment programs. In
a systematic review, Holloway et al. (2005) examined the outcomes of various
interventions in reducing drug-related crimes. Although the subject population
did not specifically have SUDs, drug-related crimes are often considered a
proxy for drug use. The authors found that both parole and probation were effective justice interventions in reducing criminal behavior.

In a 2019 study, participants sent for more enhanced treatment had more successful outcomes compared with probationers and parolees sanctioned to jail time when they committed substance-use-related community supervision violations (Boman et al. 2019). Another study examined specific substances involved in the SUDs of persons on probation and parole (Moore et al. 2022). The authors found more cocaine use in metropolitan areas and more methamphetamine use in nonmetropolitan areas, suggesting that interventions should be tailored to specific issues raised by these differences (Moore et al. 2022). Binswanger et al. (2020) showed community overdoses at alarming rates for those individuals under correctional supervision, with nearly a third (approximately 28%) on probation and about 13% on parole. These findings highlight the critical need for naloxone and overdose prevention strategies for people under this type of monitoring (Binswanger et al. 2020).

Taken together, studies examining SUDs and correctional community supervision demonstrate the relevance of examining the role of probation and parole in combination with treatment systems to help reduce morbidity and mortality and pursue best practices along the SIM. Moreover, although some interventions at the community supervision level appear to be promising, these programs may represent an opportunity that has not been fully taken advantage of, given the lack of replication studies.

# Conclusions

Legally mandated treatment for SUDs in criminal justice contexts, which is distinct from civil contexts, has shown some promise. By melding treatment goals with some of the criminal justice goals, one enters very complex waters. Applying the principles of therapeutic jurisprudence can, in the best of circumstances, serve a goal of assisting individuals in receiving fair treatment. Programs may be built to divert individuals with SUDs toward needed treatment rather than warehousing them in carceral settings where treatment is not available. At the same time, coercive elements of care are risky endeavors, and they are all too often applied inequitably across vulnerable populations. The SIM provides a framework that can help clinicians and legal professionals systematically examine the availability of programs in particular jurisdictions. The SIM can also be used as a tool to promote diversion to appropriate treatments at all steps along the criminal-legal continuum, thereby facilitating good care while unburdening the criminal system. For those already incarcerated, programs that yield effective outcomes and enhanced discharge services can tip the balance toward health and recovery when they return to their communities from incarceration.

# Key Points

- Therapeutic jurisprudence, the basis for drug courts, combines the power of the courts with elements of substance use disorder (SUD) treatment.

- Police officers have substantial discretionary authority to offer qualified individuals prebooking SUD treatment, and more programs are needed to achieve this goal.

- SUD treatment and overdose prevention during probation and parole can have a substantial positive impact.

- Effective programs in prison, along with community treatment follow-up, can enhance positive response rates in terms of addiction relapse and recidivism to the legal system.

- Medications for addiction are essential components of care before and during incarceration and detention and upon reentry following a jail stay or prison sentence; in this way, continuity of treatment should follow the person regardless of the setting in which they are found.

# References

Abreu D, Parker TW, Noether CD, et al: Revising the paradigm for jail diversion for people with mental and substance use disorders: Intercept 0. Behav Sci Law 35(5–6):380–395, 2017 29034504

American Academy of Psychiatry and the Law: Ethics guidelines for the practice of forensic psychiatry. May 2005. Available at: https://www.aapl.org/ethics.htm. Accessed November 13, 2018.

Belenko S: Research on drug courts: a critical review. Nat Drug Court Institute Rev 1(1):1–42, 1998

Bennett T, Holloway K: The causal connection between drug misuse and crime. Br J Criminol 49(4):513–531, 2009

Binswanger IA, Nguyen AP, Morenoff JD, et al: The association of criminal justice supervision setting with overdose mortality: a longitudinal cohort study. Addiction 115(12):2329–2338, 2020 32267585

Boman JH 4th, Mowen TJ, Wodahl EJ, et al: Responding to substance-use-related probation and parole violations: are enhanced treatment sanctions preferable to jail sanctions? Crim Justice Stud 32(4):356–370, 2019 34017218

Bonfine N, Munetz MR, Simera RH: Sequential intercept mapping: developing systems-level solutions for the opioid epidemic. Psychiatr Serv 69(11):1124–1126, 2018 30185122

Brad H. v City of New York, 712 N.Y.S.2d 336 (Sup. Ct. 2000)

Brinkley-Rubinstein L, McKenzie M, Macmadu A, et al: A randomized, open label trial of methadone continuation versus forced withdrawal in a combined US prison and jail: findings at 12 months post-release. Drug Alcohol Depend 184:57–63, 2018a 29402680

Brinkley-Rubinstein L, Zaller N, Martino S, et al: Criminal justice continuum for opioid users at risk of overdose. Addict Behav 86:104–110, 2018b 29544869

Bronson J, Stroop J, Zimmer S, et al: Drug Use, Dependence, and Abuse Among State Prisoners and Jail Inmates, 2007–2009 (NCJ 250546). Washington, DC, U.S. Department of Justice, June 2017. Available at: https://bjs.ojp.gov/content/pub/pdf/dudaspji0709.pdf. Accessed November 11, 2023.

Broussard B, McGriff JA, Demir Neubert BN, et al: Characteristics of patients referred to psychiatric emergency services by crisis intervention team police officers. Commun Ment Health J 46(6):579–584, 2010 20140754

Collins SE, Lonczak HS, Clifasefi SL: Seattle's Law Enforcement Assisted Diversion (LEAD): program effects on recidivism outcomes. Eval Program Plann 64:49–56, 2017 28531654

Commonwealth v Eldred, 101 N.E.3d 911 (Mass. 2018)

Compton MT, Bakeman R, Broussard B, et al: The police-based crisis intervention team (CIT) model: II. Effects on level of force and resolution, referral, and arrest. Psychiatr Serv 65(4):523–529, 2014 24382643

Duke AA, Smith KMZ, Oberleitner LMS, et al: Alcohol, drugs, and violence: a meta-meta-analysis. Psychol Violence 8(2):238–249, 2018

Freudenberg N, Ramaswamy M, Daniels J, et al: Reducing drug use, human immunodeficiency virus risk, and recidivism among young men leaving jail: evaluation of the REAL MEN re-entry program. J Adolesc Health 47(5):448–455, 2010 20970079

Gordon MS, Kinlock TW, Schwartz RP, et al: A randomized controlled trial of prison-initiated buprenorphine: prison outcomes and community treatment entry. Drug Alcohol Depend 142:33–40, 2014 24962326

Gordon MS, Kinlock TW, Schwartz RP, et al: A randomized clinical trial of buprenorphine for prisoners: findings at 12-months post-release. Drug Alcohol Depend 172:34–42, 2017 28107680

Gratton J, Cole R, Furrer C, et al: Jail Diversion for Persons With Co-Occurring Disorders. Portland, OR, NPC Research, 2001

Hagan MP, Cho ME, Jensen JA, et al: An assessment of the effectiveness of an intensive treatment program for severely mentally disturbed juvenile offenders. Int J Offender Ther Comp Criminol 41(4):340–350, 1997

Hamilton Z: Do Reentry Courts Reduce Recidivism? Results From the Harlem Parole Reentry Court. New York, Center for Court Innovation, 2010. Available at: http://www.courtinnovation.org/sites/default/files/Reentry_Evaluation.pdf. Accessed November 11, 2023.

Hartford K, Carey R, Mendonca J: Pre-arrest diversion of people with mental illness: literature review and international survey. Behav Sci Law 24(6):845–856, 2006 17171772

Ho T, Carey SM, Malsch AM: Racial and gender disparities in treatment courts: do they exist and is there anything we can do to change them? J Advancing Justice 1:5–34, 2018

Hora PF, Schma WG, Rosenthal JT: Therapeutic jurisprudence and the drug treatment court movement: revolutionizing the criminal justice system's response to drug abuse and crime in America. Notre Dame L Rev 74(2):439, 1999

Holloway K, Bennett T, Farrington D: The effectiveness of criminal justice and treatment programs in reducing drug-related crime: a systematic review. Home Office Online Report, 2005. Available at: https://www.crim.cam.ac.uk/sites/ www.crim.cam.ac.uk/files/olr2605.pdf. Accessed November 11, 2023.

Hora PF, Schma WG, Rosenthal JTA: Therapeutic jurisprudence and the drug treatment court movement: revolutionizing the criminal justice system's response to drug abuse and crime in America. Notre Dame Law Rev 74(2):439–537, 1999

Huddleston W, Marlowe DB: Painting the Current Picture: A National Report on Drug Courts and Other Problem-Solving Court Programs in the United States. Washington, DC, National Drug Court Institute, 2011. Available at: https://www.ndci.org/ wp-content/uploads/2016/05/Painting-the-Current-Picture-2016.pdf. Accessed February 23, 2022.

Hyatt JM, Lobmaier PP: Medication assisted treatment (MAT) in criminal justice settings as a double-edged sword: balancing novel addiction treatments and voluntary participation. Health Justice 8(1):7, 2020 32172481

Inciardi JA, Martin SS, Butzin CA: Five-year outcomes of therapeutic community treatment of drug involved offenders after release from prison. Crime Delinq 50(1):88–107, 2004

Kelly JF, Finney JW, Moos R: Substance use disorder patients who are mandated to treatment: characteristics, treatment process, and 1- and 5-year outcomes. J Subst Abuse Treat 28(3):213–223, 2005 15857721

Kinlock TW, Gordon MS, Schwartz RP, et al: A randomized clinical trial of methadone maintenance for prisoners: results at 1-month post-release. Drug Alcohol Depend 91(2–3):220–227, 2007 17628351

Kinlock TW, Gordon MS, Schwartz RP, et al: A randomized clinical trial of methadone maintenance for prisoners: results at 12 months postrelease. J Subst Abuse Treat 37(3):277–285, 2009 19339140

Knight K, Simpson DD, Hiller ML, et al: Three-year reincarceration outcomes for in-prison therapeutic community treatment in Texas. Prison J 79(3):337–351, 1999

Koetzle D, Listwan SJ, Guastaferro WP, et al: Treating high-risk offenders in the community: the potential of drug courts. Int J Offender Ther Comp Criminol 59(5):449–465, 2015 24363291

Kopak AM, Gleicher L: Law enforcement deflection and pre-arrest diversion programs: a tale of two initiatives. J Advancing Just 3:37–56, 2020

Krawczyk N, Picher CE, Feder KA, et al: Only one in twenty justice-referred adults in specialty treatment for opioid use receive methadone or buprenorphine. Health Aff (Millwood) 36(12):2046–2053, 2017 29200340

Kubiak SP, Arfken CL, Swartz JA, et al: Treatment at the front end of the criminal justice continuum: the association between arrest and admission into specialty substance abuse treatment. Subst Abuse Treat Prev Policy 1:20, 2006 16879743

Lattimore PK, Broner N, Sherman R, et al: A comparison of prebooking and post booking diversion programs for mentally ill substance-using individuals with justice involvement. J Contemp Crim Just 19(1):30–64, 2003

Lee JD, McDonald R, Grossman E, et al: Opioid treatment at release from jail using extended-release naltrexone: a pilot proof-of-concept randomized effectiveness trial. Addiction 110(6):1008–1014, 2015 25703440

Lincoln T, Johnson BD, McCarthy P, et al: Extended-release naltrexone for opioid use disorder started during or following incarceration. J Subst Abuse Treat 85:97–100, 2018 28479011

Lipari RN, Park-Lee E, Van Horn S: America's Need for a Receipt of Substance Use Treatment in 2015. Rockville, MD, Center for Behavioral Health Statistics and Quality, Substance Abuse and Mental Health Services Administration, September 29, 2016. Available at: https://www.samhsa.gov/data/sites/default/files/report_2716/ShortReport-2716.pdf. Accessed November 11, 2023.

Magura S, Lee JD, Hershberger J, et al: Buprenorphine and methadone maintenance in jail and post-release: a randomized clinical trial. Drug Alcohol Depend 99(1–3):222–230, 2009 18930603

Martin SS, Butzin CA, Saum CA, et al: Three-year outcomes of therapeutic community treatment for drug involved offenders in Delaware: from prison to work release to aftercare. Prison J 79(3):294–320, 1999

Maston CT, Bureau of Justice Statistics: Criminal Victimization in the United States, 2007—Statistical Tables (NCJ No. 22769). Washington, DC, U.S. Department of Justice, March 2, 2010. Available at: https://bjs.ojp.gov/library/publications/criminal-victimization-united-states-2007-statistical-tables. Accessed November 11, 2023.

Miller JM, Miller HV, Barnes JC: Outcome evaluation of a family based jail reentry program for substance abusing offenders. Prison J 96(1):53–78, 2016

Miller TR, Levy DT, Cohen MA, et al: Costs of alcohol and drug-involved crime. Prev Sci 7(4):333–342, 2006 16845591

Mitchell O, Wilson D, Egger A, et al: Assessing the effectiveness of drug courts on recidivism: a meta-analytic review of traditional and non-traditional drug courts. J Crim Just 40(1):60–71, 2012a

Mitchell O, Wilson D, MacKenzie DL: The effectiveness of incarceration-based drug treatment on criminal behavior: a systematic review. Campbell Syst Rev 8(1):1–76, 2012b

Moore J, Renn T, Veeh C: The metropolitan context of substance use and substance use disorders among US adults on probation or parole supervision. Subst Abus 43(1):161–170, 2022 33848449

Morabito MS, Socia K, Wik A, et al: The nature and extent of police use of force in encounters with people with behavioral health disorders. Int J Law Psychiatry 50:31–37, 2017 28029437

Munetz MR, Griffin PA: Use of the sequential intercept model as an approach to decriminalization of people with serious mental illness. Psychiatr Serv 57(4):544–549, 2006 16603751

National Association of Drug Court Professionals: Defining Drug Courts: The Key Components (NCJ 205621). Washington, DC, U.S. Department of Justice, Bureau of Justice Assistance, 1997. Available at: https://www.ojp.gov/pdffiles1/bja/205621.pdf. Accessed November 10, 2023.

National Association of Drug Court Professionals: Adult drug court best practice standards, Vol. 1 2018. Available at: https://allrise.org/publications/adult-drug-court-best-practice-standards/. Accessed November 10, 2023.

National Treatment Court Research Center: What are drug courts? 2023. Available at: https://ndcrc.org/what-are-drug-courts/. Accessed January 2, 2023.

Novak KJ, Engel RS: Disentangling the influence of suspects' demeanor and mental disorder on arrest. Policing 28(3):493–512, 2005

Perry AE, Darwin Z, Godfrey C, et al: The effectiveness of interventions for drug-using offenders in the courts, secure establishments and the community: a systematic review. Subst Use Misuse 44(3):374–400, 2009 19212928

Pesce v Coppinger, 355 F. Supp. 3d 35 (D. Mass. 2018)

Peters RH, Young MS, Rojas EC, et al: Evidence-based treatment and supervision prac-tices for co-occurring mental and substance use disorders in the criminal justice system. Am J Drug Alcohol Abuse 43(4):475–488, 2017 28375656

Pinals DA, Carey CJPM: The courts' role in combatting the opioid crisis: using the se-quential intercept model (SIM) as a place to start. National Judicial Opioid Task Force, May 2019. Available at: https://www.ncsc.org/__data/assets/pdf_file/0028/64729/The-Courts-Role-in-Combating-the-Opioid-Crisis-Using-the-SIM_Final.pdf. Accessed November 11, 2023.

Prendergast ML: Interventions to promote successful re-entry among drug-abusing pa-rolees. Addict Sci Clin Pract 5(1):4–13, 2009 19369913

Rich JD, McKenzie M, Larney S, et al: Methadone continuation versus forced withdrawal on incarceration in a combined US prison and jail: a randomised, open-label trial. Lancet 386(9991):350–359, 2015 26028120

Rossman SB, Rempel M, Roman JK, et al (eds): The Multi-Site Adult Drug Court Eval-uation: The Impact of Drug Courts, Vol. 4. Washington, DC, Urban Institute Justice Policy Center, 2011. Available at: https://www.ojp.gov/pdffiles1/nij/grants/237112.pdf. Accessed November 11, 2023.

Rothbard A, Alterman A, Rutherford M, et al: Revisiting the effectiveness of methadone treatment on crime reductions in the 1990s. J Subst Abuse Treat 16(4):329–335, 1999 10349606

Saucier R, Wolfe D, Dasgupta N: Review of case narratives from fatal overdoses associ-ated with injectable naltrexone for opioid dependence. Drug Saf 41(10):981–988, 2018 29560596

Scott RL: Evaluation of a mobile crisis program: effectiveness, efficiency, and consumer satisfaction. Psychiatr Serv 51(9):1153–1156, 2000 10970919

Shafer MS, Arthur B, Franczak MJ: An analysis of post-booking jail diversion program-ming for persons with co-occurring disorders. Behav Sci Law 22(6):771–785, 2004 15386559

Sharma A, O'Grady KE, Kelly SM, et al: Pharmacotherapy for opioid dependence in jails and prisons: research review update and future directions. Subst Abuse Rehabil 7:27–40, 2016 27217808

Steadman HJ, Naples M: Assessing the effectiveness of jail diversion programs for per-sons with serious mental illness and co-occurring substance use disorders. Behav Sci Law 23(2):163–170, 2005 15818607

Steadman HJ, Deane MW, Borum R, et al: Comparing outcomes of major models of po-lice responses to mental health emergencies. Psychiatr Serv 51(5):645–649, 2000 10783184

U.S. General Accounting Office: Drug Courts: Overview of Growth, Characteristics, and Results (GAO/GGD-97–106). Washington, DC, U.S. General Accounting Office, July 1997. Available at: https://www.gao.gov/assets/ggd-97–106.pdf. Accessed No-vember 11, 2023.

Waddell EN, Springer SA, Marsch LA, et al: Long-acting buprenorphine vs. naltrexone opioid treatments in CJS-involved adults (EXIT-CJS). J Subst Abuse Treat 128:108389, 2021 33865691

Wakefield v Thompson, 177 F.3d 1160 (1999)

Wakeman SE: Why it's inappropriate not to treat incarcerated patients with opioid ago-nist therapy. AMA J Ethics 19(9):922–930, 2017 28905733

Welsh WN: A multisite evaluation of prison-based therapeutic community drug treatment. Crim Just Behav 34(11):1481–1498, 2007

Westerberg VS, McCrady BS, Owens M, et al: Community-based methadone maintenance in a large detention center is associated with decreases in inmate recidivism. J Subst Abuse Treat 70:1–6, 2016 27692182

Wexler DB, Winick BJ: Therapeutic jurisprudence as a new approach to mental health law policy analysis and research. Univ Miami Law Rev 45(5):979–1004, 1991

Wexler H, Melnick G, Lowe L, et al: Three-year reincarceration outcomes for Amity in-prison therapeutic community and aftercare in California. Prison J 79(3):321–336, 1999

World Health Organization: Guidelines for the Psychosocially Assisted Pharmacological Treatment of Opioid Dependence. Geneva, Switzerland, World Health Organization Department of Mental Health and Substance Abuse, 2009

# CHAPTER 10

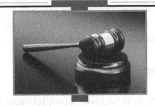

# SUBSTANCE USE DISORDERS IN CORRECTIONAL SYSTEMS

## Introduction

The U.S. correctional system encompasses a complex network of facilities and supervising entities, such as probation and parole, which manage millions of lives every day. With years of tough-on-crime and war-on-drugs policies, the populations of individuals with substance use disorders (SUDs) in correctional settings and under correctional supervision reflect a significant proportion of those within corrections overall. It is helpful when working with individuals with SUDs under correctional supervision to understand some of the ways in which correctional systems work and how case law has helped shape practices. There is growing interest in recognizing the legal issues involved for individuals with SUDs in correctional settings who may not have access to the full array of services needed to treat their disorders. This chapter reviews correctional systems and the legal and regulatory backdrop to providing substance use services to individuals in jails and prisons and for those under correctional supervision.

# FORENSIC DILEMMA

A 33-year-old man is admitted to a local jail. He has a 10-year history of opioid use disorder (OUD) and a 15-year history of alcohol use disorder. He has been admitted for a charge related to stealing from family to support his drug use. Upon his arrest, the man becomes concerned that he will not have access to heroin in jail, and he conceals an undetected package containing the drug in a body cavity. On intake, he is not asked about a history of suicidal ideation or substance use, and he is not referred to a qualified mental health professional. Approximately 2 days into his stay, the man becomes very restless and is feeling very ill, likely because of withdrawal. Officers examining his cell note that he is trying to mix a powder in some fashion, and they pull him out of his cell, confiscate the powder, and place him in administrative segregation for a disciplinary hearing.

Consider the following:

1. Is there a responsibility to do a more complete assessment of this man with regard to suicide risk and SUDs?
2. Can a jail inmate access substance use treatment?
3. What can happen to an inmate or detainee found with an illegal substance?
4. What are trends in legal cases that could have helped him get more immediate treatment?

In correctional settings, screening at intake for suicidal risk and substance use issues can be critical to ensure that an individual receives needed care. The requirements for suicide risk screening, at least, have been a source of litigation, and a failure to complete such screening can result in liability. With that requirement, jails have typically put in place receiving screening at the front door and then further screening and assessments as needed. That said, putting such procedures in practice can be difficult, and individuals with positive screens need to be referred in a timely way for further assessment. Also, certain initial screenings may be conducted by correctional officials, and these officials must know where to turn if they identify issues during screening.

As for substance use treatment, jails typically have detoxification protocols with various comfort medications available, and there are typically services for pregnant women that provide methadone or buprenorphine and naloxone (Suboxone). For individuals experiencing alcohol withdrawal, the health services unit of a jail generally provides monitoring. Increasingly, jails are examining ways to add medications for opioid use disorder (MOUD) as a treatment modality, but progress has been challenged by regulatory, logistic, and other barriers, including fears that inmates will divert medications from proper use to misuse by others in the facility.

If an inmate is alleged to possess an illegal substance in the facility, there would generally be a disciplinary review and sometimes a hearing with a cor-

**Table 10–1.** Correctional populations in the United States, 2019

| Category | Population |
|---|---|
| Total under correctional supervision | 6,344,000 |
| Total incarcerated | 2,086,600 |
| Jails | 734,500 |
| Prisons | 1,430, 800 |
| Community supervision | 4,357,700 |
| Probation | 3,492,900 |
| Parole | 878,900 |

*Source.* Adapted from Minton et al. 2021.

rectional officer. If the allegation is borne out, the inmate would likely be sentenced to serve in restrictive housing (something inmates often refer to as "the hole"). There should still be access to care in those settings, but this is not a uniform practice, and increasingly, jail standards are highlighting this issue.

Legal case trends have examined whether jails are sufficiently accommodating individuals who have exhibited SUDs, among other conditions. As shown in this chapter, prisoners are the only group within the United States with a constitutionally based right to treatment under the principles of the Eighth Amendment of the U.S. Constitution, which encompasses the right to be free from cruel and unusual punishment. Pretrial inmates are generally considered to be required to have access to treatment under the due process clause of the Fourteenth Amendment. This case law has typically not centered around SUDs, but failure to treat SUDs in carceral settings is an area of increased litigation and attention.

# Correctional Issues in Addiction Psychiatry

This chapter expands on information from Chapter 9 ("Substance Use Disorders and Specialty Courts, Jail Diversion, and Alternatives to Incarceration Programs") and focuses on correctional issues themselves. Correctional populations in the United States include approximately 6.3 million Americans, according to 2019 Bureau of Justice Statistics data (Minton et al. 2021). Approximately 2 million of those individuals are incarcerated, with 1.4 million held in prison and the remaining 734,000 held in local jails. Individuals under community supervision are even more numerous, with almost 4.4 million people on either probation or parole (see Table 10–1).

In a 2017 report by the Bureau of Justice Statistics examining data from 2007 to 2009, Bronson and colleagues (2017) noted that the prevalence of individuals with SUDs was much higher among incarcerated people than the general population. Specifically, they found that whereas 5% of the general population had symptoms that met DSM-IV (American Psychiatric Association 1994) criteria for drug dependence or abuse, 58% of state prisoners and 63% of sentenced jail inmates had symptoms that met similar criteria. Furthermore, the authors noted that 17% of state prisoners and 19% of sentenced jail inmates regularly used heroin and opiates, and 42% of state prisoners and 37% of sentenced jail inmates were using drugs at the time of their offenses. In another study, more than 80% of state prison and local jail inmates had a history of using an illegal drug (Belenko et al. 2013).

As noted in Chapter 2, policies and laws have contributed to the high prevalence of individuals with SUDs in correctional settings and under correctional supervision in the community. The war on drugs from the mid-1970s to the 1990s contributed to sweeping laws across the country that included strict mandatory minimum sentences to punish the manufacture, use, and distribution of drugs, along with other offenses (American Civil Liberties Union 2015). Although those laws have largely affected male offenders, the population of women inmates is growing. One review reported that from 2009 to 2018, the number of women in city and county jails increased by 23%; arrests for women also increased, primarily for drug-related offenses (Herring 2020). Mandatory minimum sentencing created strict parameters on holding people in carceral settings and resulted in prison overcrowding, and the passage of recent laws related to substance use has lowered correctional populations. For example, Proposition 47, a California law that reduced penalties associated with certain drug-related offenses, among others, was passed in 2014, and jail populations declined subsequently. At the same time, individuals who had other types of charges but may have been released early because of overcrowding were held, creating a shift in who remained in jail (Bird et al. 2016).

Overall, the high prevalence rates of substance use and SUDs among the criminal-legal population warrants scrutiny of public policies. At the same time, these prevalence rates demonstrate the need for understanding how SUDs are managed in correctional settings, case law regarding the provision of services, and emerging legal and regulatory issues pertaining to individuals with SUDs in correctional settings.

# Contexts for Clinical Services: Describing Correctional Systems

Correctional facilities fall along a continuum that follows criminal case processing but also relates to management, financing, and authority. These various settings encompass different sizes and populations. This is important for

**Table 10–2.** Typical makeup of adult state and local correctional facilities

| Facility | Length of stay | Management |
|----------|----------------|------------|
| Lock-up | Up to 72 hours | Municipality |
| Jail | Pretrial and up to 1 year | County |
| Prison | Longer than 1 year | State |

individuals with SUDs, who may move from one carceral setting to another or may move from a community setting into a facility that serves a function for the criminal system (see Table 10–2).

An individual who is arrested may or may not be taken into custody. For individuals not taken into custody immediately, a criminal complaint may be formally filed with a requirement for them to appear in court. For those taken into custody, the site where they are taken would most likely be a lock-up facility. These are often small and run by local municipalities, and they house only a few cells where individuals are grouped together, awaiting the opening of court on the next business day after their arrest. An individual with an acute medical or psychiatric condition may be brought to the local emergency department for evaluation and clearance. What this clearance entails is often undefined, but it typically involves evaluation for dire medical conditions that cannot wait for treatment (Dunlop and Pinals 2021).

The first court appearance is typically called the *arraignment*, which is when formal charges are presented. After that, an individual who remains in custody would be sent to a jail. In some communities, the local lock-up is essentially the county jail space. In general, however, jails are places that have a variety of populations. They are most often run at the county level by a sheriff, but a few states (such as Connecticut) have one correctional system combining jail- and prison-type functions. The populations primarily, but not exclusively, include pretrial inmates, or detainees, and individuals who are sentenced for crimes generally punishable by less than 1 year. The duration of stay may be very short, and there is a great deal of movement in and out of jails daily as individuals are brought in, released, or leave for court appearances and then return. Individuals also may be brought back to jail after violations of community supervision. Although jail sentences are usually shorter than prison sentences, the time spent in a jail or house of correction can be years for pretrial populations and individuals facing consecutive sentences.

Prisons are state-run facilities where individuals are sent to serve out their sentences on felony-level charges involving, in most jurisdictions, sentences of longer than 1 year. Generally, prisons are large facilities and can hold thousands of individuals. Because people are sentenced to prison for longer periods of time than jail, mental health services are delivered at all levels of care—from outpatient-equivalent to hospital levels, all within the facilities. Substance use services are also delivered, but this aspect of care is evolving.

It should be noted that there are also other carceral environments. These include the Federal Bureau of Prisons, which is a network of facilities across the United States where individuals charged with federal crimes are sent both pretrial and for sentencing, and even for some forms of treatment. Military correctional facilities are distinct from other systems. Juvenile facilities house young people, although states have different upper and lower age limits for who can be served in a juvenile detention or commitment facility, in contrast with being sent elsewhere. An entire review of these types of facilities is beyond the scope of this chapter. Suffice it to say that addiction issues run rampant throughout these various facilities, which current policies and protocols are attempting to address.

Other aspects of correctional supervision involve community-based supervision through probation, parole, or both. Probation generally encompasses a court order for community supervision. It can be a pretrial supervision, part of a sentence, or a sentence unto itself (e.g., a person can be ordered to 1 year of probation). Administrative probation and risk/needs probation can be divided between cases with less intensive oversight and more intensive oversight, respectively. Also, conditions of probation are determined by the sentencing judge, often based on the recommendation of the probation department. The probation officer upholds the court order and reports back to the judge if there are infractions.

Parole is generally a community supervision provision following a term of sentence. There is usually an independent parole board. In some states, parole can be its own agency; in others, it is subsumed under the state correctional system. An individual may have to serve a portion of their sentence in a carceral setting, after which they can be eligible for parole; this is when a parole board determines whether they should be granted release under parole supervision. In some cases, an individual may serve the maximum allowable sentence, which would then mean that they would be released from prison without parole supervision.

Outcomes for parole or probation violations can vary, ranging from addressing the violation programmatically if the violation is technical (e.g., failure to show for a probation appointment, a positive test result for a substance) to further criminal sanction if the violation is nontechnical by virtue of involvement in a new crime. An important aspect of managing violations is that the individual may end up back in jail or prison. Thus, probation and parole serve as conduits both from carceral settings and back into them.

There are several considerations regarding legal issues pertaining to individuals with SUDs under correctional supervision. With regard to probation and parole, there are increasing concerns about the provisions of the Americans With Disabilities Act of 1990 (ADA) and whether individuals receive proper accommodations for their disabilities. The Legal Action Center (2022c) produces resources to help attorneys and others ensure that an individual with an SUD would not be discriminated against in court processes.

A 2018 legal case specifically examined whether being on probation could require an individual to remain drug free—and penalize relapse—as a public safety measure and as part of the conditions of probation. In *Commonwealth v. Eldred* (2018), the Massachusetts Supreme Judicial Court held that the probation requirement of this nature was permissible. Commentaries expressing concern about the ultimate court ruling included concerns that the very nature of OUD, the condition that Julie Eldred exhibited, created an inability to control her use (Harvard Law Review 2019).

In this case, Eldred had stolen some $250 worth of jewelry in part to pay for her heroin and was found guilty of larceny with a sentence of 1 year of probation (Harvard Law Review 2019). Part of her probation was a requirement to remain drug free. When Eldred was found to have a positive drug screen for fentanyl during the course of her probation, the judge was notified by the probation officer. Her situation was then reviewed for whether this finding should result in detention in jail. The judge who presided over the probation violation proceeding preliminarily ordered Eldred into inpatient treatment, but this was not immediately available and instead she was held in the state prison. During this period, Eldred contested the probation violation finding, claiming that her OUD compromised her volitional capacity to remain substance free. There were several advocate groups who wrote amicus briefs (friend of the court briefs to help inform the deciding judge) on behalf of Eldred's position, including the Massachusetts Medical Society. Some of the comments cited the unconstitutional nature of criminalizing addiction, as noted in *Robinson v. California* (1962). Still, Eldred's probation violation carried forth.

The Eldred case was appealed to the Massachusetts Supreme Judicial Court. The justices ruled unanimously, noting that a requirement for remaining drug free was allowable and that a defendant could be held in a custodial setting during the pendency of the case hearing. The justices found that the probation terms were "reasonably related" to the sentencing goals in light of the underlying crime (*Commonwealth v. Eldred* 2018). They noted that this was not the same as *Robinson*, because the defendant was not being punished for relapsing or for the "status" of being an addict. Instead, they wrote, Eldred was being punished related to her underlying offense of larceny. The Massachusetts Supreme Judicial Court noted further that the brain science available had not evolved to the point where one could say the addiction precluded total control of drug use.

The *Eldred* case generated much discussion prior to the ruling, as a ruling in the opposite direction could have widely changed the nature of probation and its requirements. Advocates have raised concerns that the Massachusetts Supreme Judicial Court missed an opportunity to recognize more advancing brain science about the compromised ability of an individual with an SUD to exert control in some cases in their return to substance use (Harvard Law Review 2019). At the same time, public safety arguments and findings by the court were considered important in balancing the purpose of the drug testing and the risk of missing a significant community threat by not taking seriously such testing and its results.

Even in the domain of parole, legal cases are starting to be heard. For example, in *U.S. v. Massachusetts Parole Board* (2021), a settlement agreement was reached with the Massachusetts Parole Board and the U.S. Attorney for the District of Massachusetts. In this case, the parole board had been requiring parolees with OUD to take naltrexone (marketed as Vivitrol), without considering further assessment by a health care provider or allowing for the determination that the best treatment might be an alternative medication. With the settlement agreement, the parole board agreed to modify its parole condition orders so that people were not mandated to take certain kinds of MOUD.

# Conditions of Confinement and Constitutional Right to Treatment: Case Law

Over the last several decades, more attention has been paid to health care provided within jails and prisons, sometimes framed as an examination of *conditions of confinement*. Administrators and clinicians treating people with SUDs in a place of confinement should understand their legal obligation for providing care.

In *Estelle v. Gamble* (1976), a prison inmate filed a lawsuit in federal court alleging a violation of his civil rights under 42 U.S.C. § 1983. He claimed that the failure to address his back injury constituted cruel and unusual punishment under the Eighth Amendment. When this case was heard before the U.S. Supreme Court, it was determined that deliberate indifference to a prisoner's illness or injury would violate the Eighth Amendment constitutional right that all people are entitled to under U.S. law. Although the facts of the particular case did not clearly rise to the level of deliberate indifference to the court, which remanded the case back to the local court, the precedent established a clear expectation for prisoner health care, making prisoners the only class of people who have a constitutionally based right to treatment.

In *Bowring v. Godwin* (1977) a year later, the *Estelle* ruling was extended to mental health care when a federal appeals court held that an inmate is entitled to mental health care if a physician or other health care provider deems it medically necessary, and that there was no real distinction between the right to medical care and the right to psychological or psychiatric care. The court noted further that this right attaches specifically when the symptoms exhibited reflect a serious disease or injury, which can be cured or alleviated with treatment, and when the potential for harm to the prisoner due to delay or denial of care would be substantial.

A related case, *Bell v. Wolfish* (1979), extended the constitutional protections to pretrial inmates under the rubric of expectations for individuals who are detained. This case established a different constitutional approach to the notion of conditions of confinement for pretrial inmates compared with how *Estelle* tackled a right to health care for prison inmates. In *Bell*, the U.S. Supreme Court examined practices within the federal pretrial detention center (Metropolitan Correctional Center) that involved double-bunking inmates in cells meant for single inmates, restrictions on books being received, the practice of performing body cavity searches after contact visits with the inmates, and the requirement that pretrial detainees needed to stay outside of their cells during cell inspections. The U.S. Supreme Court reviewed the pretrial detainee's right to be free from punishment, noting that they should not be held in custody for punishment as a sentenced inmate would be. Thus the evaluation of conditions or restrictions invokes analysis of deprivation of liberty without due process of law (Fourteenth Amendment issues) when the conditions or restrictions were for punishment rather than a legitimate nonpunitive governmental objective. This could also involve examining whether conditions or restrictions were purposeless or arbitrary and therefore could be interpreted as a form of punishment. This ruling and logic apply to the provision of health care and mental health care, in that deprivation of needed care could amount to such punishment by causing needless suffering (Metzner 2002). The court acknowledged that correctional administrators have difficult roles in maintaining institutional security that can justify restrictions and practices to preserve internal order and maintain institutional security. With regard to SUDs, as discussed further later in this chapter, it is noteworthy that in prescribing an inmate a controlled substance, legitimate security issues exist, including diversion and other misuse. This then becomes an area of complex evolving law and scrutiny that requires various balancing tests.

In *Ruiz v. Estelle* (1980), an inmate of the Texas Department of Corrections filed suit under the provisions of 42 U.S.C. § 1983 for relief from violation of his constitutional rights in the Eighth and Fourteenth Amendments. Similar lawsuits by other inmates resulted in joining cases into one legal case. The inmates challenged a number of issues, including their lack of access to appropriate health care and the conditions of confinement. The case called for specific elements of constitutionally required minimally adequate elements of services including the following:

- Systematic screening and evaluation
- Treatment

- Participation by trained mental health professionals
- An accurate, complete, and confidential record
- Safeguards against psychotropic medications
- A suicide prevention program

As noted by Metzner (2002), this wave of landmark legislation has been the foundation that allows inmates to litigate pursuant to 42 U.S.C. § 1983, which is a civil rights code that the U.S. Supreme Court interpreted to allow claims regarding conditions of confinement for prisoners and jail inmates.

In another landmark legal case regarding correctional health care, two cases were consolidated and heard by the U.S. Supreme Court in what became known as *Brown v. Plata* (2011a, 2011b). In this case, the court held that the over-crowded conditions within the California prison system violated inmates' Eighth Amendment right to be free from cruel and unusual punishment. The judicial decision rested its analysis on the finding that the overcrowding compromised inmates' access to appropriate physical health and mental health care. Although this case was not about the treatment of SUDs, the same issues could apply because these are considered health conditions that can require medically necessary treatments. As a result of the *Brown* decision, the California prison system moved to redistribute inmates to various settings, including releasing those on parole that could be released and moving many others to their local jails (Newman and Scott 2012).

Finally, the federal appellate case of *Madrid v. Gomez* (1995) examined seg-regation for discipline. The court found segregation for discipline permissible for general inmates, as long as it did not constitute systemic psychological deprivation and as long as vulnerable populations were segregated only under rare exceptions and were given specific programming when they were segre-gated. Among the vulnerable populations were individuals with known mental illness, traumatic brain injury, intellectual and developmental disabilities, and severe personality challenges. It is noteworthy that individuals with significant SUDs were not separately identified. It remains to be seen as to whether placing individuals with SUDs in segregation (which can occur especially when they are found to have diverted or acquired illegal drugs) who may have acute symp-toms of withdrawal or intoxication or associated mood or behavioral dysregu-lation could lead to further legal challenges. Here again, screening, assessment, monitoring, and programming, as well as quality improvement efforts, would be needed.

With regard to advancing practices particularly related to MOUD, the court decisions just described set the stage for growing expectations that if the com-munity standard of care is to provide SUD treatment (including medications when needed and as available), then this would be the same standard in prisons and jails. Therefore, situations are increasing where access to MOUD is needed across settings.

# Relevant Federal Legislation

The health care of inmates in jails and prisons has been affected not only by court cases but also by several pieces of federal law. For example, the Civil Rights of Institutionalized People Act (1980) authorizes the U.S. attorney general through the U.S. Department of Justice to bring suit on behalf of the United States to halt practices that cause systemic problems for those confined in these institutions. This process does not provide redress for an individual issue; rather, the U.S. Department of Justice will review patterns or practices on a broader scale. Cases have been raised in many jurisdictions, and one data source indicated that in less than 20 years after the law's passage, the Civil Rights Division of the U.S. Department of Justice had investigated more than 300 institutions under the act. Watchdog groups monitor this work and help inform the public of these activities in an effort to improve the conditions for incarcerated individuals.

The Prison Litigation Reform Act (1996) established more procedural requirements before inmates can file for litigation, and it limited the ability of courts to order relief (Metzner 2002). Some have called for the Prison Litigation Reform Act to be repealed (Fenster and Schlanger 2021), citing concerns that it diminishes the ability of incarcerated individuals to file and prevail in civil rights litigation. For example, the law requires filing fees, and it allows cases to be dismissed on technical grounds, among other provisions. It was passed originally in an effort to curtail frivolous lawsuits filed by incarcerated people. Despite some authors calling for its repeal, the act is still on the books and can impact an individual inmate who is seeking redress regarding not getting needed treatment.

Protections of disabled prisoners also fall under Section 504 of the Rehabilitation Act (1973) and Title II of the Americans With Disabilities Act (1990; ADA). The former applies to any entity that is within a federal executive agency, such as the Federal Bureau of Prisons, as well as any program that receives federal funding. The ADA protects people with disabilities receiving public services, including those of local and state governments.

Several cases help delineate the rights of people with disabilities in the jail and prison context. In a landmark case, *Pennsylvania Department of Corrections v. Yeskey* (1998a, 1998b), Yeskey had been sentenced to serve up to 36 months in a Pennsylvania correctional facility. However, as a first-time offender, he was eligible for placement in a specialized motivational bootcamp that could have gotten him an earlier release on parole. However, he was denied entry into the bootcamp due to his medical condition of hypertension. Yeskey then sued the Pennsylvania Department of Corrections, alleging that they violated Title II of the ADA, as a public entity discriminating against an otherwise qualified individual based on his disability. The case went up to the U.S. Supreme Court, which settled the issue that state prisons fall squarely within the Title II definition of a public entity. This case has far-reaching ramifications and, ultimately, has become relevant in the considerations related to treating SUDs within carceral settings.

It is important to realize that, as pointed out by the American Civil Liberties Union (2023), the ADA defines disability as having a physical or mental impairment that substantially limits one or more of the major life activities of such individuals, a record of such an impairment, or being regarded as having such an impairment. Active drug use with illegal drugs is not covered under the ADA, but alcohol use disorder and other SUDs with any substance are covered; this can be a complicated distinction. Nevertheless, prisoners with a disability have sued to get equal access to facilities, programs, and services as others with SUDs who are not incarcerated (American Civil Liberties Union 2023). It should be noted, however, that within the structure of the ADA, an entity is not required to accommodate the person with a disability if those accommodations are unreasonable, impose "undue financial and administrative burdens," or represent a "fundamental alteration in the nature of the program" (Americans With Disabilities Act 1990). In addition, prison officials are allowed to discriminate if the participation by the person with a disability would pose health and safety risks or a "direct threat" to others (referred to as the *direct threat* exception to the requirement for accommodations). With regard to prisoners, some courts have also said that discrimination is allowable as long as the discrimination policies serve "legitimate penological interests" (American Civil Liberties Union 2023). In 2010, the U.S. Department of Justice issued prison- and jail-specific ADA regulations that require inmates with disabilities to be placed in the most integrated care setting possible (American Civil Liberties Union 2023). Now that there is increased attention on the critical importance of MOUD to save lives for individuals returning from jails and prisons to their communities, there is more focus on ADA claims involving these issues.

# Application of Newer Case Law to SUD Services in Jails and Prisons

In furthering the advances that legal cases have made in setting expectations for health care within correctional settings, organizations such as the National Commission of Correctional Health Care (2024) provide accreditation standards related to health care and mental health care in jails, prisons, and juvenile detention facilities. The American Psychiatric Association (2016) has also published guidelines for psychiatric services in jails and prisons. The elements noted in *Ruiz* have relevance to individuals with SUDs. However, aspects of the treatment of SUDs have not been a major focus of these standards until recently, especially with the recognition of the dire consequences of the opioid overdose epidemic and its association with the population of people moving in and out of correctional settings.

Even with increasing recognition of high rates of incarceration of individuals with SUDs, treatment of SUDs has been limited within correctional contexts. Such treatment primarily consists of two types: 1) acute management of withdrawal from substances with comfort measures or prophylactic measures, or 2) residential-type psychoeducation and supportive-type treatments. A primary component of SUD treatment in prisons and jails has been through federally funded residential substance abuse treatment programs, designed to "break the cycle of drug addiction and violence by decreased demand for, use and trafficking of illegal drugs" (Bureau of Justice Assistance 2021b). Authorizing federal legislation that has supported these programs dates back to 1994 (Violent Crime Control and Law Enforcement Act 1994). Additionally, individual programs for certain SUDs have been shown to help with decreasing re-offending, as seen in programs delivering alcohol use disorder treatment in a correctional facility that led to a decrease in driving while intoxicated recidivism (Miller et al. 2014).

Correctional facilities are increasingly offering MOUD, in part stemming from emerging litigation as well as expanding federal policies that require entities receiving federal dollars in grants to promote and provide these services. In a four-state study of carceral facilities in the Northwest, including 146 county jails and state prisons in Washington, Oregon, and Idaho, 90.7% of respondents provided medications for acute withdrawal from alcohol, opioids, or both; and only 5%–60% provided MOUD (Neill-Gubitz et al. 2022). A national review of residential substance abuse treatment programs reported that since 2016, it had served approximately 28,800 individuals per year through its jail- and prison-based programs, with the former serving individuals for at least 3 months and the latter for at least 6 months. In addition, as of 2019, 57% of jail-based programs and 34% of prison-based programs offered medication-assisted treatment (MAT) to eligible inmates (Bureau of Justice Assistance 2021a). The use of methadone in correctional settings to treat pregnant inmates dates back many years, but its overall use in other populations to treat OUD has been limited, other than to support total withdrawal from opioids. A 2003 survey of medical directors of all 50 states and the federal system reported that 48% of the sites used methadone, but predominantly for pregnant inmates or for short-term detoxification, and only 8% of respondents referred inmates with OUD to methadone programs after release (Rich et al. 2005).

There have been several efforts to litigate denial of access to MOUD in correctional settings. For example, in *Pesce v. Coppinger* (2018), the appellate court held that it was likely a violation of both the ADA and the Eighth Amendment to deny incarcerated people access to MOUD without an individual assessment and despite a professional's determination that MOUD was medically indicated. The Essex County Jail in Massachusetts, in its own defense, argued that MOUD would create a risk to the safety of the institution and raised concerns about diversion of illegal substances among inmates. Still, the case laid a foundation for ADA claims going forward.

In another example, *P.G. v. Jefferson County* (2021), the court held that it likely violates Title II of the ADA and the Fourteenth Amendment to deny medically necessary methadone treatment to pretrial detainees. In this case, the plaintiff alleged that the denial of methadone to all but pregnant detainees failed to provide medically necessary treatment of OUD in violation of Title II and the Fourteenth Amendment. They also noted that the defendants were likely acting with deliberate indifference to a serious medical need (Legal Action Center 2022a). Settlements with correctional facilities and systems in Maine, Massachusetts, and the Federal Bureau of Prisons have emerged and continue to grow in number, as there is increasing recognition of the significant need for MOUD among the high-risk population of incarcerated people.

In *Smith v. Aroostook County* (2019) in Maine, a federal judge in the First Circuit Court of Appeals ordered the Aroostook County Jail to provide one of their inmates access to her prescribed buprenorphine. In this case, the U.S. District Court judge heard arguments about Brenda Smith, who had been in active recovery for a decade and had been prescribed buprenorphine, which had shown positive success in reducing her need for more intensive services. This case set forth how a court might hold a jail in violation of the ADA for failure to prescribe yet another treatment for OUD.

With buprenorphine now available, many correctional systems are developing programs to offer this medication and previously offered naltrexone especially prior to release. Yet with agonist therapies showing such benefits, it is harder to justify not offering those treatments. Because of concerns about diversion of medications, the use of long-acting buprenorphine in injectable forms has grown in carceral settings. Its costs are often prohibitive, but cost alone would not be a defense in litigation. In one review of these cases and the current structures, researchers noted that the complex regulatory scheme associated with buprenorphine prescribing contributed to the difficulty of having that medication readily available within correctional facilities (Toyoshima et al. 2021). From a penological perspective, barriers to accessing MOUD have included concerns related to security as described in this chapter, given that these drugs are known to be diverted and misused in society at large and in corrections in particular. Nevertheless, the threat of litigation or court oversight for failure to provide medications for SUDs has catalyzed the beginning of change in many correctional facilities, Trends seem to be pointing to putting correctional facilities on notice that they may be subject to litigation if they do not provide MOUD in their facilities. Many addictions and forensic psychiatrists are being called to testify on cases involving this issue, and treatment providers should be aware of community standards in this regard and can support policies and programs that increase access to these medications.

# Clinical Work in Jails and Prisons

The *Ruiz* elements for care in correctional settings are relevant to the treatment of substance use. For example, timely screening within an SUD treatment facility is needed, with a clear triage assessment and referral protocol that gives patients identified as in need of care access within certain time frames. Generally, screening tools to identify the presence of SUDs can be appropriate for justice-involved populations. For example, the TCU Drug Screen 5 was shown to be effective in identifying even mild SUDs among adult and juvenile justice-involved populations (Knight et al. 2018). The Rapid Opioid Dependence Screen is another tool that has been used in correctional settings to identify individuals who may have OUD (Wickersham et al. 2015).

Generally, screening would be conducted on admission, referred to as *receiving screening*. If an individual does not screen for any mental health conditions or SUDs, then they would not be triaged as urgent and would instead require review within approximately 2 weeks. Also, it is important within jails and prisons to have a system that allows for referrals for care to be reviewed at any point in the incarceration, and inmates must have a means of making their needs known. This includes the requirement for crisis services that should be accessible as well as careful record keeping to track health care interventions.

Relapse is often part of the trajectory toward recovery for SUDs. Given this finding, it is not surprising that individuals with SUDs in jails and prisons can face challenges with their own relapse. Contrary to what some might believe, detainees and inmates can access illegal substances within jails and prisons. The possession of illegal substances within a correctional facility can result in further sanctions or disciplinary actions by prison administrators. For example, federal law speaks to punishments, including extended prison time, for inmates in federal prisons who are found to distribute, make, obtain, or possess illegal substances or other prohibited objects (18 U.S.C. § 1791). In 2017, a woman visiting her inmate boyfriend passed multiple tiny balloons filled with methamphetamine into his mouth during a kiss during a contact visit (Associated Press 2017). Two of the balloons broke in his stomach sometime later, and he died as a result. The woman was eventually sentenced to 2 years of incarceration related to drug conspiracy charges. In 2020, a federal inmate's prison sentence was extended after he was found in possession of contraband consisting of synthetic cannabinoid (U.S. Department of Justice 2020). In addition, prisoners use a wide range of recipes to make an alcoholic substance (sometimes referred to as hooch, brew, or Pruno) (Sestanovich 2014). These activities result in legalized sanctions against inmates, who may be subject to disciplinary hearings and punitive sanctions within the correctional system. One study from the Pennsylvania Department of Corrections reported that there were increased odds of receiving a severe disciplinary response to minor misconduct for women with co-occurring SUDs and mental illness compared with those with either disorder alone or with no disorders (Houser and Belenko 2015). Given the prevalence of individuals with preexisting SUDs and the risks that others might develop such disorders given the potentially broad access to substances within a correctional environment, ongoing attention is needed to identify SUDs and deliver treatment services.

# Legal Regulation of Clinical Practice in Correctional Settings

As with noncorrectional settings, some aspects of SUD care fall under legal and regulatory frameworks, including confidentiality within correctional settings. The *Ruiz* case outlined that confidential medical records were one of the six essential elements required for mental health care in a correctional setting. The National Commission on Correctional Health Care accreditation standards require medical treatment to be conducted in private unless security or safety issues require observation by a correctional officer. State laws also require privacy, as do federal laws, such as the Health Insurance Portability and Accountability Act of 1996 (HIPAA) and 42 C.F.R. Part 2 with regard to SUDs.

One challenge within corrections is the determination of whether the environment is a covered entity in which disclosure of personal health information is protected by HIPAA. As one author pointed out, this determination can be "vexing" and may require the input of legal counsel (Goldstein 2012). Regardless, there are noted exceptions within HIPAA for inmates. HIPAA requires that covered entities provide adequate notice to individuals regarding uses and disclosures of protected health information that a covered entity may make, but this notice is specifically carved out for inmates in HIPAA. Thus, correctional systems can opt to provide greater notice than the law requires (Goldstein 2012). As Goldstein pointed out, covered entities are permitted to disclose protected health information to a correctional institution official with lawful custody of an inmate for the purpose of providing health care and for the health and safety of other inmates and staff at the facility or to people transporting inmates between institutions. Goldstein (2012) provided the example of a nurse notifying officers about an inmate's injuries. She pointed out, however, that once an inmate is released and there are not overarching security issues, these exceptions do not apply.

In 42 C.F.R. Part 2, which is the separate privacy law that covers substance use treatment, there are greater restrictions than HIPAA that generally require individual consent to release information. Exceptions may include when a valid court order authorizes such disclosure of information. The Part 2 provisions, however, do not create the same carved-out exceptions for inmates (Goldstein 2012). There are allowances for disclosures for participation in programs that are a condition of the disposition after criminal proceedings (e.g., participation in drug courts), if the individuals who will receive the information have a need for it to effectuate monitoring of patient progress and with the patient's consent (Goldstein 2012).

Of course, there are legal exceptions to clinical confidentiality even outside of correctional settings, as is seen with mandated reporting requirements. Hanson (1999) argued that the correctional setting is unique in that there is a balancing of security and treatment that changes perspectives on interpretation of operating statutes in correctional contexts. She noted many examples in which otherwise confidential information may be examined by prison administrators, including inmate grievances regarding their medical or mental health care and when an individual poses a security breach such as planning for escape or possession of contraband. HIPAA and 42 C.F.R. Part 2 constitute a "floor" for protection of individual privacy, and state laws can be even more protective or restrictive. Overall, for clinicians working with individuals with SUDs within correctional contexts, it is important to understand local policies and practices and the interpretation of these confidentiality requirements. It is always permissible to share information with patient consent, and there should be ongoing efforts 1) to work across programs to determine what information would be important to share and for what purpose and 2) to develop collaborative strategies for engaging patients in understanding the potential benefits and risks to them to help make informed decisions about information sharing.

# Medications and Drug Diversion in Correctional Settings

With the promulgation of MAT within correctional settings, much attention has been paid to concerns about diversion of drugs that have misuse potential. This issue is not new, however. Prescribers within correctional systems have long known about a multitude of substances that have potential for misuse and could signal individuals who have some underlying or overt SUDs. For example, Keller (2017) identified six categories of substances that have abuse potential and are known within correctional settings as having value for diversion. Although there has been a great deal of focus on buprenorphine and methadone, other substances that have garnered scrutiny and attention include benzodiazepines legitimately prescribed for anxiety, stimulants used primarily for ADHD, stimulant laxatives, antihistamines, antidiarrheal agents, and others, to name a few.

There are legitimate concerns about nonmedical uses and black markets for these types of substances. An issue brief on this subject from the Substance Abuse and Mental Health Services Administration and Bureau of Justice Assistance (2019) identified common diversion techniques of avoiding swallowing medications and storing them on one's person (including within body cavities), selling urine containing a substance, or regurgitating medication after it is swallowed. The agency recommended creating safeguards to prevent this type of activity, including developing dedicated staff to support MOUD, using multidisciplinary teams, creating a patient-centered approach to care, providing staff training, and ensuring safe administration of medications, to name a few. As noted earlier in this chapter, when these issues emerge, it is important to identify the root causes, including the potential that purchasers and distributors have an SUD in need of treatment.

# Reentry Planning

Individuals with SUDs, especially those with co-occurring mental health conditions, who are moving from correctional environments to community settings often fare worse than others without these conditions. Two leading studies highlighted the critical nature of reentry planning. For example, Binswanger and colleagues (2007) found that the risk of death among prison inmates is 12.7 times higher within 2 weeks of release than for state population residents, with leading causes of death including drug overdose and suicide as well as cardiovascular events and homicide. A 2018 study of North Carolina inmates reported that at 2 weeks, 1 year, and complete follow-up after release, inmates' respective opioid overdose risk was 40, 11, and 8.3 times as high as general North Carolina residents (Ranapurwala et al. 2018). Opioid overdose risk was greatest for those who were male, ages 26–50 years, White, who had two prior prison terms, and who had received both mental health and SUD treatment while in prison.

Although not part of the *Ruiz* requirements, other legal cases have examined discharge planning (Metzner 2002). One is *Wakefield v. Thompson* (1999), in which the U.S. Ninth Circuit Court of Appeals ruled in favor of the plaintiff and found that states must provide outgoing prisoners with a sufficient supply of medications to ensure enough time for them to consult a doctor and obtain a new supply. *Brad H. v. City of New York* (2000) highlighted the importance of discharge planning in examining the discharge of people with disabilities from Rikers Island (Barr 2003). More recently, COVID-19 outbreaks in correctional settings have heightened scrutiny of who is staying in prison and who should be eligible for release. A significant settlement agreement resulted in the early reentry of 3,500 people from North Carolina prisons (*N.C. State Conference of NAACP v. Cooper* 2021; *North Carolina NAACP v. Cooper* 2021) in cooperation with local reentry centers to provide individuals with appropriate reentry services.

Models for enhancing the chance of successful reentry have been developed, including a framework known as the APIC (Assess, Plan, Identify, and Coordinate) model that has been widely promulgated. The APIC model breaks out tasks along its four dimensions, including identification of required programs responsible for postrelease services (Osher et al. 2002; Substance Abuse and Mental Health Services Administration 2017). Using this framework, other more focused models have emerged with wraparound supports, such as MISSION (Maintaining Independence and Sobriety through Systems Integration, Outreach, and Networking)–Criminal Justice, which uses a case manager and peer along with an amalgamation of evidence-based practices (Hanna et al. 2020), and efforts to enhance access to MOUD before and after release (Berk et al. 2022).

From a legal perspective, federal legislation addresses certain barriers and opportunities for inmates. For example, the Fair Housing Act (1968) places restrictions on individuals with certain criminal records to access specific housing supports (Legal Action Center 2014). State policies can thwart efforts of returning citizens with proper supports. For example, according to a report from the Hamilton Project, at the time of their survey, 12 states placed restrictions on access to Temporary Assistance for Needy Families or Supplemental Nutrition Assistance Program benefits for individuals with felony convictions (Whitmore Schanzenbach et al. 2016). The Legal Action Center (2022b) highlighted laws such as voting rights restrictions and lack of ability to seal and expunge records as creating barriers for successful reentry. Others have highlighted that individuals with past drug or felony convictions can be ineligible for public housing, which can further the cycle of rearrest (Taber et al. 2023). Thus, legal and policy barriers, as well as limited access to treatment providers upon release, can disproportionately affect individuals with SUDs returning from incarceration.

Despite these barriers, there are also efforts in legislation to improve access to proper supports. For example, the Workforce Innovation and Opportunity Act (2014), effective in 2016, provides federal funding to states that helps develop employment opportunities for disadvantaged people, including those with criminal records (Council of State Governments 2017). The U.S. Department of Justice has promulgated an overview of offender reentry that lays out elements that should be considered in reentry planning (Office of Justice Programs 2018). The Biden administration has also described efforts to make modifications and enhancements to opportunities for individuals coming out of incarceration with commitments to "second chances," including diverting individuals who have used illegal drugs out of incarceration, as well as other goals that remain to be realized as of this writing (The White House 2021). There is also discussion of whether laws will eventually allow Medicaid funding to cover some aspects of care as individuals are released from jails and prisons. Practitioners working with individuals with SUD in correctional settings would do well to stay attuned to advances in legislation that may shift options for patients in care.

# Class Action Litigation and the Role of the Psychiatrist and the Mental Health Professional

Class action litigation is the process in which a group of individuals who are similarly situated are considered as a "class" in litigation. In the prison context, this usually involves litigating about constitutional violations and deprivation of some aspects of their rights. In prison litigation cases, class action litigation has helped move the needle on standards of care expected within systems. Although litigation is not the only approach or always the best approach to system reform (e.g., legislation and policy can also be helpful), the strategy may both benefit the plaintiff class members and help transition toward improved practices overall with far-reaching impact. The examples highlighted in this chapter reflect these types of legal cases. These cases often involved the expertise of mental health professionals who had experience with correctional psychiatry and could review systems across a variety of standards and expectations. According to Metzner (2002), class action litigation can be seen as having three basic phases: 1) the liability phase, in which constitutional deficiencies are determined to exist or not; 2) the remedial phase, in which a remedy is identified for those deficiencies identified; and 3) the implementation phase, in which the remedial plan is implemented. The mental health expert can play a role in all three phases, such as evaluating the prison mental health system in litigation (Metzner and Dubovsky 1986) and monitoring the remedial plan (Metzner 2009). Not all prison- and jail-related litigation involves the certification of a class, and there are plenty of individual cases that take specific situations one by one. As SUD services become increasingly scrutinized within correctional environments, knowledge of SUDs and the law as they relate to correctional system expectations will assist courts and parties to litigation in developing better trends and best practices.

# Conclusions

The legal regulation of practice with regard to SUDs in correctional institutions is a unique area for further development. Much of correctional psychiatric practice has evolved with a lens on mental illnesses more broadly, and systems are constantly examining their laws and policies related to aspects of care, with increased interest in broadening SUD treatment. Litigation cases are also arising related to access to treatments for SUDs, with a particular focus on MOUD. However, these cases rest on well-established constitutional rights as well as rights of people with disabilities to be free from discrimination. There is a role for knowledgeable treatment providers as well as forensic and correctional experts with SUD policy and treatment expertise to help inform these practices and legal advances. Given penological interests and prison and jail safety priorities that can present challenges for getting people the care they require, there are unique considerations for practitioners practicing in correctional environments. This chapter offers an overview for individuals seeking to better understand where law and SUD issues intersect in correctional psychiatry.

# Key Points

- A majority of state and federal prisoners have symptoms that meet criteria for a substance use disorder (SUD).

- Correctional facilities must treat SUDs as a risk factor for suicidal behavior and provide the appropriate assessments.

- Jails, which usually hold pretrial detainees for a short period of time and receive only local funding, must nonetheless provide basic mental health and addiction evaluations and services.

- Judges must address violations of probation or parole, and often the best clinical response to an SUD-related violation is treatment rather than legal sanction.

- Release from incarceration is a particularly vulnerable time for those with SUDs, making clinical follow-up extremely important.

# References

American Civil Liberties Union: Know your rights: disability rights. October 2023. Available at: https://www.aclu.org/know-your-rights/disability-rights. Accessed June 12, 2024.

American Civil Liberties Union: Overcrowding and overuse of imprisonment in the U.S. May 2015. Available at: https://www.ohchr.org/sites/default/files/Documents/Issues/RuleOfLaw/OverIncarceration/ACLU.pdf. Accessed March 11, 2022.

American Psychiatric Association: Diagnostic and Statistical Manual of Mental Disorders, 4th Edition. Washington, DC, American Psychiatric Association, 1994

American Psychiatric Association: Psychiatric Services in Correctional Facilities, 3rd Edition. Arlington, VA, American Psychiatric Association, 2016

Americans With Disabilities Act of 1990 (P.L. 101–336), 104 Stat. 328 § 12131

Associated Press: Woman jailed after inmate boyfriend dies from meth-laden kiss. Daily News, November 22, 2017. Available at: https://www.nydailynews.com/news/crime/woman-jailed-inmate-boyfriend-dies-meth-laden-kiss-article-1.3649783. Accessed March 11, 2022.

Barr H: Transinstitutionalization in the courts: Brad H. v City of New York, and the fight for discharge planning for people with psychiatric disabilities leaving Rikers Island. Crime Delinq 49(1):97–123, 2003

Belenko S, Hiller M, Hamilton L: Treating substance use disorders in the criminal justice system. Curr Psychiatry Rep 15(11):414, 2013 24132733

Bell v Wolfish, 441 U.S. 520 (1979)

Berk J, Del Pozo B, Rich JD, et al: Injecting opioid use disorder treatment in jails and prisons: the potential of extended-release buprenorphine in the carceral setting. J Addict Med 16(4):396–398, 2022 34954747

Binswanger IA, Stern MF, Deyo RA, et al: Release from prison: a high risk of death for former inmates. N Engl J Med 356(2):157–165, 2007 17215533

Bird M, Tafpya S, Grattet R, et al: How Has Proposition 47 Affected California's Jail Population? San Francisco, CA, Public Policy Institute of California, March 2016. Available at: https://www.ppic.org/wp-content/uploads/content/pubs/report/R_316MB3R.pdf. Accessed March 8, 2022.

Bowring v Godwin, 551 F.2d 44 (4th Cir. 1977)

Brad v City of New York, 185 Misc. 2d 420 (N.Y. Sup. Ct. 2000)

Bronson J, Stroop J, Zimmer S, et al: Drug Use, Dependence, and Abuse Among State Prisoners and Jail Inmates, 2007–2009. Washington, DC, Bureau of Justice Statistics, U.S. Department of Justice, June 2017. Available at: https://bjs.ojp.gov/content/pub/pdf/dudaspji0709.pdf. Accessed March 11, 2022.

Brown v Plata, 131 S. Ct. 1910 (2011a)

Brown v Plata, 563 U.S. 493 (2011b)

Bureau of Justice Assistance: Activity Report: Residential Substance Abuse Treatment Programs Medication-Assisted Treatment (FYS 2016–2019). Washington, DC, U.S. Department of Justice, June 2021a. Available at: https://bja.ojp.gov/sites/g/files/xyckuh186/files/media/document/rsat-medication-assisted-treatment-fy-2016–2019.pdf. Accessed February 22, 2022.

Bureau of Justice Assistance: Residential Substance Abuse Treatment for State Prisoners Program. Washington, DC, U.S. Department of Justice, 2021b. Available at: https://bja.ojp.gov/program/residential-substance-abuse-treatment-state-prisoners-rsat-program/overview. Accessed on March 11, 2022.

Civil Rights of Institutionalized People Act, 42 U.S.C. § 1997 (1980)

Commonwealth v Eldred, 101 N.E.3d 911 (Mass. 2018)

Council of State Governments: The Workforce Innovation and Opportunity Act. Washington, DC, Council of State Governments, May 2017. Available at: https://csg justicecenter.org/publications/the-workforce-innovation-and-opportunity-act-what-corrections-and-reentry-agencies-need-to-know/. Accessed March 11, 2022.

Dunlop JG, Pinals DA: The psychiatric emergency care of prisoners, in Emergency Psychiatry: Principles and Practice, 2nd Edition. Edited by Glick RL, Zeller SL, Berlin JS. Philadelphia, PA, Wolters Kluwer, 2021, pp 449–458

Estelle v Gamble, 429 U.S. 97 (1976)

Fair Housing Act, 42 U.S.C. 3601 (1968)

Fenster A, Schlanger M: Slamming the Courthouse Door: 25 Years of Evidence for Repealing the Prison Litigation Reform Act. Northampton, MA, Prison Policy Initiative, April 2021. Available at: https://www.prisonpolicy.org/reports/PLRA_25.html. Accessed February 20, 2022.

Goldstein MM: Health Information Privacy in the Correctional Environment. Oakland, CA, Community Oriented Correctional Health Services, April 2012. Available at: https://publichealth.gwu.edu/departments/healthpolicy/DHP_Publications/pub_uploads/dhpPublication_C199DFF7–5056–9D20–3D2099CBB55AC369.pdf. Accessed February 22, 2022.

Hanna J, Kubiak S, Pasman E, et al: Evaluating the implementation of a prisoner re-entry initiative for individuals with opioid use and mental health disorders: application of the consolidated framework for implementation research in a cross-system initiative. J Subst Abuse Treat 108:104–114, 2020 31285078

Hanson AL: Confidentiality in Corrections: Fact or Fiction? American Academy of Psychiatry and the Law Newsletter, September 1999. Available at: https://www.aapl.org/docs/newsletter/N243Confidentiality_corrections.htm. Accessed February 22, 2022.

Harvard Law Review: Commonwealth v Eldred: Massachusetts Supreme Judicial Court holds drug-free probation requirement enforceable for defendant with substance use disorder. May 10, 2019. Available at: https://harvardlawreview.org/2019/05/commonwealth-v-eldred/. Accessed October 29, 2023.

Herring T: Since You Asked: What Role Does Drug Enforcement Play in the Rising Incarceration of Women? Northampton, MA, Prison Policy Initiative, November 10, 2020. Available at: https://www.prisonpolicy.org/blog/2020/11/10/women-drug-enforcement/. Accessed March 8, 2022.

Houser K, Belenko S: Disciplinary responses to misconduct among female prison inmates with mental illness, substance use disorders, and co-occurring disorders. Psychiatr Rehabil J 38(1):24–34, 2015 25664757

Keller J: Medications at high risk for diversion and abuse in correctional facilities. Jail Medicine, April 14, 2017. Available at: https://heliometrics.net/medications-at-high-risk-for-diversion-and-abuse-in-correctional-facilities-corrections-com. Accessed June 12, 2024.

Knight DK, Blue TR, Flynn PM, et al: The TCU Drug Screen 5: identifying justice-involved individuals with substance use disorders. J Offender Rehabil 57(8):525–537, 2018 31666789

Legal Action Center: Equal Housing Opportunity: National Blueprint for Reentry, 2nd Edition. National H.I.R.E. Network, July 2014. Available at: https://www.lac.org/assets/files/Recommendations-to-promote-the-successful-reentry-of-individuals-with-criminal-records-through-housing.pdf. Accessed February 22, 2022.

Legal Action Center: Cases Involving Discrimination Based on Treatment With Medication for Opioid Use Disorder (MOUD). U.S. Department of Justice, January 12, 2022a. Available at: https://www.lac.org/assets/files/Cases-involving-denial-of-access-to-MOUD.pdf. Accessed February 20, 2022.

Legal Action Center: Alternatives to incarceration and reentry. Available at: https://www.lac.org/work/priorities/restoring-opportunities/alternatives-to-incarceration-and-reentry. Accessed March 8, 2022b.

Legal Action Center: MAT/MOUD Advocacy Toolkit. November 2022c. Available at: https://www.lac.org/resource/mat-advocacy-toolkit. Accessed February 16, 2024.

Madrid v Gomez, 889 F. Supp. 1146 (N.D. Cal. 1995)

Metzner JL: Class action litigation in correctional psychiatry. J Am Acad Psychiatry Law 30(1):19–29, discussion 30–32, 2002 11931366

Metzner JL: Monitoring a correctional mental health care system: the role of the mental health expert. Behav Sci Law 27(5):727–741, 2009 19544449

Metzner JL, Dubovsky SL: The role of the psychiatrist in evaluating a prison mental health system in litigation. Bull Am Acad Psychiatry Law 14(1):89–95, 1986 3697521

Miller JM, Miller HV, Tillyer R: Effect of Prison-Based Alcohol Treatment: A Multi-Site Process and Outcome Evaluation. Washington, DC, National Institute of Justice, April 2014. Available at: https://www.ncjrs.gov/pdffiles1/nij/grants/246125.pdf. Accessed March 8, 2022.

Minton TD, Beatty LG, Zeng Z: Correctional Populations in the United States, 2019—Statistical Tables. Washington, DC, Bureau of Justice Statistics, U.S. Department of Justice, July 2021. Available at: https://bjs.ojp.gov/sites/g/files/xyckuh236/files/media/document/cpus19st.pdf. Accessed March 8, 2022.

National Commission of Correctional Health Care: Standards. 2024. Available at: https://www.ncchc.org. Accessed April 14, 2024.

N.C. State Conference of NAACP v Cooper, 1:18CV1034 (M.D.N.C. Aug. 17, 2021)

Neill-Gubitz H, Graves JM, Barbosa-Leiker C: Availability of health care services and medications for opioid use disorder in carceral facilities in Washington, Oregon, and Idaho. J Health Care Poor Underserved 33(1):407–418, 2022 35153230

Newman WJ, Scott CL: Brown v Plata: prison overcrowding in California. J Am Acad Psychiatry Law 40(4):547–552, 2012 23233477

North Carolina NAACP v Cooper, File No. 20 CVS 500110 (Wake Cty. Sup. Ct. 2021)

Office of Justice Programs: An Overview of Offender Reentry. Washington, DC, National Institute of Justice, U.S. Department of Justice, 2018. Available at: https://www.ojp.gov/pdffiles1/nij/251554.pdf. Accessed February 22, 2022.

Osher F, Steadman JH, Barr H: A Best Practice Approach to Community Re-Entry From Jails for Inmates with Co-Occurring Disorders: The APIC Model. Delmar, NY, The National GAINS Center, 2002

Pennsylvania Department of Corrections v Yeskey, 524 U.S. 206 (1998a)

Pennsylvania Department of Corrections v Yeskey, 524 U.S. 206, 118 S. Ct. 1952 (1998b)

Pesce v Coppinger, 355 F. Supp. 3d 35 (D. Mass. 2018)

P.G. v Jefferson County, Case No. 5:21-cv-388 (DNH/ML) (N.D.N.Y. 2021)

Prison Litigation Reform Act, 42 U.S.C. 1997e (1996)

Ranapurwala SI, Shanahan ME, Alexandridis AA, et al: Opioid overdose mortality among former North Carolina inmates: 2000–2015. Am J Public Health 108(9):1207–1213, 2018 30024795

Rehabilitation Act of 1973 (P.L. 93–112), 97 Stat. 355 (codified as amended at 29 U.S.C. § 701)

Rich JD, Boutwell AE, Shield DC, et al: Attitudes and practices regarding the use of methadone in US state and federal prisons. J Urban Health 82(3):411–419, 2005 15917502

Robinson v California, 370 U.S. 660, 82 S. Ct. 1417 (1962)

Ruiz v Estelle, 503 F. Supp. 1265 (S.D. Tex. 1980)

Sestanovich C: Prison moonshine. The Marshall Project, 2014. Available at: https://www.themarshallproject.org/2014/12/30/prison-moonshine. Accessed March 7, 2022.

Smith v Aroostook County, 922 F.3d 41 (1st Cir. 2019)

Substance Abuse and Mental Health Services Administration: Guidelines for Successful Transition of People with Mental or Substance Use Disorders from Jail and Prison: Implementation Guide. Rockville, MD, Substance Abuse and Mental Health Services Administration, 2017. Available at: https://store.samhsa.gov/sites/default/files/d7/priv/sma16–4998.pdf. Accessed November 12, 2023.

Substance Abuse and Mental Health Services Administration; Bureau of Justice Assistance: MAT Inside Correctional Facilities: Addressing Medication Diversion. Rockville, MD, Substance Abuse and Mental Health Services Administration, August 2019. Available at: https://store.samhsa.gov/sites/default/files/d7/priv/pep19-mat-corrections.pdf. Accessed November 12, 2023.

Taber N, Marin JA, Bae J, et al: Public housing eligibility for people with conviction histories. Cityscape 25(2), 2023. Available at: https://www.huduser.gov/portal/periodicals/cityscape/vol25num2/ch4.pdf. Accessed June 20, 2024.

Toyoshima T, McNiel DE, Schonfeld A, et al: The evolving medicolegal precedent for medications for opioid ese disorder in U.S. jails and prisons. J Am Acad Psychiatry Law 49(4):545–552, 2021 34341145

U.S. Department of Justice: Federal Inmate Gets More Time Possessing Contraband. Pittsburgh, PA, U.S. Attorney's Office, Western District of Pennsylvania, 2020. Available at: https://www.justice.gov/usao-wdpa/pr/federal-inmate-gets-more-time-possessing-contraband. Accessed on March 11, 2022.

U.S. v Massachusetts Parole Board, DJ 204–36–241 (D. Mass 2021)

Violent Crime Control and Law Enforcement Act of 1994 (P.L. 103–322)

Wakefield v Thompson, 177 F.3d 1160 (9th Cir. 1999)

The White House: A Proclamation on Second Chance Month, 2021. March 13, 2021. Available at: https://www.whitehouse.gov/briefing-room/presidential-actions/2021/03/31/a-proclamation-on-second-chance-month-2021/. Accessed March 6, 2022.

Whitmore Schanzenbach D, Nunn R, Bauer L, et al: Twelve Facts About Incarceration and Prisoner Reentry. Washington, DC, Brookings Institution, October 21, 2016. Available at: https://www.brookings.edu/research/twelve-facts-about-incarceration-and-prisoner-reentry/. Accessed February 22, 2022.

Wickersham JA, Azar MM, Cannon CM, et al: Validation of a brief measure of opioid dependence: the Rapid Opioid Dependence Screen (RODS). J Correct Health Care 21(1):12–26, 2015 25559628

Workforce Innovation and Opportunity Act of 2014 (P.L. 113–128)

# PART 4

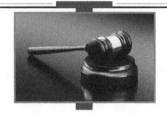

# SPECIAL TOPICS

# CHAPTER 11

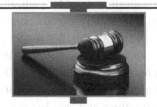

# Special Topics in Law and Addiction

## Introduction

Patients (and forensic evaluees) rightly look to clinicians to help distinguish between exciting new treatments for addiction and the unhelpful, or even dangerous, modalities sometimes promoted for addiction treatment. The ever-increasing wave of cannabis decriminalization and legalization in the United States presents numerous dilemmas for addiction professionals. These challenges include parsing any apparently good effects of the substance, identifying the bad effects, and remaining familiar with the rapidly changing legal contexts that affect the lives of those who use cannabis. Fairly or not, addiction clinicians are often regarded as *de facto* experts on the substance itself as well as on the downstream effects of its use.

The authors thank Steve Woolworth, Ph.D., for his review of this section.

Similarly complicated are FDA-approved and non-approved uses of substances such as kratom and the hallucinogenic form of ketamine. (Although esketamine is legally prescribed and dispensed, illicit use of ketamine remains common.) These substances vary in terms of their effects and dangerousness, but they share with cannabis an uncertainty as to the actual content in a sample bought illicitly or from a nonlicensed entity (this variation in actual content is one cogent argument for legalization of these substances). Awareness of the legal structures for clinical use and research involving these substances is important.

Prescription opioid medications used for pain, although highly effective in the right clinical situation, have rightly gained a reputation for lethality in overdose and have caused significant mortality simply by being overprescribed. Both in their interactions with pain medicine prescribers and in their own prescription of medications for opioid use disorder (MOUD), addiction clinicians must be aware of the clinical aspects of the medications they recommend or prescribe and the legal structures and case law that surround their use. This chapter reviews various aspects of these conundrums.

## FORENSIC DILEMMA

A 23-year-old woman twists her ankle while stocking shelves in the big-box store where she works and is escorted to an urgent care center by her supervisor. A urine drug screen (UDS) is a mandatory part of the evaluation for any work-related injury, and the employee discloses that she has a medical marijuana card and, in fact, smokes marijuana most days.

Consider the following:

1. What should the supervisor do?
2. What are the Americans With Disabilities Act (ADA) implications of the employee's disclosure?

At the urgent care center, the employee declines the UDS as part of her evaluation. She requests care for her twisted ankle, but says she sees no relevance to the UDS.

3. Does a late Δ-9-tetrahydrocannabinol (THC) screen have any relevance?
4. What are the obligations of the urgent care physician vis-à-vis a UDS?

The medical examination reveals a tendon strain only, and the employee is released with an ankle wrap, a recommendation to take ibuprofen, and a follow-up appointment with an orthopedist if her discomfort has not improved after 3 days.

5. Should the workplace physician allow the employee to return to work?
6. Who should the supervisor inform about the employee's disclosure?

This is a complicated situation, and the responses of the work supervisor and workplace physician should be governed by state law and the workplace drug policy. Generally speaking, the work supervisor should inform the company's attorney or human resources department of the disclosure but no one else. The presence of a medical marijuana card likely represents protected health information under the Health Insurance Portability and Accountability Act of 1996 (HIPAA). The employee may well be protected under the ADA, but that would be determined by a hearing, long after the afternoon's events have unfolded. In addition, the employee's refusal to have a UDS that same day is probably irrelevant in regard to THC, because THC remains in fat stores for days to weeks after use: a test done several days later will yield a similar result. The urgent care physician has no obligations regarding the UDS; they can offer the UDS but cannot and should not pressure the employee to take the test. All parties would be better off waiting until a forensic-level chain-of-custody UDS can be done.

After the workplace physician receives notification from the company attorney or human resources department, the physician might examine the employee for intoxication, withdrawal, or any other condition that might render her presently unfit to return to work. The workplace physician may bar the employee from returning to work only if there are demonstrable safety concerns. The flow of information should be carefully controlled and structured in the company drug policy and managed by the attorney or human resources department.

# Forensic Implications of COVID-19 for People With Substance Use Disorders

Although the COVID-19 pandemic has correlated with worsening U.S. rates of substance use disorders (SUDs), governmental attempts to adjust treatment regulations have to some extent mitigated the damage. These modifications, although necessarily fluid as the pandemic progressed, allowed clinicians to effectively treat SUDs while avoiding breaching regulations and therefore facing legal liability. In addition, some of the regulatory changes forced by the circumstances of the pandemic may turn out to be advantageous and will likely be codified into law after the COVID-19 public health emergency has passed.

A particularly devastating marker of COVID-19's apparent effect on substance users was the increase in opioid overdose deaths during the pandemic. In the 12 months before April 2021, 100,306 overdose deaths occurred in the United States, compared with 78,056 in the previous 12 months (Centers for Disease Control and Prevention 2021). Although fentanyl- and methamphetamine-fueled overdose rates had been creeping up in the previous few years, the 28.5% increase was unprecedented and directly linked to the COVID-19 pandemic. Unsurprisingly, studies of alcohol use also revealed an increase. In one social media study of 5,850 respondents, 29% reported that they had increased their alcohol use since the beginning of the pandemic (Capasso et al. 2021).

The reasons for this worsening picture for SUDs during the COVID-19 pandemic are myriad and likely build on one another. They include social isolation, which denies substance users the support that they need to achieve and maintain sobriety; the society-wide stressors that substance users address with their habitual agent of choice; and the shutdown of services needed for emergency response to addiction and for outpatient and inpatient treatment, which can mitigate the physical and emotional damage that substance users face (National Institute on Drug Abuse 2022). As the pandemic worsened and morphed into waves of novel variants, public health authorities put into effect regulations and rules to support social distancing and, out of necessity, closed places where people gather, including addiction treatment facilities.

In the face of these public health measures, the U.S. Department of Health and Human Services (HHS) relaxed enforcement of HIPAA regulations with the specific intent of getting patients with COVID-19 treated safely but also allowing patients to safely receive treatments for all types of maladies. In a communication last updated in January 2021, the HHS made official its intention to eschew enforcement of HIPAA, even (startlingly) for clinicians who used specific communication methods previously banned as non-HIPAA compliant:

> During the COVID-19 national emergency, which also constitutes a nationwide public health emergency, covered health care providers subject to the HIPAA rules may seek to communicate with patients, and provide telehealth services, through remote communications technologies....[A] covered health care provider may provide similar telehealth services in the exercise of their professional judgment to assess or treat any other medical condition, even if not related to COVID-19, such as a sprained ankle, dental consultation or psychological evaluation, or other conditions....Under this Notice, covered health care providers may use popular applications that allow for video chats, including Apple FaceTime, Facebook Messenger video chat, Google Hangouts video, Zoom, or Skype, to provide telehealth. (U.S. Department of Health and Human Services 2021)

In addition to relaxed confidentiality rules, many states modified licensure requirements, including medical licensure, for the purpose of providing care for patients with COVID-19 and for those who could not access care because of the prevalence of the virus and the dearth of available treatment facilities. Although directed at medical care, these changes in licensure requirements clearly benefited clinicians treating people with addiction and dual diagnoses. New York State, for instance, extended previous permissions for clinicians licensed in other states through March 1, 2022, to allow "certified clinical laboratory technicians, certified histological technicians, licensed clinical social workers, licensed master social workers, podiatrists, physical therapists, physical therapist assistants, mental health counselors, marriage and family therapists, creative arts therapists, psychoanalysts, and psychologists" to practice within New York State without civil or criminal penalty related to lack of licensure (New York State 2021).

This official relaxation of rules about confidentiality, telehealth, and in some instances, medical licensure represented a golden opportunity for the promulgation of telehealth to individuals with SUDs who could not, or would not, access an in-person treatment facility. Although telehealth for addiction treatment was arguably a good idea that was a long time coming, the pandemic clarified for many the absolute necessity of telehealth for the treatment of SUDs in the COVID-19 era and beyond. A few obvious challenges exist for the practitioner: cameras cannot reveal the gait of a seated patient, the commotion that patient may make in the waiting room, or the alcohol-laden breath they bring into the consultation room. A new standard of care is being developed for telehealth modalities, and it will certainly focus on maintaining the patient's confidentiality, dignity, and right to informed consent as well as possibly even (or especially) over the internet. Clinicians who treat individuals with SUDs should stay abreast of the innovations and guidelines in mental health treatment and modify them for practice with those with SUDs. Table 11–1 lists some excellent suggestions for providing effective, and private, telehealth services.

The COVID-19-related federal relaxation of confidentiality rules and the decision by many states to waive specific state medical license requirements were matched by an easing of regulations in the nation's jails and prisons, allowing for quicker and more effective treatment of SUDs. Approximately one in three incarcerated people has received an SUD diagnosis, and 9%–13% were using opioids before they were incarcerated (Krawczyk et al. 2017). Unfortunately, correctional settings today still struggle to provide MOUD (see Chapter 10).

Early indications of a seismic change in a *de facto* anti-opioid use disorder (anti-OUD) bias show that barriers to MOUD fell quickly in the face of a desperate situation faced by incarcerated people at risk of COVID-19, OUD, and other SUDs. In a study of the volume of buprenorphine and methadone supplied to various institutions, including prisons and jails, researchers found that the availability of MOUD increased 471.3% between January 2018 and October 2020, with the majority of that increase happening after the pandemic's inception in March 2020 (Dadiomov et al. 2022). There was, unfortunately, no similar increase in MOUD use in hospitals, clinics, and long-term care facilities, and data showed that MOUD use decreased slightly in those facilities. One jail system, the Hennepin County Jail system in Minneapolis, Minnesota, capitalized on the COVID-19-induced 43% reduction in their population and the relaxed public federal telemedicine guidelines. It began initiating patients on buprenorphine without an in-person visit and instituting a program to taper medication

**Table 11–1.** Telehealth in the treatment of substance use disorders

Have available on-site physical examination, including blood pressure and gait assessment

Have available drug or alcohol screening

Establish a clean and professional-looking office space

Have reliable internet

Plan for connecting if video drops (e.g., telephone call)

Place the camera at eye level

Ensure patient privacy

*Source.*   Adapted from Oesterle et al. 2020.

for interested patients to their preference of a maintenance dosage or complete taper. These newfound abilities to provide patient-specific OUD care were described as follows:

> [These] are examples of policy changes and clinical creativity during a pandemic during which physical distancing is critical yet clinicians must continue to treat opioid withdrawal symptoms. The taper policy, while not dependent on the continuation of relaxed federal telemedicine regulations, makes patient care efficient: it is a practice that jail clinicians intend to continue beyond the current pandemic. (Duncan et al. 2021, p. 2)

# Cannabis and the Law

Although the prevailing cultural ethos in favor of the medicalization and subsequent state-level decriminalization of cannabis in the United States is inarguable, the legal ramifications of these changes are confusing for individuals who decide to use cannabis and for employers, law enforcement officers, and physicians who choose to recommend the substance for therapeutic purposes. Because numerous states have legalized the personal use of marijuana, despite the substance remaining on the prohibited federal Schedule I, practical concerns such as employment matters and cannabis (discussed in Chapter 4), the liability of physicians who recommend cannabis use, and regulations on impaired driving and cannabis become quite relevant. Even if recent initiatives to reschedule cannabis to  to Schedule III of the Controlled Substances Act succeed (DEA 2024), individuals subject to drug testing  and those doing the testing would be well advised to avoid making any changes absent explicit  guidance from their employer on the subject of cannabis. Legal sanctions would likely survive the change to Schedule III for physicians who commit malpractice in their recommendation for cannabis or drivers who are arrested for intoxication with cannabis. By way of comparison, the medication buprenorphine is presently listed under Schedule III of the CSA, and that placement is no defense to driving while intoxicated charges (Kuhlman et al. 2022) or criminal charges for illegal drug distribution (United States v Sriramloo Kesari MD 2022).

Because cannabis contains several different compounds and is not approved by the FDA as a medication, the public perception that a physician "prescribes" cannabis is simply inaccurate. Although physicians definitively cannot prescribe cannabis, a 2002 U.S. Court of Appeals case (*Conant v. Walters* 2002), flowing from the 1996 legalization of cannabis in California and Arizona, upheld as free speech the right of physicians to "recommend" cannabis and prevented the government from punishing them for doing so or holding the physician responsible for what the patient does subsequent to the office visit.

Using this legal theory, most state medical marijuana regulations require a physician's recommendation that the patient take cannabis for a particular indication. The original California statute requires the following:

> that medical use is deemed appropriate and has been recommended by a physician who has determined that the person's health would benefit from the use of marijuana in the treatment of cancer, anorexia, AIDS, chronic pain, spasticity, glaucoma, arthritis, migraine, or any other illness for which marijuana provides relief. (Compassionate Use Act 1996)

Notwithstanding the cursory evaluations sometimes offered by physicians online, by telephone, or in cannabis dispensaries, published advice to physicians who are called on to make cannabis recommendations contains fairly standard guidelines for helping potential patients assess the risks and benefits of taking a particular substance. Although medical recommendations will likely become less relevant as the legal use of cannabis for any (or no) reason spreads, a medical exemption may remain important in the employment context or as a defense to possession of larger amounts than would be considered legal, or in those jurisdictions where recreational use has still not been decriminalized.

One early publication on physician recommendations for cannabis emphasized that 1) the patients should have failed more conventional strategies for treatment of a particular condition, and 2) a detailed informed consent discussion should be held, including discussion of the specific risks of cannabis use (Voth 2001). In addition, it may be advisable for a physician to do the following when recommending cannabis: conduct an assessment of addiction or the potential for addiction, seek pulmonary function testing (for cannabis smokers) and ongoing drug testing, and ensure that the physician has the proper state and federal licensure to make the medical recommendations for its use.

Some have also recommended that physicians test the actual THC potency in the preparations that the patient ingests, but it would be impractical for any physician to regularly test the actual cannabis that a patient is ingesting. This impracticality points out one source of liability for the recommending physician: the unregulated nature of the substances being sold as cannabis, which the physician has recommended. One comprehensive outline of the potential malpractice liabilities for physicians who recommend cannabis identified a few likely candidates for malpractice actions (Marlowe 2016). A breach of the duty of care might be alleged, despite the fact that the physician is not recommending a standard course of treatment and would likely not be held responsible for harm related to a contaminated or too-potent cannabis preparation. A duty of care has been established as soon as the doctor-patient relationship begins, and any advice that the doctor gives (even about off-label use of substances) could reasonably be construed as part of the doctor-patient relationship. There is considerable disagreement in the medical literature as to whether cannabis preparations are reasonable treatments for even the few FDA-approved indications, and there is no agreement at all as to whether cannabis is a reasonable treatment for the wide variety of conditions it is actually used for, including psychiatric conditions. A physician accused of being complicit in a poor outcome would have a great deal of difficulty marshalling a defense for such a recommendation. In addition to a simple breach-of-duty allegation, a physician who did not fulfill the state's specific educational requirements for a cannabis-prescription certificate or who does not have a well-documented physician-patient relationship might be held liable on those grounds. Finally, as part of the informed consent process, physicians must provide patients with all material information about the treatment being offered: this is a very high bar, given that unregulated cannabis is a very controversial treatment, with uncertain ingredients. Given these potential pitfalls, physicians who recommend cannabis would do well to carefully consider their obligations, provide complete information, and carefully document all aspects of the patient-physician relationship.

One particular risk of cannabis use is driving while impaired, and liability for this would accrue to the user and (possibly) the physician who recommended the cannabis. Driving under the influence of cannabis is, unfortunately, relatively common but hard to assess. According to 2018 CDC data, 12 million U.S. adults (4.7% of the population) acknowledged driving under the influence of cannabis during the previous year, compared with 2.3 million adults (0.9% of the population) who said they had driven while impaired by other drugs (Azofeifa et al. 2019). These numbers compare to the approximately 20.5 million adults (8% of the population) who said that they had driven while impaired by alcohol in the previous year.

Cannabis has been described as causing a less certain driving impairment than alcohol, because the effect on driving is mitigated by tolerance, differences in the way the cannabis is ingested, and variable absorption of THC. Often alcohol and marijuana are used together, and the sum of the driving impairment is greater than the impairment conferred by each substance alone (Sewell et al. 2009). However, police officers' assessment of intoxication by cannabis is problematic because cannabis intoxication is often less obvious than it would be for alcohol intoxication, and users may ingest edibles or lozenges and therefore avoid any smoke. Although training programs on how to recognize driving under the influence of cannabis exist for law enforcement officials, they are subjective by necessity and are not focused on measuring cannabis levels, because most jurisdictions do not have definitive regulations on a legal limit for cannabis, much less equipment for measuring cannabis levels. One manualized program for assessing cannabis intoxication (National Traffic Law Center 2022), sponsored by the National District Attorneys Association, teaches how to obtain legal cannabis in order to give course participants a chance to observe and assess the impairing effects of cannabis.

State laws that set limits for driving while intoxicated by cannabis vary widely, as might be expected by the uncertain science of cannabis-related impairment. As of July 2021, 33 states had no cannabis-specific drugged driving law, 11 states had zero-tolerance laws for any THC levels found, 4 states codified a THC level of 5 ng/cc as intoxication, and 2 states (Nevada and Ohio) classified a THC level of 2 ng/cc as intoxication (Responsibility.org 2021).

Presumably, legal challenges to these state laws will elucidate a national consensus, as there is for alcohol, regarding what level of THC constitutes presumptive intoxication. However, given the long period of time that cannabis can result in a positive urine toxicology result (around 30 days in heavy users), the zero-tolerance paradigm for any THC in a urine toxicology screen is unlikely to stand up to legal challenge.

In addition to an eventual consensus on the identification of THC intoxication for the sake of determination of driving under the influence and given the failure of cannabis prohibition, there is a need for consensus on legal boundaries for the use of THC products and the treatment of individuals who are damaged by the substance. Like alcohol, THC will probably have agreed-upon age limits that are imposed nationwide and vigorously enforced. Perhaps some profits from the nascent cannabis industry will be directed toward those who are harmed by the substance.

# Forensic Issues With the Clinical Use of Opioids

## TREATMENT OF PAIN AND CRIMINALIZED EXCESSIVE PRESCRIBING

The liability of the pharmaceutical industry, such as Purdue Pharma and the Sackler family (who developed and marketed prescription opioid medications), for at least some aspects of the prescription opioid epidemic has been explored in popular books (Keefe 2021) and television shows (Dopesick 2021). Individual physicians have also been held legally responsible for addiction, overdose, and other damages caused to their patients by the prescription of opioid medications.

The most egregious cases of opioid addiction and overdose in the practice of medicine are caused by clinical work so far outside the usual scope of practice that they are prosecuted by federal law enforcement agencies as criminal matters. For instance, a dedicated health care fraud unit consisting of 80 prosecutors is tasked with prosecuting cases against those who illegally prescribe, distribute, or divert prescription opioids (U.S. Department of Justice 2021). These health care fraud units, which focus on regions that have been particularly hard-hit by the opioid crisis (such as Appalachia), deploy "strike forces." These strike forces consist of personnel from the Federal Bureau of Investigation, Internal Revenue Service, local offices of the U.S. attorney general, and other agencies in an attempt to identify potential bad actors via suspicious billing patterns and then investigate and arrest those who are, in fact, breaking the law and contributing to opioid-induced morbidity and mortality. Fifteen strike forces exist across the country, and they have charged more than 4,200 defendants who billed Medicare, in aggregate, more than $19 billion (U.S. Department of Justice 2021).

One recent conviction obtained by the federal health care fraud unit involved Delaware physician Patrick Titus, who was convicted of 13 counts of unlawfully distributing and dispensing controlled substances and 1 count of maintaining a drug-involved premises (*United States of America v. Patrick Titus* 2018; U.S. Department of Justice 2021). The 58-year-old internist ran a pain clinic and was shown in court to have prescribed multiple opioids, including fentanyl, morphine, methadone, and oxycodone, without providing any meaningful medication evaluation or care, and he prescribed them to some patients he knew had an SUD and to others who he knew were diverting the medication. Titus's 2018 indictment resulted in a 2-week trial in 2021 and a sentence of 20 years in prison.

This federal indictment was not Titus's first brush with the law. Local Delaware records reveal that Titus had previously been held accountable for dangerous and illegal prescribing practices: in 2011, his Delaware Controlled Substance Registration was suspended because his medical practice did the following:

> present(ed) an imminent danger to the public…[because he] …overprescribed controlled substances to patients in amounts that exceed safe therapeutic levels without conducting proper medical examinations; without contacting patients' primary care or other treating physicians; without requesting medical records or ordering tests; without establishing any legitimate medical basis or need for medication; and without taking reasonable and necessary precautions to pre-

vent illegal diversion of controlled substances. (Delaware Department of State 2011)

A similar criminal case and verdict occurred for Dr. Xiulu Ruan, but Ruan's conviction was overturned by the U.S. Supreme Court. Ruan owned a pain management clinic and pharmacy in Mobile, Alabama, and was accused of prescribing and dispensing large numbers of opioid medications, including the instant-release fentanyl preparation Subsys, for the treatment of neck, back, and joint pain. In addition to the aberrant prescriptions, Ruan was accused of accepting kickbacks from a dispensary management company, participating in a RICO (Racketeer Influenced and Corrupt Organizations) conspiracy, and illegally billing Medicare $3,649,092. He was convicted in 2017 and sentenced to 21 years in prison. A U.S. Drug Enforcement Administration (DEA) spokesman underlined the main reason for their pursuit of Ruan and others like him: "Opiate abuse is a major problem in Alabama and throughout the nation. The diversion of prescription pain killers contributes to the widespread abuse of opiates and is a gateway to heroin addiction, which is devastating our local communities" (Southern District of Alabama U.S. Attorney's Office 2017).

In their appeal to the U.S. Supreme Court (*Ruan v. United States* 2022), Ruan's attorneys argued that their client was exercising his best professional judgment and, in legal terms, both "reasonably believed" and "subjectively intended" that his prescriptions would fall within the realm of usual professional practice. An apparent split between the Eleventh Circuit Court's reliance on the "generally accepted medical standards" test and the Second, Fourth, and Sixth Circuits' reliance on the "good faith" test supported this appeal to the court. Although Ruan's attorneys noted some support for Ruan's practice from his own expert witnesses, they relied on the public policy argument that granting latitude in medical practice is important for the best care of patients:

> Depriving physicians of a meaningful good faith defense to [Controlled Substances Act] charges leads to just such overdeterrence and chills the practice of pain medicine. As this Court explained in *Moore*, "Congress understandably was concerned…that physicians be allowed reasonable discretion in treating patients and testing new theories" 423 U.S. at 143…. "[L]atitude must therefore be given to doctors trying to determine the current boundaries of acceptable medical practice…." The Supreme Court's decision in this matter hinged on the observation that Dr. Ruan was lawfully prescribing the opiates and practicing in "subjective good faith," in the sense that he was "not intending to facilitate[e] addiction or recreational drug abuse. (*Ruan v. United States* 2022)

The court ruled that although Ruan may have been functioning as a "bad doctor," he was nonetheless entitled to defense under the CSA: the conviction was overturned.

Although the two criminal cases just described show massive and apparently intentional overprescriptions of opioids, patient deaths, apparent financial chicanery, and collusion between practitioners, many more civil matters are brought against practitioners whose alleged misdeeds are merely acts of carelessness, practice below the minimum standard of care, or failure to comply with all aspects of the relevant regulations. Regardless, liability can ensue, and prescribers and dispensers of controlled substances must register with the DEA, maintain this registration, and comply with all relevant regulations.

In one typical case, anesthesiologist Pramila Byahatti had her New Jersey medical license permanently suspended because of her practice of indiscriminately prescribing narcotics to her patients. Byahatti regularly saw 45 patients during 6.5-hour clinics and prescribed high dosages of fentanyl, oxycodone, and other opioids. According to the consent order she signed, Byahatti concurred with the medical board's observation that she "failed to perform appropriate medical and mental health assessments, order appropriate diagnostic testing, monitor patients' use of [controlled dangerous substances] medications, and appropriately screen for possible substance abuse issues, all while maintaining insufficient medical records." (State of New Jersey Office of the Attorney General 2020, p. 2)

Table 11–2 presents a useful summary of red flags for atypical prescribing and dispensing policies. Note that all of these must be interpreted in light of the relevant clinical situation.

# CASE LAW IN SUPPORT OF MEDICATIONS FOR THE TREATMENT OF OPIOID USE DISORDER

In contrast to the criminal cases against physicians who prescribe opioids for the treatment of pain as just described, a growing body of civil cases support the use of MOUD, including methadone and buprenorphine. The following cases are examples of a generalizing support for the use of MOUD in the criminal legal system and the avoidance of discrimination against patients with OUD in employment and health care.

In an important Massachusetts case (*Pesce v. Coppinger* 2018a, 2018b), Pesce, whose symptoms had been stable with methadone treatment for several years, faced incarceration in a Massachusetts facility that provided no MOUD. The plaintiff's physician noted the efficacy of this treatment for Pesce's condition, cited medical literature on the high rate of overdose for those with OUD in general, and described Pesce's numerous overdose events and failed attempts at different types of treatment. The defendant prison system claimed that safety and diversion concerns made the provision of MOUD within the jail system burdensome and practically impossible. The judge granted summary judgment to Pesce, writing that denying this effective and life-sustaining treatment would

**Table 11–2.** Red flags for narcotic misuse or diversion

Intoxication or symptoms associated with heavier use (agitation, psychosis, shortness
   of breath, palpitations)
Demands for a particular, usually fast-acting, medication
Repeated lost prescriptions
Multiple prescribers
Discordant pill count
Prescription issued by physicians outside of their scope of practice
Prescriptions paid for by cash
Patients who travel long distances to fill prescriptions

*Source.*   Adapted from Cote 2016; F. Levin, personal communication, 2022.

likely be found a violation of the ADA and was in addition tantamount to a violation of the Eighth Amendment as "cruel and unusual punishment." (This
case is also addressed in Chapter 10.)

The U.S. Equal Employment and Opportunity Commission (EEOC)
brought a case in 2018 against Appalachia Wood Products (*EEOC v. Appalachian Wood Products, Inc.* 2018) for discriminating against a job applicant because he was prescribed buprenorphine/naltrexone. In addition to illegally
inquiring about the applicant's medication use, the employer then failed to consider whether the applicant would actually be impaired from performing the
requisite duties. In a finding citing the opioid epidemic and clearly designed to
support the treatment of OUD using MOUD, the EEOC found that the defendant company in fact violated the ADA with its medication question (before a
job offer) as well as its failing to contemplate the specific effects of MOUD on
the applicant or considering him for a non-safety-sensitive position. The defendant company was ordered to pay the applicant a monetary settlement, create
nondiscretionary employment policies, provide ADA training to its employees,
report to the EEOC regarding any further complaints of disability discrimination, and post a workplace notice of the settlement.

In a particularly egregious pattern by a health care facility, the EEOC found that
Selma Medical Associates regularly refused to evaluate patients who were prescribed Suboxone (U.S. Department of Justice 2019). The decision read, "Selma
Medical regularly turns away prospective new patients who are treated with narcotic controlled substances such as Suboxone"; it was unclear whether the clinic
turned away patients who take opioids, was unprepared to prescribe Suboxone, or
simply preferred not to treat pain patients. Whatever the intent, Selma was found to
have discriminated against a person with an SUD because they imposed eligibility
criteria that would exclude such patients from treatment or even evaluation. The
clinic agreed with the U.S. Department of Justice to pay a monetary settlement to
one patient they had turned away and to modify their policies and practices to avoid
any future discrimination against people with OUD.

In another example of federal protection for MOUD and the patients who receive it, the EEOC settled an ADA discrimination suit against Massachusetts General Hospital after the hospital declined to consider a patient with cystic fibrosis for a lung transplant because the (potential) patient was prescribed Suboxone (U.S. Department of Justice 2020). It appears that the hospital's reflexive refusal to consider the patient for a transplant, without following their usual practice of consulting specialists when there is a question of appropriateness, was a particular aggravating factor in this matter, as the settlement agreement notes that no addiction or pain specialists were consulted. Massachusetts General Hospital, in the settlement agreement, agreed to pay a monetary settlement to the potential transplant recipient, who had in the meantime received a successful transplant elsewhere. In addition, the hospital agreed to cease discrimination on the basis of an OUD diagnosis, draft and adopt a policy to that effect, and train its entire staff about this nondiscrimination requirement.

# Non-FDA-Approved Substances in the Treatment of SUDs and Other Psychiatric Conditions

Treating SUDs using molecules that are close analogs of the addicting substances is neither new nor original, as patients who have been helped by methadone, buprenorphine, or off-label use of synthetic THC can attest. So, it should not be surprising that publications about the use of hallucinogens as potential treatments for SUD have prompted patient requests for these substances, an increased number of scientific studies, and clinician interest in prescribing or at least recommending them. Given the lack of definitive clinical data or FDA approval, clinicians must decide whether the liability risk in recommending hallucinogens is worth the potential benefits to their patients. Although lysergic acid diethylamide (LSD) has a history of being investigated by U.S. intelligence agencies for nefarious reasons (Treaster 1977), modern research strives for scientific objectivity and relevance.

Although there are a few scientific reports about LSD and psilocybin in the treatment of SUDs (Bogenschutz and Johnson 2016), ibogaine, a naturally occurring indole alkaloid, has long been put forward as an addiction treatment. Advocates assert that a single administration of ibogaine can cure a patient's addictive behaviors. More measured assessments of ibogaine acknowledge that although some data indicate rapid effectiveness in the treatment of SUDs, this must be weighed against (controversial) reports of lethal side effects (including arrythmias and seizures) and the lack of any medical consensus about the clinical use of ibogaine and noribogaine in human subjects (Köck et al. 2022).

Although ibogaine is still ensconced on federal Schedule I ("no current accepted medical use and a high potential for abuse"), ibogaine clinics outside of the United States operate as *de facto* addiction treatment facilities. For example, several facilities in Mexico cater to U.S. medical travelers and tourists. Because of the lack of well-controlled studies about ibogaine, its use has been characterized as a "vast, uncontrolled experiment" (Vastag 2005). Although ibogaine proponents cite some observational clinical trials with promising results (Noller et al. 2018) and dismiss the reports of deaths as incidental rather than caused by ibogaine, the treatment remains below the minimum standard of care in the United States.

A 15-subject pilot study of psilocybin as a facilitating agent, along with standard cognitive-behavioral therapy, reported that abstinence rates were substantially higher than in subjects in other studies using cognitive-behavioral therapy alone or other medications. In addition to improved abstinence rates, 13 of the participants reported that their experience with psilocybin was "among the five most meaningful and spiritually significant experiences of their lives" (Johnson et al. 2017).

Although most hallucinogenic substances that remain on the federal Schedule I are not appropriate for clinical use, burgeoning interest and research has led to numerous state regulations specifically allowing their use in research and some clinical environments. Use of agents like MDMA (3,4-methylenedioxymethamphetamine), LSD, psilocybin, and ayahuasca has garnered significant public interest, generated by descriptions of the science and practical aspects of hallucinogens for end-of-life use and intrapsychic exploration. One such example is journalist Michael Pollan's *How to Change Your Mind: What the New Science of Psychedelics Teaches Us About Consciousness, Dying, Addiction, Depression, and Transcendence* (Pollan 2018). The widespread use of ketamine (as distinct from FDA-approved esketamine) as an off-label treatment for depression, anxiety, and end-of-life dread is promoted by some modestly positive studies (Shiroma et al. 2020) and large national chains of ketamine infusion centers (e.g., Mindbloom). One ketamine infusion facility described its services in glowing, if vague, terms:

> For appropriate conditions ketamine can be an exceptionally effective option, often helping when other treatments have been exhausted....Data analysis of our own results shows about 70% effectiveness for patients, which we think is impressive both for its high efficacy and for the fact that we treat many patients that do not meet limited criteria of academic studies. Many patients know whether the treatments are a good option for them after the first infusion....Doing your own research is an important part of deciding to pursue infusion therapy treatment. (Lone Star Infusion 2023)

The opioid analog kratom (7-hydroxymitragynine) can be used for pain and mood symptoms but is often used by people with OUD to avoid withdrawal effects. Kratom is legally available in many U.S. jurisdictions and is usually in-

gested as a tea by individuals who feel that the easy availability, natural provenance, and unique method of intake make it harmless. However, growing
concern about dependence on the substance has generated detoxification programs at many facilities, and six states have banned kratom entirely from the gas
stations and other venues where it is usually sold. In 2020, the Wisconsin legislature briefly considered lifting its 2013 ban on kratom; however, it decided not
to on the basis of testimony from law enforcement officials and the president of
the Wisconsin Society of Addiction Medicine, who noted that kratom has never
been proven safe or effective for the treatment of OUD and that there are FDA-
approved medications for treating OUD (Beck 2022). Although there have been
reports of deaths related to kratom (Gershman et al. 2019; U.S. Food and Drug
Administration 2018), advocates for the substance point out that most of these
deaths involved kratom in combination with other dangerous substances. Like
all non-FDA-approved substances, of course, substances labeled "kratom" may
contain kratom of varying potency or no kratom at all, making it difficult if not
impossible for physicians to identify a standard of care for off-label detoxification from other opioids.

In a cultural moment strikingly similar to the last 20 years of the move toward cannabis legalization and decriminalization, advocates have pushed legislatures, sometimes successfully, to expand availability of hallucinogenic agents
for clinical purposes. For instance, in May 2019, the Denver, Colorado, elector-
ate (barely) passed Ordinance 301, a psilocybin mushroom initiative designed
to make possession of psilocybin mushrooms a low law enforcement priority
and directed the city to avoid spending resources on enforcing penalties for
possession. Although the ballot initiative cited sources noting psilocybin's association with lower rates of opioid problems and violent crime, the ballot initiative was designed not for medical treatments with psilocybin, but to protect the
"personal use and possession of psilocybin" (Denver Psilocybin Mushroom Decriminalization Initiative 2022).

A much broader ordinance, Washington, D.C. Initiative 81 (Entheogenic
Plants and Fungus Measure), passed with 76% of the votes cast. The initiative
directed local police to "treat the non-commercial cultivation, distribution,
possession, and use of entheogenic plants and fungi among the lowest law enforcement priorities." Entheogenic plants were defined as "ibogaine, dimethyl-
tryptamine, mescaline, psilocybin, or psilocyn" (Council of the District of
Columbia 2021).

Although it is unclear what effect, if any, these local ordinances will have on
overall enforcement, it is certainly striking that drug legalization advocates in
two jurisdictions that were early adopters of cannabis legalization have chosen to
propose legalized "recreational use" first, without even the fig leaf of medical use.

For researchers who evaluate the medical use of hallucinogenic substances,
ethical and legal frameworks are highly structured in the medical literature and

codified at the federal level. The DEA has attempted to simplify research applications for Schedule I substances, including hallucinogens, by providing a web portal for researchers to upload their protocols, qualifications to do the research, and information on the institution supporting the research (U.S. Drug Enforcement Administration 2018). One institution that has developed numerous protocols for evaluating the therapeutic efficacy of hallucinogens has developed a list of safeguards, summarized in Table 11–3, against the particular risks of research on human subjects using hallucinogens (Johnson et al. 2008).

# Legal Issues Related to Needle and Syringe Exchange Programs and Supervised Injection Facilities

Although ample, replicated evidence shows that needle and syringe exchange programs (NSEPs) for people who inject drugs decrease rates of bloodborne infections and overdose mortality (Fernandes et al. 2017; Kaplan and O'Keefe 1993; Ng et al. 2017; Ruiz et al. 2016), these programs have faced stiff political resistance that has begun to shift only in the last several years. Institutions such as the World Health Organization, the American Medical Association, and the CDC have gone on the record with their unqualified support for NSEPs as early adopters and exemplars of the harm reduction model (Abbasi 2017; American Medical Association 2020; World Health Organization 2004).

Opponents to NSEPs have historically raised three major objections: 1) that the programs signal official support for drug use, 2) that the programs would actually increase drug use with damaging effects to public health, and 3) that the programs themselves would corrupt children (Weinmeyer 2016). In perhaps the most famous comment on the subject by a politician, Senator Jesse Helms (R-N.C.) said in 1988 that the programs are essentially the government saying, "It's not only all right to use drugs, but we'll give you the needles." Senator Helms backed up his rhetoric with sponsorship of a prohibition of federal funds supporting NSEPs codified in Section 300ee-5 of the Public Health and Welfare Act (42 U.S.C. § 300ee-5 [1988]). Importantly, however, Helms's amendment contained a provision allowing for future federal funding of NSEPs if the U.S. Surgeon General determined that the NSEPs in fact reduced "drug abuse" and decreased HIV infection.

Starting with Amsterdam's experiments with needle exchange programs in 1984 (Witteveen and Schippers 2006) and an innovative, community-based initiative in Tacoma, Washington, in 1988 (Sherman and Purchase 2001), NSEPs convincingly demonstrated that their clients experienced fewer HIV and hepatitis C virus infections, decreased their drug use, and often gained access to addiction treatment programs and other necessary public services. It

**Table 11–3.** Hallucinogen research safety guidelines

Exclude potential subjects with personal or family history of psychotic disorders
Establish trust between subjects and treatment monitors before the session
Carefully prepare subject
Ensure safe physical session environment
Monitor for hallucinogen persisting perception disorder in follow-up contacts

*Source.* Adapted from Johnson et al. 2008.

was not until 2009 that the Obama administration lifted the federal ban on funding for NSEPs—only to be reversed by the fiscal year 2012 omnibus spending bill, which again banned federal funding of NSEPs. Despite the political back and forth, NSEPs eventually prevailed, supported by congress members from both parties who were dealing with the devastating effects of the opioid epidemic and became willing to accept NSEPs because of their demonstrated good effects on public health, including reducing spread of bloodborne infections related to injection drug use. Republican politicians, including Senator Mitch McConnell and (eventually) then-Senator Mike Pence, came out in support of NSEPs, allowing federal funding for NSEP major expenses like staffing, transportation, outreach, and addiction treatment, although the (relatively minor) expense of the needles themselves was still banned for public funding (Centers for Disease Control and Prevention 2022; Ungar 2016).

As of March of 2022, 43 U.S. states had NSEPs, with a total of 402 separate facilities, although that total is self-reported and possibly a low estimate (Kaiser Family Foundation 2022). The clinical and public health efficacy of NSEPs, along with their political support, is essentially unchallenged at this point. Yet NSEPs may still be a low-hanging fruit in prevention efforts related to intravenous drug use. Facilities that allow safe injection on their premises, and even teach safe injection techniques, are arguably even more effective for their benefits to public health and their ability to treat and prevent opioid overdose. The debate over safe injection spaces, like the original disputes about NSEPs, becomes ensnared in public debates about abstinence versus harm reduction approaches to engaging with people who inject drugs (Lofaro and Miller 2021). It is hoped that the policymakers and clinicians engaging in this debate will remain focused on addressing the morbidity and mortality flowing from the ongoing opioid epidemic and thus make policy decisions grounded in evidence and science.

# Conclusions

SUDs present a variety of unique issues for practitioners at the mental health and law interface. With the shifting policies related to COVID-19, practitioners have faced an evolving legal and regulatory landscape. The decriminalization of marijuana and the expansion of research looking at psychedelics and other substances raise new questions about balancing risk and benefits without causing harms. The use of telepsychiatry is a growing industry that creates new challenges in working with individuals with addiction. Worries about legal involvement underlie some clinicians' reluctance to treat patients with addiction or get involved with addicted patients at all. Although patients with addiction or a dual diagnosis are indeed often involved with the law and take or are prescribed potentially dangerous substances, the thoughtful clinician can practice well above the minimum standard of care by understanding the somewhat disparate narratives about off-label substances and opioid prescribing issues described in this chapter.

# Key Points

- Changes in psychiatric practice during COVID-19, such as telepsychiatry, may have unexpected benefits for patients with substance use disorders.

- Opioid prescriptions, whether for pain or for the treatment of opioid use disorder (OUD), can be done judiciously and with a minimum of legal risk.

- The Americans With Disabilities Act provides significant protections for patients who receive medications for OUD (MOUD).

- MOUD, both in correctional institutions and in medical clinics, is supported by a growing corpus of case law.

- Needle and syringe exchange programs have a growing and legally supported role in the treatment of those who use injection drugs.

# References

Abbasi J: CDC says more needle exchange programs needed to prevent HIV. JAMA 317(4):350, 2017

American Medical Association: AMA urges states to adopt new Maine needle, syringe exchange policy. Press Release, April 10, 2020. Available at: https://www.ama-assn.org/press-center/press-releases/ama-urges-states-adopt-new-maine-needle-syringe-exchange-policy/. Accessed May 2, 2022.

Azofeifa A, Rexach-Guzmán BD, Hagemeyer AN, et al: Driving under the influence of marijuana and illicit drugs among people aged >16 years—United States, 2018. MMWR Morb Mortal Wkly Rep 68(50):1153–1157, 2019 31856145

Beck M: Assembly lawmakers abandon vote on bill legalizing herbal supplement kratom after objection from police and doctors. Milwaukee Journal Sentinel, February 23, 2022. Available at: https://www.jsonline.com/story/news/politics/2022/02/23/wisconsin-lawmakers-take-up-legalizing-kratom-over-objection-cops-doctors/6907304001/. Accessed on February 23, 2022.

Bogenschutz MP, Johnson MW: Classic hallucinogens in the treatment of addictions. Prog Neuropsychopharmacol Biol Psychiatry 64:250–258, 2016 25784600

Capasso A, Jones AM, Ali SH, et al: Increased alcohol use during the COVID-19 pandemic: the effect of mental health and age in a cross-sectional sample of social media users in the U.S. Prev Med 145:106422, 2021 33422577

Centers for Disease Control and Prevention: Drug Overdose Deaths in the US Top 100,000 Annually. Atlanta, GA, Centers for Disease Control and Prevention, November 17, 2021. Available at: https://www.cdc.gov/nchs/pressroom/nchs_press_releases/2021/20211117.htm. Accessed February 24, 2022.

Centers for Disease Control and Prevention: Federal funding for syringe services programs. Available at: https://www.cdc.gov/ssp/ssp-funding.html. Accessed March 12, 2022.

Compassionate Use Act of 1996, Calf. Health Saf. Code §11362.5

Conant v Walters, 309 F.3d 629, 639 (9th Cir. 2002)

Cote LP: DEA decisions: evidence of "red flags" of drug diversion. DEA Chronicles, November 13, 2016. Available at: https://www.deachronicles.com/2016/11/dea-decisions-evidence-of-red-flags-of-drug-diversion. Accessed March 9, 2022.

Council of the District of Columbia: B23-1033 - Initiative No. 81 - Entheogenic Plant and Fungus Policy Act of 2020. 2021. Available at: https://lims.dccouncil.gov/Legislation/B23-1033. Accessed May 5, 2024.

Dadiomov D, Trotzky-Sirr R, Shooshtari A, et al: Changes in the availability of medications for opioid use disorder in prisons and jails in the United States during the COVID-19 pandemic. Drug Alcohol Depend 232:109291, 2022 35033953

Delaware Department of State: State prohibits three from prescribing controlled substances. Press Release, December 9, 2011. Available at: https://sos.delaware.gov/newsroom/state-prohibits-three-prescribing-controlled-substances/. Accessed March 8, 2022.

Denver Psilocybin Mushroom Decriminalization Initiative: Available at: https://library.municode.com/co/denver/codes/code_of_ordinances?nodeId=TITIIREMUCO_CH28HURI_ARTXPUSAENPREN_S28-302ENPRSIMU. Accessed May 5, 2024.

Dopesick, Created by Danny Strong. Hulu, 2021

Drug Enforcement Administration: 21 CFR Part 1308 Docket No. DEA-1362; A.G. Order No. 5931-2024. Schedules of Controlled Substances: Rescheduling of Marijuana. Available at: https://www.dea.gov/sites/default/files/2024-05/Scheduling%20NPRM%20508.pdf. Accessed May 25, 2024.

Duncan A, Sanders N, Schiff M, et al: Adaptations to jail-based buprenorphine treatment during the COVID-19 pandemic. J Subst Abuse Treat 121:108161, 2021 33371945

EEOC v Appalachian Wood Products, Inc., Case No. 3:18-cv-00198 (W.D. Pa., 2018)

Fernandes RM, Cary M, Duarte G, et al: Effectiveness of needle and syringe programmes in people who inject drugs—an overview of systematic reviews. BMC Public Health 17(1):309, 2017 28399843

Gershman K, Timm K, Frank M, et al: Deaths in Colorado attributed to kratom. N Engl J Med 380(1):97–98, 2019 30601742

Johnson M, Richards W, Griffiths R: Human hallucinogen research: guidelines for safety. J Psychopharmacol 22(6):603–620, 2008 18593734

Johnson MW, Garcia-Romeu A, Griffiths RR: Long-term follow-up of psilocybin-facilitated smoking cessation. Am J Drug Alcohol Abuse 43(1):55–60, 2017 27441452

Kaiser Family Foundation: Sterile syringe exchange programs. 2022. Available at: https://www.kff.org/hivaids/state-indicator/syringe-exchange-programs/?current Timeframe=0&sortModel=%7B%22colId%22:%22Location%22,%22sort%22: %22asc%22%7D. Accessed March 12, 2022.

Kaplan EH, O'Keefe E: Let the needles do the talking! Evaluating the New Haven Needle Exchange. J Appl Anal 23(1):7–26, 1993

Keefe PR: Empire of Pain: The Secret History of the Sackler Dynasty. New York, Doubleday, 2021

Köck P, Froelich K, Walter M, et al: A systematic literature review of clinical trials and therapeutic applications of ibogaine. J Subst Abuse Treat 138(1):108717, 2022 35012793

Krawczyk N, Picher CE, Feder KA, et al: Only one in twenty justice-referred adults in specialty treatment for opioid use receive methadone or buprenorphine. Health Aff (Millwood) 36(12):2046–2053, 2017 29200340

Kuhlman JJ, Harris C, Wright T: Buprenorphine prevalence in DUID cases in southwestern Virginia: case studies and observations. J Anal Toxicol 46(1):89–98, 2022

Levin F: Personal communication, March 9, 2022.

Lofaro RJ, Miller HT: Narrative politics in policy discourse: the debate over safe injection sites in Philadelphia, Pennsylvania. Contemp Drug Probl 48(1):75–95, 2021

Lone Star Infusion: Ketamine assisted psychotherapy. Available at: https://www.lonestarinfusion.com/contents/treatments/treatments-pain. Accessed November 12, 2023.

Marlowe D: Malpractice liability and medical marijuana. The Health Lawyer, American Bar Association, Health Law Section, December 2016. Available at: https://flboardofmedicine.gov/forms/malpractice-liability-medical-marijuana.pdf. Accessed on May 4, 2022.

National Institute on Drug Abuse: COVID-19 and Substance Use. Bethesda, MD, National Institutes of Health. Available at: https://nida.nih.gov/drug-topics/comorbidity/covid-19-substance-use. Accessed on May 4, 2022.

National Traffic Law Center: Cannabis Impairment Detection Workshop Handbook. Arlington, VA, National District Attorneys Association, 2022. Available at: https://www.responsibility.org/wp-content/uploads/2020/11/FAAR_4090-Cannabis-Impairment-Detection-Workshop-Handbook_V-3-002.pdf. Accessed March 6, 2022.

New York State: Executive Order: No. 4. Declaring a Statewide Disaster Emergency due to Health Care Staffing Shortages in the State of New York. Governor Katy Hochul, September 27, 2021. Available at: https://www.governor.ny.gov/executive-order/no-4-declaring-statewide-disaster-emergency-due-healthcare-staffing-shortages-state. Accessed March 19, 2022.

Ng J, Sutherland C, Kolber MR: Does evidence support supervised injection sites? Can Fam Physician 63(11):866, 2017 29138158

Noller GE, Frampton CM, Yazar-Klosinski B: Ibogaine treatment outcomes for opioid dependence from a twelve-month follow-up observational study. Am J Drug Alcohol Abuse 44(1):37–46, 2018 28402682

Oesterle TS, Kolla B, Risma CJ, et al: Substance use disorders and telehealth in the COVID-19 pandemic era: a new outlook. Mayo Clin Proc 95(12):2709–2718, 2020 33276843

Pesce v Coppinger, Civ. A. No. 18-cv-11972-DJC (D. Mass. 2018a)

Pesce v Coppinger, 355 F. Supp. 3d 35, 35–49 (D. Mass. 2018b)

Pollan M: How to Change Your Mind: What the New Science of Psychedelics Teaches Us About Consciousness, Dying, Addiction, Depression, and Transcendence. New York, Penguin Press, 2018

Responsibility.org: National Drunk Driving Statistics Map. 2021. Available at: https://www.responsibility.org/alcohol-statistics/state-map/issue/marijuana-drug-impaired-driving-laws. Accessed March 6, 2022.

Ruan v United States, 142 S. Ct. 2370, 2374–82 (2022)

Ruiz MS, O'Rourke A, Allen ST: Impact evaluation of a policy intervention for HIV protection in Washington DC. AIDS Behav 20(1):22–28, 2016 26336945

Sewell RA, Poling J, Sofuoglu M: The effect of cannabis compared with alcohol on driving. Am J Addict 18(3):185–193, 2009 19340636

Sherman SG, Purchase D: Point defiance: a case study of the United States' first public needle exchange in Tacoma, Washington. Int J Drug Policy 12(1):45–57, 2001 11275503

Shiroma PR, Thuras P, Wels J, et al: A randomized, double-blind, active placebo-controlled study of efficacy, safety, and durability of repeated vs single subanesthetic ketamine for treatment-resistant depression. Transl Psychiatry 10(1):206, 2020 32591498

Southern District of Alabama U.S. Attorney's Office: Dr. Couch and Dr. Ruan sentenced to 240 and 252 months in federal prison for running massive pill mill. Press Release, May 26, 2017. Available at: https://www.justice.gov/usao-sdal/pr/dr-couch-and-dr-ruan-sentenced-240-and-252-months-federal-prison-running-massive-pill. Accessed March 8, 2022.

State of New Jersey Office of the Attorney General: Board of Medical Examiners permanently revokes license of physician who traveled weekly from Rhode Island to prescribe large quantities of opioid pain medications to New Jersey patients without a medical basis. Echoes Sentinel, October 28, 2020. Available at: https://www.newjerseyhills.com/echoes-sentinel/news/state-revokes-warren-doctors-license-for-prescribing-large-quantities-of-pain-meds/article_c908e683-e186-5eb4-88ab-765de45428ce.html#:~:text=The%20doctor%2C%20Pramila%20Byahatti%2C%20who,examinations%2C%20properly%20monitoring%20their%20intake. Accessed March 9, 2022.

Treaster JB: Researchers say that students were among 200 who took LSD in tests financed by CIA in early '50's. The New York Times, August 9, 1977. Available at: https://www.nytimes.com/1977/08/09/archives/researchers-say-that-students-were-among-200-who-took-lsd-in-tests.html. Accessed November 12, 2023.

Ungar L: Funding ban on needle exchanges effectively lifted. USA Today, January 7, 2016. Available at: https://www.usatoday.com/story/news/nation/2016/01/07/funding-ban-needle-exchanges-effectively-lifted/78420894/. Accessed March 14, 2022.

United States of America v Patrick Titus, 18–45 (D. Del. 2018)

United States of America v Sriramloo Kesari MD, 21 U.S.C. 841(a)(1); 21 U.S.C. 846, 2019. Available at: https://www.justice.gov/criminal/criminal-vns/file/1204851/dl. Accessed May 25, 2024

U.S. Department of Health and Human Services: Notification of Enforcement Discretion for Telehealth Remote Communications During the COVID-19 Nationwide Public Health Emergency. Washington, DC, U.S. Department of Health and Human Services, January 21, 2021. Available at: https://www.hhs.gov/hipaa/for-professionals/special-topics/emergency-preparedness/notification-enforcement-discretion-telehealth/index.html. Accessed February 26, 2022.

U.S. Department of Justice: Settlement agreement between the United States of America and Selma Medical Associates. Inc., under the Americans With Disabilities Act (DJ No 202-80-64). Press Release, January 31, 2019. Available at: https://www.ada.gov/selma_medical_sa.html. Accessed May 2, 2022.

U.S. Department of Justice: Settlement agreement between the United States of America and Massachusetts General Hospital under the Americans With Disabilities Act (DJ No 202-36-304). Press Release, August 7, 2020. Available at: https://www.ada.gov/mass_gen_hosp_sa.html. Accessed May 2, 2022.

U.S. Department of Justice: Health Care Fraud Unit. August 2021. Available at: https://www.justice.gov/criminal-fraud/health-care-fraud-unit. Accessed March 8, 2022.

U.S. Drug Enforcement Administration: DEA speeds up application process for research on Schedule I drugs. Press Release, January 18, 2018. Available at: https://www.dea.gov/press-releases/2018/01/18/dea-speeds-application-process-research-schedule-i-drugs. Accessed March 5, 2022.

U.S. Food and Drug Administration: Statement from FDA Commissioner Scott Gottlieb, MD, on the agency's scientific evidence on the presence of opioid compounds in kratom, underscoring its potential for abuse. Press Release, February 6, 2018. Available at: https://www.fda.gov/news-events/press-announcements/statement-fda-commissioner-scott-gottlieb-md-agencys-scientific-evidence-presence-opioid-compounds. Accessed May 2, 2022.

Vastag B: Addiction research. Ibogaine therapy: a "vast, uncontrolled experiment." Science 308(5720):345–346, 2005 15831735

Voth EA: Guidelines for prescribing medical marijuana. West J Med 175(5):305–306, 2001 11694470

Weinmeyer R: Needle exchange programs status in US politics. AMA J Ethics 18(3):252–257, 2016 27002996

Witteveen E, Schippers G: Needle and syringe exchange programs in Amsterdam. Subst Use Misuse 41(6–7):835–836, 2006 16809172

World Health Organization: Policy Brief: Provision of Sterile Injecting Equipment to Reduce HIV Transmission. Geneva, Switzerland, World Health Organization, 2004. Available at: https://apps.who.int/iris/bitstream/handle/10665/68711/WHO_HIV_2004.03.pdf?sequence=1andisAllowed=y. Accessed March 10, 2022.

# INDEX

*Page numbers printed in **boldface** type refer to tables and figures.*